T0248999

Encyclopedia of Endocrinology: Modern Concepts

Volume II

Encyclopedia of Endocrinology: Modern Concepts
Volume II

Edited by **Joy Foster**

FOSTER
A C A D E M I C S

New Jersey

Published by Foster Academics,
61 Van Reypen Street,
Jersey City, NJ 07306, USA
www.fosteracademics.com

Encyclopedia of Endocrinology: Modern Concepts
Volume II
Edited by Joy Foster

International Standard Book Number: 978-1-63242-145-6 (Hardback)

This book contains information obtained from authentic and highly regarded sources. Copyright for all individual chapters remain with the respective authors as indicated. A wide variety of references are listed. Permission and sources are indicated; for detailed attributions, please refer to the permissions page. Reasonable efforts have been made to publish reliable data and information, but the authors, editors and publisher cannot assume any responsibility for the validity of all materials or the consequences of their use.

The publisher's policy is to use permanent paper from mills that operate a sustainable forestry policy. Furthermore, the publisher ensures that the text paper and cover boards used have met acceptable environmental accreditation standards.

Trademark Notice: Registered trademark of products or corporate names are used only for explanation and identification without intent to infringe.

Printed in the United States of America.

Contents

Preface

The aim of the book is to provide basic as well as advanced trends with an analytical focus on endocrine disorders. Apart from covering a variety of topics including adrenal tumors and metabolic bone disease, this book also discusses more specific issues which have not yet been fully elucidated. These include molecular pathways involved in thyrotropin beta gene regulation or monogenic phosphate balance disorders. This book will provide an opportunity to readers from distinct backgrounds to attain knowledge and clarify areas of uncertainty and controversies in several topics of endocrine disorders.

Significant researches are present in this book. Intensive efforts have been employed by authors to make this book an outstanding discourse. This book contains the enlightening chapters which have been written on the basis of significant researches done by the experts.

Finally, I would also like to thank all the members involved in this book for being a team and meeting all the deadlines for the submission of their respective works. I would also like to thank my friends and family for being supportive in my efforts.

Editor

Part 1

Adrenal Glands

Adrenal Cortex Tumors and Hyperplasias

Duarte Pignatelli[1,2,3]
[1]Endocrinology, Hospital S. João, Porto
[2]Faculty of Medicine of the University of Porto
[3]IPATIMUP, University of Porto
Portugal

1. Introduction

The adrenal cortex tumors include both malignant adrenal cortex cancers (ACC) and benign masses (ACT) that can be either secreting, of one of the hormones normally produced in the adrenal cortex (Cushing's syndrome if the hypersecretion is of cortisol or Conn's syndrome if it is aldosterone) or non-secretory (Incidentalomas).

The outer part of the adrenal glands, the adrenal cortex, is responsible for regulating important body functions including blood sugar levels, body water and salt levels, and consequently blood pressure and kidney functions, the immune system, the inflammatory response, the physiological response to stress, and, finally, sexual and reproductive functions.

The three different parts of the adrenal cortex, *zona glomerulosa*, *zona fasciculata* and *zona reticularis*, are responsible for producing different hormones namely mineralocorticoids, glucocorticoids, and androgens (and eventually also estrogens). The *glomerulosa* secretes aldosterone, and gives rise to Primary Aldosteronism (PA)/Hyperaldosteronism that can result either from an adenoma (Conn's syndrome) or from bilateral hyperplasia (BAH). The *zona fasciculata* secretes cortisol and adenomas that produce this hormone are associated to a distinct syndrome called Cushing's syndrome. Finally the adrenal cortex *reticularis* zone is supposed to produce adrenal androgens (namely dehydroepiandrosterone – DHEA and dehydroepiandrosterone sulfate – DHEA-s) that can in turn be either converted into testosterone or aromatized to estrogen in peripheral organs like the adipose tissue. In spite of the fact that normally this peripheral conversion is more important than the local production, there are adrenal cortex tumors that can produce testosterone directly, the Androgen-secreting tumors as well as adrenocortical carcinomas expressing aromatase and producing estrogens, the Estrogen-secreting tumors.

The majority of adrenocortical tumors (ACT) are benign and silent (non-secreting adenomas or incidentalomas) since they do not ever result in hormone secretion. Its true incidence is still unknown because it is probable that many of these cases still go undiagnosed. However, it is estimated that they are present in at least 3% of the adult population (especially over 50 years of age) (National Institutes of Health, 2002; Grumbach et al., 2003). Most of these tumors are discovered incidentally due to the widespread availability of imaging studies for intra-abdominal diseases. This is the reason why they are designated as Incidentalomas.

In summary, only a minority of the adrenocortical benign tumors (about 15%) are hormone-secreting adenomas, responsible for Cushing's syndrome, primary aldosteronism (Conn's syndrome) or even sometimes virilization.

Adrenocortical carcinoma is a rare, highly malignant tumor usually associated with a poor prognosis which may occur either in children or adults. This is a malignancy with an heterogeneous presentation and despite probably still underestimated it has an expected incidence of about 1-2 cases per 1 million population per year (Wajchenberg et al., 2000; Dackiw et al., 2001; Kebebew et al., 2006). Although the adrenocortical carcinomas may occur and develop at any age, two different disease peaks were identified, one before the age of five and the other in the fifth decade of life (Wajchenberg et al., 2000; Ng & Libertino, 2003).

2. Adrenal cortex cancer

The evaluation and categorization of adrenocortical neoplasms remain among the most challenging areas in adrenal pathology (Lau & Weiss, 2009), since the pathological diagnosis of ACC, which is based on gross and microscopic criteria, is still full of areas of subjectivity. Moreover, in the absence of the gold standards that constitute the appearance of metastases, local invasion or recurrence, the diagnosis of malignancy may represent a great difficulty for both clinicians and pathologists.

Several multiparametric systems have been developed to assess this malignancy (Aubert, 2005). Among them, the Weiss system (Weiss, 1984), first introduced 25 years ago, and based on nine microscopic criteria, appears to be the most employed scoring methodology, because of its simplicity and reliability.

This system provides specific guidelines for differentiating adrenocortical adenoma from adrenocortical carcinoma and is considered the standard for determining malignancy in tumors of the adrenal cortex. However, considerable advances in the understanding of the pathology of adrenocortical neoplasias have occurred since delineation of the Weiss system, offering alternative approaches in the contemporary assessment of adrenocortical tumors (Lau & Weiss, 2009). In a recent study based on whole genome gene analysis the authors proposed a molecular assay for the classification and prognosis of adrenocortical tumors (Giordano et al., 2009). There were many genetic expression differences between ACC and ACT and normal adrenals. There were in fact 879 genes over expressed and 1011 under expressed in ACC that could differentiate ACC from ACT and normal adrenals. The most significant ones were related to cell proliferation, as would be expected. But the reality is that such systems are still very expensive and add very little to the diagnostic power of the morphological analyses. Therefore, in most adrenocortical tumors, the morphological approach considering the probability of malignancy in adrenal masses > 6 cm and that of being benign in tumors < 4 cm, together with the postoperative assessment by the Weiss system, brings sufficient elements to establish the differential diagnosis between a benign and a malignant tumor (Tissier, 2010).

The Weiss system, which, as previously was said, is currently the most popular scoring system, combines nine morphological parameters, of which three are structural ("dark" cytoplasm, diffuse architecture, necrosis), three are cytological (atypia, mitotic count, atypical mitotic figures) and three are related to invasion (of sinusoids, veins and tumor capsule) (Volante et al., 2008). The nine histological criteria are:

- High nuclear grade (grades 3 or 4) (High Nuclear/Cytoplasm ratio; marked variation of nuclear characteristics; giant cells with hyperchromatic nuclei; visible nucleoli)
  1. Small roundish nuclei; without nucleoli
  2. Larger nuclei, more irregular in shape and with visible nucleoli (at 400x magnification)
  3. Irregular nuclei, with larger size, with visible nucleoli (at 100x)
  4. enormous cells with polylobulated nuclei
- Mitoses (>5 per 50 HPF vs. <6)
- Abnormal mitoses (absent vs. present)
- Clear cells ($\leq$25% vs. >25%)
- Diffuse architecture (>33% vs. $\leq$33% of the area) (cells unorganized in trabecular or alveolar structures)
- Necrosis (present vs. absent)
- Venous invasion (present vs. absent)
- Sinusoidal invasion (present vs. absent)
- Capsular invasion (present vs. absent)

1. Nuclear grade: nuclear grade III and IV based on criteria of Fuhrman (Fuhrman et al., 1982).
2. Mitotic rate: greater than 5/50 HPF (x400 objective). According to Weiss, "mitosis was evaluated by counting 10 random high-power-fields in the area of the greatest numbers of mitotic figures on the five slides with greatest number of mitoses. If less than five slides were available for a case, a correspondingly greater number of fields per slide were used to make fifty high power-fields."
3. Atypical mitotic figures: "mitosis was regarded as atypical when it definitely showed an abnormal distribution of chromosomes or an excessive number of mitotic spindles."
4. Cytoplasm: presence of $\leq$25% "clear or vacuolated cells resembling the normal *zona fasciculata*."
5. Diffuse architecture: diffuse architecture was present "if greater than one-third of the tumor formed patternless sheets of cells." Trabecular, columnar, alveolar or nesting organizations were regarded as non-diffuse patterns.
6. Necrosis: necrosis was "regarded as present when occurring in at least confluent nests of cells."
7. Venous invasion: Weiss defined a vein as an "endothelial-lined vessel with smooth muscle as a component of the wall."
8. Sinusoid invasion: a sinusoid was defined as "endothelial-lined vessel in the adrenal gland with little supportive tissues." Only sinusoids located within the tumor were considered.
9. Invasion of tumor capsule: "invasion of the capsule was accepted as present when nests or cords of tumor extended into or through the capsule, with a corresponding stroma reaction."

Fig. 1. Weiss classification

Tumors are classified as malignant when they meet 4 or more of these histological criteria. However, it must be stated that there are still some difficulties and subjectivity in the application of this system. Also, whether the presence of 3 criteria represents malignancy, is still controversial (Aubert et al., 2005). But, despite the referred limitations and subjectivity the Weiss classification is still the most reliable and most used criteria system.

Other markers not included in the Weiss scores are now perfectly identified as being associated with the risk of recurrence and lower survival. Ki67 expression ≥ 10% for instance is associated with much less chances of survival at 5 years. The same can be said about a high expression of   SF-1. The immuno-histochemistry of these two factors is now routine in most pathology labs. (Fassnacht et al., 2011; Sbiera et al., 2010; Terzolo et al., 2001)

2.1 Adrenal cortex cancer pathogenesis

Molecular studies support the fact that uncontrolled cell proliferation is probably the most important factor in the development of cancers and ACC is no exception. ACC consist of monoclonal populations of cells (Beuschlein et al., 1994) while for instance adrenocortical macronodular hyperplasias are usually polyclonal. It is a basic rule that the mutations that give rise to cancer development are deletions of tumor suppressor genes or amplifications of oncogenes. The increase in cell proliferation induced by growth factors like the IGFs, bFGF or TGF β1 (Feige et al., 1991; Mesiano et al., 1991; Mesiano et al., 1993) leads to the development of polyclonal tumors but also renders the cells more susceptible to mutations in tumor suppressor genes or in oncogenes and if these mutations give those cells a genetic advantage, cancer development may ensue. Genomic instability is the basis of gross chromosomal alterations and aneuploidy (Giordano et al., 2009).

Most cases of adrenocortical cancers appear to be sporadic and only a small percentage of patients present ACC as a component of one of the known hereditary cancer syndromes, such as the Li-Fraumeni's syndrome, the Beckwith-Wiedemann syndrome or the Multiple Endocrine Neoplasia type 1 (Koch et al., 2002; Sidhu et al., 2004; Libé & Bertherat, 2005; Kjellman et al., 1999; Schulte et al., 2000; Heppner et al., 1999).

One important difference between these two forms of adrenocortical carcinomas (either sporadic or part of an hereditary syndrome) is the current degree of knowledge about its tumorigenesis (Soon et al., 2008).   For sporadic adrenocortical malignant tumors the molecular mechanisms underlying its development are still far from completely understood (Sidhu et al, 2002). One hypothesis refers the possible evolution of adrenocortical cancers from adrenal adenomas (Bernard et al., 2003); however long-term follow-up data of incidentally discovered adrenal neoplasms do not support that hypothesis (Barzon et al., 2003; Bernini et al., 2005).

The study and investigation of the pathophysiology of ACC is not only crucial for the understanding of these malignant tumors but also for the development of more sensitive means of diagnosis and better ways of treatment. And despite the fact that knowledge of these tumors has greatly evolved in the last decades, the understanding of the genes and pathways underlying the development of adrenal cortex cancers has been slow. Many genes and pathways are thought to play an important role in their development but frequently their biological plausibility is still missing.

Hereditary tumor syndrome	Gene (*locus*)	Prevalence of ACT
Li-Fraumeni syndrome (LFS)	*TP53* (17p13), HIC-1 (17p13), *hCHK2* (22q12.1)	ACC 3%-4%
Beckwith-Wiedemann syndrome (BWS)	*IGF-II, H19, CDKN1C (p57kip2), KCNQ1* (11p15)	ACC 5%
Multiple Endocrine Neoplasia 1 (MEN-1)	*Menin gene* (11q13)	ACT 25-50%; ACC rare
Congenital Adrenal Hyperplasia (CAH)	*Mostly CYP21B* (6p21.3)	ACT in up to 82%; ACC (rare) vs Hyperplasia (usual)

- In LFS there is a germline mutation of the tumor suppressor gene TP53 in more than 70% of the families. Tumors associated with this syndrome include breast carcinoma; soft tissue sarcoma; brain tumors; osteosarcoma; leukemia and ACC. Mutations in Checkpoint Kinase 2 gene (hCHK2) encoding a kinase that phosphorylates TP53 were identified in some of these tumors but not in ACC (Libé & Bertherat, 2005).
- In BWS there is, on the contrary, deregulation of the imprinted IGF-II locus at 11p15. The IGF-II gene is maternally imprinted and so it's expressed only from the paternal allele. H19 and p57kip2 are paternally imprinted. In cases of paternal isodisomy, IGF-II is over-expressed and H19 and p57kip2 are under-expressed! BWS is a syndrome of "overgrowth" that includes many tumors like the renal' Wilms tumor, ACC, neuroblastoma and hepatoblastoma (Libé & Bertherat, 2005).
- In MEN-1 the germline mutation is in the Menin gene (90% of the families). This gene is also a tumor suppressor gene and it is located in chromosome 11 (11q13). LOH at 11q13 exist in more than 90% of ACC (Kjellman et al., 1999; Schulte et al., 2000; Heppner et al., 1999)

Adapted from Soon P. et al., (2008). Molecular markers and the pathogenesis of adrenocortical cancer. The Oncologist 13: 548-561

Table 1. Hereditary tumor syndromes, responsible genes and associated ACT prevalence

In **sporadic ACC** it has been reported that hyper-expression of the insulin-like growth factor II **(IGF-II)** is observed in the vast majority of cases (Boulle et al., 1998; Gicquel et al., 1994; Gicquel et al., 1997; Gicquel et al., 2001; Ilvesmaki et al., 1993). Together with the increase of this growth factor there is also an increased expression of its receptor (IGF-IR) in most ACC (Weber et al., 1997). The over-expression of IGF-II is probably related to adrenal cancer cell proliferation, through the IGF-I receptor (Fottner et al., 2001 and Logié et al., 1999).

The IGF-II overexpression is the result of changes at the 11p15 locus (Gicquel et al., 1994; Gicquel et al., 1997). LOH at 11p15 is much more frequent in ACC (78,5%) than in ACT (9,5%) (Gicquel et al., 2001). It is associated with a higher risk of tumor recurrence, and correlates with Weiss score. Thus, according to Gicquel and colleagues, 11p15 alterations could be used as a biological marker for confirming ACC malignancy after surgical removal of the tumor (Gicquel et al., 2001).

The 11p15 region is organized in a telomeric domain containing the IGF-II gene and H19 and a centromeric domain including the CDKN1C (p57kip2) (DeChiara et al., 1991; Hao et al., 1993; Lee et al., 1995; Matsuoka et al., 1995). Genetic and epigenetic changes in the imprinted 11p15 region resulting in low p57kip2 and H19 and elevated IGF2 mRNA expression levels have been reported in sporadic ACCs (Gicquel et al., 1994; Gicquel et al., 1997). The IGF-II system, in the adrenal gland, is responsible for growth-promoting and differentiating functions during the fetal period (Mesiano et al., 1993), but its role has been largely documented in adrenocortical malignant tumors, also in adult patients (Gicquel et al., 2001). In fact, several studies have been successful in showing the strong overexpression of IGF-II in malignant adrenocortical tumors (in approximately 90% of the cases) (Boulle et al., 1998; Gicquel et al., 1994; Gicquel et al., 1997; Gicquel et al., 2001; Ilvesmaki et al., 1993a).

Inactivating mutations of the **TP53 gene** located at the 17p13 locus are another genetic alteration that is frequently encountered in ACC. TP53 is one of the most relevant tumor suppressor genes, frequently mutated in human cancers. The TP53 mutations are thought to happen late in the evolution of sporadic malignant adrenocortical tumors. Mutations in the exons 5-8 are found more frequently in ACC than in ACT (Hollstein et al., 1991; Reincke et al., 1994). The germline mutations in TP53 have been observed in 50-80% of children diagnosed with sporadic ACC (Libé & Bertherat, 2005; Wagner et al., 1994; Varley et al., 1999). In southern Brazil where the prevalence of ACC in children is 10 times greater than in the rest of the world, there is a particular mutation at exon 10 of TP53 (Arginine 337 Histidine) in most of the cases (Ribeiro et al., 2001; Latronico et al., 2001).

Considering TP 53 gene mutations in sporadic ACC in adults, its frequency has been reported in different proportions in diverse studies ranging from 25% to 70%. (Ohgaki et al., 1993; Reincke et al., 1994; Barzon et al., 2001; Lin et al., 1994) Loss of Heterozigoty (LOH) at 17p13 was reported in 95% of ACC and only in 30% of ACT (Gicquel et al., 2001) and therefore this can also be used as a marker of malignancy.

Other reported molecular studies have suggested that genetic alterations of the **Wnt signaling pathway** may also be associated with the development of adrenocortical tumors. In fact the activation of the Wnt signaling pathway is the most prevalent defect in adrenocortical tumorigenesis particularly due to the fact that it is not only present in malignant lesions but in benign adrenocortical adenomas as well (Tissier et al., 2005).

The Wnt family includes a group of growth factors involved in developmental and homeostatic processes. Some regulatory genes in this pathway (including the down regulators of β-catenin, GSK3, Axin and APC, and β-catenin itself) can be mutated in primary human cancers (Polakis et al., 2000). In all of them the common denominator is the activation of gene transcription by β-catenin (via the transcription factors TCF and LEF).

β-catenin has a dual function in the cell: cell-adhesion (conjugated with E-cadherin) and transcriptional regulation. When the regulators of β-catenin are down-regulated the transcriptional function is increased and the adhesion is reduced and both of these alterations lead to the progression of malignancies (Brembeck et al., 2006).

Genetic alterations in the Wnt pathway conducting to β-catenin accumulation in the cytoplasm have been correlated with the pathogenesis of different types of cancer

(Gordon & Nusse, 2006). Curiously, in adrenocortical tumors, the accumulation of β-catenin has been found in both benign and malignant situations although with a slightly higher prevalence in adrenal cortex cancer (Tissier et al., 2005). It is a fact that β-catenin mutations are the most frequent genetic defects reported in adrenocortical adenomas and in these benign ACT it is mostly the non-secretory adenomas that have these mutations (Tissier et al., 2005). According to that study, abnormal cytoplasmic and/or nuclear accumulation of β-catenin was found in 38% of the adrenocortical adenomas (ACA) and in 77% of the ACC, but mutations in the β-catenin gene were found with similar frequencies of in both ACA and ACC (27% *vs.* 31%) (Tissier et al., 2005). These somewhat opposite results suggest that other components of the Wnt signaling pathway, such as the adenomatous polyposis coli (APC) or axin, may be contributing to the pathogenesis of ACC (Tissier et al., 2005).

2.2 Adrenal cortex cancer – Diagnosis and clinical presentation

Adrenocortical tumors can be classified as functional, when their hormonal secretions result in clinical consequences, or nonfunctional tumors, when they do not secrete hormones in a sufficient level to produce clinical consequences. About 50 to 60% of the adrenocortical carcinomas are functional, therefore, associated with hormonal secretion (Ng & Libertino, 2003; Allolio & Fassnacht, 2006). The most frequent presentation among adults is the Cushing's syndrome alone (45%) or the association of Cushing's syndrome with a virilization syndrome, with over-production of both glucocorticoids and androgens (25%) (Ng & Libertino, 2003; Wajchenberg et al., 2000). Other forms of functional tumors include the virilization syndrome alone and the feminization syndrome. Thus, signs and symptoms of adrenocortical tumors may vary significantly according to their origin and depending on the type of hormones that are released. Cortisol excess can be associated to symptoms such as centripetal obesity, protein wasting with skin thinning and striae, muscle atrophy (myopathy), osteoporosis, psychiatric disturbances, impaired defense against infections, diabetes, hypertension and gonadal dysfunction in men and women. In the case of aggressive malignant ACC weight loss may be observed. Androgen over-secretion is associated with various manifestations in women like hirsutism, menstrual abnormalities, infertility and eventually virilization, while excess of estrogen, although not so common, can present as gynecomastia in men. It is most important to characterize the adrenocortical carcinoma's secretory profile in order to establish its origin and better guide its treatment and follow-up (Libé et al., 2007).

Due to the elevated possibility of non-specific symptoms, both symptomatic and apparently asymptomatic patients should be evaluated.

According to the European Network for the Study of Adrenal Tumors (ENSAT), both should be studied with the following laboratory tests to determine the secretory activity of the tumor (Fassnacht & Allolio, 2009):

- fasting blood glucose and HbA1c;
- serum potassium;
- adrenal androgens (DHEA-s, androstenedione, testosterone, 17-OH progesterone);
- serum estradiol in men and postmenopausal women;
- cortisol and adrenocorticotropic hormone (ACTH) both fasting and around midnight (in the serum or in the saliva);

- fasting serum cortisol at 8 AM following a 1 mg dose of dexamethasone on the previous day at bedtime;
- 24-hour urinary free cortisol.

After careful hormonal assessment, imaging studies, by means of computerized tomography (CT), magnetic resonance imaging (MRI) or 18 F-fluorodeoxyglucose positron emission tomography (FDG-PET), are the next essential exams both to localize and delimitate the tumor and to distinguish benign adenomas from adrenocortical carcinomas (Boland et al., 1998; Hamrahian et al., 2005; Szolaret al., 2005; Caoili et al., 2002; Groussin et al., 2009; Minn et al., 2004; Metser et al., 2006 Wajchenberg et al., 2000). Despite sometimes being considered a controversial position, several studies have shown that the size and the appearance of the tumor remains one of the best indicators of malignancy (most molecular studies add only a little to the accuracy of malignancy identification by the mere determination of tumor size). In a study from the National Italian Study Group on Adrenal Tumors including 887 patients with adrenal incidentalomas, adrenocortical carcinomas were significantly associated with mass size, with 90% being more than 4 cm in diameter when discovered (Angeli et al., 1997). According, to a study by Sturgeon and colleagues at the University of California (San Francisco) including 457 ACC cases, a size of ≥ 4 cm makes the likelihood of malignancy double (to 10%) while in tumors ≥ 8 cm it gets more than ninefold higher (47%) (Sturgeon et al., 2006).

However, because of the growing evidence of adrenocortical cancers diagnosed with a diameter between 4 and 6 cm (Sturgeon et al., 2006; Grumbach et al., 2003; Herrera et al., 1991; Mantero et al., 2000) and since it seems evident that during their early stages of development, carcinomas have to be small, it becomes clear that surgical intervention would be most beneficial the smaller and more localized the tumor would be.

Overall, prognosis does improve for patients with smaller adrenocortical tumors at the time of diagnosis. In a retrospective review of 62 ACC cases (Henley et al., 1983) patients with stages I to III lesions who underwent curative resections had significantly longer survival rates. In another study done by Fassnacht and colleagues, the five year survival significantly improved (82% *vs* 18%) for patients with smaller tumors (stages I and II, confined to the adrenal gland) vs. metastatic disease, stage IV (Fassnacht et al., 2009).

As general rules, one could say that the prognosis is better in the case of young children, in smaller and localized tumors specially if nonfunctioning and in which a complete resection can be achieved.

Despite the importance of evaluating an adrenal mass size and appearance, this should not be the only parameter guiding diagnosis and posterior treatment, since radiographic features are often of strong predictive value (Dunnick et al., 1996). MRI and CT images may in fact be useful in helping to define what will be the histological type of the adrenal tumor:

On unenhanced CT scanning, the measurements of Hounsfield units (HU) are of great value in differentiating malignant from benign adrenocortical tumors. The Hounsfield scale is a semi-quantitative method of measuring x-ray attenuation. Despite the fact that around 30% of adenomas do not contain large amounts of lipid, being indistinguishable from non-adenomas, adrenal masses with < 10 HU on unenhanced CT are almost certainly benign tumors (Grumbach et al., 2003). Therefore, this seems to be the consensus cut-off for distinguishing adrenocortical carcinomas from benign adrenal tumors, according to several studies (Boland et al., 1998; Hamrahian et al., 2005). However, in those cases of benign tumors with poor intracytoplasmatic lipid concentration a better discrimination can be obtained by searching for a delayed contrast clearance in contrast-enhanced CT. In this case, tumors measuring > 10HU in a unenhanced CT, that show a contrast washout of less than 50% after 10- to 15-min of contrast-enhanced CT and also a delayed attenuation of more than 35HU, are suspicious for malignancy (Szolar et al., 2005; Caoili et al., 2002).

The use of MRI for differentiating benign and malignant adrenocortical tumors is equally effective to CT scan. But since MRI is more expensive and less standardized, CT scan remains the primary adrenal imaging procedure,

The utilization of the PET scanning with fluorodeoxyglucose (FDG) has been successful in identifying unilateral adrenal tumors with higher suspicion for malignancy, due to the greater reported uptake of FDG by malignant tumors compared to the benign adrenocortical tumors (Groussin et al., 2009; Maurea et al. 2001; Minn et al., 2004). The use of integrated PET-CT can further improve the capacity to distinguish between malignant and benign tumors by increasing the quality of the image. This improvement is also due to the combination of CT attenuation measurements with the intensity of FDG uptake, as described by the standardized uptake value (SUV) for the adrenal lesion (Metser et al., 2006; Caoili et al., 2007).

In what concerns **fine-needle aspiration biopsy** (FNA) one must stress that usually it is not successful in distinguishing between malignant and benign tumors and there are doubts about the risk of disseminating a carcinoma through the abdominal cavity; it can however be of some utility in differentiating an adrenal tumor from a metastasis to the adrenal and in evaluating staging for a known cancer (Jhala et al., 2004; Kocijancic et al., 2004).

2.3 Adrenal cortex cancer staging

The first staging system published by the World Health Organization (WHO) dates from in 2004 (DeLellis, 2004), and was based on different staging systems, such as the Sullivan modification of the Macfarlane system (Sullivan, 1978). The AJCC (American Joint Committee on Cancer)/UICC (International Union Against Cancer) developed a TNM staging system with the same definitions for the first time in 2009, being published on the AJCC/UICC Cancer Staging Manual, Seventh Edition. A simplified classification system was recently proposed by the European network ENSAT in which stage III includes cases with lymph nodes metastasis, infiltration of surrounding tissues and venous tumor thrombosis and stage IV only cases with distant metastases (Fassnacht et al., 2009).

Tumor clinical staging is most dependent of clinical examination and radiographic imaging in order to evaluate the size of the primary tumor and the extent of local and distant disease. Since disease-free and overall survival rates seem to be strongly related with tumor staging, resection of the primary tumor and examination of local extension of the disease and regional lymph nodes involvement should be performed for a better pathologic tumor staging.

The following table describes the AJCC/UICC anatomic stages and prognostic groups:

Stage	T	N	M	Description
Stage I	T1	N0	M0	Tumor 5 cm or less in greatest dimension, no extra-adrenal invasion.
Stage II	T2	N0	M0	Tumor greater than 5 cm, no extra-adrenal invasion.
Stage III	T1	N1	M0	Tumor 5 cm or less in greatest dimension, no extra-adrenal invasion but with metastasis in regional lymph node(s).
	T2	N1	M0	Tumor greater than 5 cm, no extra-adrenal invasion but with metastasis in regional lymph node(s).
	T3	N0	M0	Tumor of any size with local invasion, but not invading adjacent organs*.
Stage IV	T3	N1	M0	Tumor of any size with local invasion, but not invading adjacent organs* plus metastasis in regional lymph node(s).
	T4	N0	M0	Tumor of any size with invasion of adjacent organs*.
	T4	N1	M0	Tumor of any size with invasion of adjacent organs* plus metastasis in regional lymph node(s).
	Any T	Any N	M1	Tumor of any size and with or without invasion of adjacent organs and lymph nodes, but with distant metastases.

Adapted from Edge, SB., Byrd, DR., Compton, CC., Fritz, AG., Greene, FL., Trotti, A. (Eds.). (2010). AJCC Cancer Staging Manual, 7th Ed. Springer, Chicago.
*Adjacent organs include kidney, diaphragm, great vessels, pancreas, spleen and liver.

Table 2. AJCC/UICC anatomic stages and prognostic groups

2.4 Adrenal cortex cancer treatment

For being a very rare and aggressive carcinoma the prognosis for patients with adrenocortical cancer is poor, also due to usually not being diagnosed in the early stages of the disease (Ng & Libertino, 2003; Harrison et al., 1999). Its rarity is one of the main reasons for the lack of robust clinical studies on the most efficacious treatments (Decker et al., 1991; Bukowski et al., 1993; Khan et al., 2000). Several studies and clinical trials, however, have shown that this trend in prognosis is changing and in fact patients with this type of carcinoma are living longer as progresses are being made in its treatment (Berruti et al., 2005; Adam et al., 2006; Allolio et al., 2004; Terzolo et al., 2007; van Ditzhuijsen et al, 2007; Fassnacht et al., 2011).

Currently, the only potentially curative treatment for adrenal cortex carcinomas is total resection of the tumor at the time of initial evaluation (Allolio et al., 2006; Dackiw et al., 2001). However, in a study of Haak and colleagues with 96 patients, the overall five-year survival rate after total resection was only 49% (Haak et al., 1994). This happens probably due to the presence of hidden micrometastases that will only become apparent some months to years later (Allolio & Fassnacht, 2006; Stojadinovic et al., 2002). In fact, many patients may develop distant metastases two or more years after the diagnosis date (Abiven et al., 2006).

Therefore, surgery in these patients must be as extensive as possible, with lymphadenectomy associated. One should be very careful to avoid capsular damage and the spill of malignant cells that may result in the development of metastasis (Terzolo et al., 2007; van Ditzhuijsen et al., 2007). Nowadays, open adrenalectomy is the most consensual operation type, since laparoscopy is associated with greater risk of malignant cells spread and therefore higher risk of recurrence or dissemination (Schteingart et al., 2005; Gonzalez et al., 2005; Cobb et al., 2005). Studies have also shown that whenever total resection is not possible, maximal debulking is associated with a decrease in excess of hormone production and with better overall survival when compared with non-surgical treatments (Ng & Libertino, 2003; Luton, et al., 1990).

Whenever surgery is not feasible or is unable to completely remove the tumor, mitotane (Lysodren), an adrenocorticolytic drug, was shown to be effective, either as a primary therapy or as an adjuvant therapy (Henley et al., 1983; Dackiw et al., 2001; Berruti et al., 2005; Terzolo et al., 2007; Luton et al 1990; Hahner & Fassnacht, 2005)· Mitotane has a specific effect on adrenal cells resulting in their lysis (Hahner & Fassnacht, 2005).

As a primary treatment for unresectable tumors, mitotane is especially beneficial in improvement of symptoms associated with hypercortisolism. However this benefit tends to last for short periods of time, and is associated to inconsistent survival rates (Henley et al., 1983; Baudin et al., 2001).

In what concerns the adjuvant use of mitotane therapy, its benefits have been questioned mainly due to the lack of data from controlled clinical trials and even from large prospective studies with consistent assessments of dosing and tumor variability (Kendrick et al., 2001; Kopf et al., 2001). Despite the lack of robust data, several retrospective analyses have reported higher recurrence-free survival when compared to control groups and tumor regression rates of around 30% also being associated with a better control of hormone excess (Allolio & Fassnacht, 2006; Terzolo et al., 2007). Treatment with mitotane has especially good results in patients previously submitted to tumor resection, who begun therapy right after surgery and who are submitted to regular monitoring of mitotane plasma levels (Daffara et al., 2008).

When considering recurrent or advanced adrenocortical cancer, aggressive resection of local or distant disease is still considered to be an effective therapy method capable of increasing overall survival (Schteingart et al., 1982; Meyer et al., 2004). However, in these cases the use of cytotoxic drugs such as mitotane alone or in combination with other chemotherapeutic agents has to be utilized (Allolio & Fassnacht, 2006).

Mitotane is recommended even in patients with unresectable advanced disease, since several studies have reported the effectiveness of this drug in producing objective improvements in the majority of treated patients, despite its low impact on survival. Moreover, it has been demonstrated that cytotoxic activity of chemotherapeutic agents is increased when combined with mitotane in human adrenal carcinoma cells in vitro (Bukowski et al., 1993; Abraham et al., 2002). Despite the modest results found in the few prospective trials published until now, the combination of mitotane with different chemotherapeutic regimens resulted in overall response rates varying between 14 to 49% (Berruti et al., 2005; Khan et al., 2000; Abraham et al., 2002; Bonacci et al., 1998).

Other regimens of chemotherapy without mitotane have been also evaluated in a few clinical trials but showed modest response rates, revealing the need for the development of more and better drugs and well-designed prospective trials (Schlumberger et al., 1988; Quinkler et al., 2008; Khan et al., 2004).

One must be conscious that progresses in this cancer treatment are limited and slow. More clinical trials and large prospective studies are necessary to better support physicians' choices of treatment. An example of those trials was the recently concluded "First International Randomized trial in locally advanced and Metastatic Adrenocortical Carcinoma Treatment" (FIRM-ACT), an international clinical study comparing the efficacy of etoposide, doxorubicin and cisplatin (EDP) plus mitotane versus streptozotocin plus mitotane in patients with metastatic adrenocortical cancer. This sufficiently large prospective study gave support to the use of the first therapeutic combination (EDP+mitotane) in these conditions (Fassnacht et al., 2011).

The use of radiation therapy or radiofrequency ablation are the least studied hypothesis. They are mainly beneficial in patients with unresectable local tumors with local symptoms or symptomatic metastasis (Schteingart et al., 2005; Polat et al., 2009; Magee et al., 1987). Their impact in patients' survival is still unknown and needs further investigation (Wood et al., 2003; Mayo-Smith et al., 2004).

In the future one may expect that the understanding of the specific molecular alterations in these malignant cells can identify suitable therapeutical targets that may significantly improve the prognosis for these patients.

3. Primary hyperaldosteronism/Conn's syndrome

The synthesis of aldosterone by the adrenal glands occurs in the *zona glomerulosa*. The major conditions for the production of this hormone such as the low concentration of 17-alpha-hydroxylase and the ability to add an hydroxyl group at the 18-carbon position and its subsequent oxidation to an aldehyde, only occur in the *zona glomerulosa* and this processing is mediated by a single multifunctional cytochrome P450 - CYP11B2 or Aldo Synthase (White et al., 1987; White, 1994; Ulick et al., 1992; Holland & Carr, 1993).

The aldosterone-producing adenoma was first described by Conn in 1954 (Conn, 1955; Young, 2007a), who also established for the first time the relationship between adrenal aldosterone-producing tumors, hypertension, and hypokalemia (Gittler & Fajans, 1995). In addition to the aldosterone-producing adenoma (APA), other subtypes of primary aldosteronism (PA) have been described over the subsequent four decades (Conn, 1955; Conn, 1964; Gitler & Fajans, 1995; Young, 2007a; Stowasser, 2009). The most common is the bilateral idiopathic hyperaldosteronism (IHA) which represent approximately 70% of all PA cases (while APA, approximately 30%). Other forms include unilateral hyperplasia or primary adrenal hyperplasia (caused by hyperplasia of the *zona glomerulosa* of only one adrenal gland), familial hyperaldosteronism type I (glucocorticoid-remediable aldosteronism - GRA) caused by the existence of an hybrid gene composed of the CYP11B1 promoter and CYP11B2 gene in which aldosterone is produced in response to ACTH and hence responds to glucocorticoid mediated suppression of ACTH, familial hyperaldosteronism type II (the familial occurrence of aldosterone-producing adenoma or bilateral idiopathic hyperplasia or both), and also the familial or sporadic occurrence of APA due to a mutation in the gene of the K^+ channel (KCNJ5) (Choi et al., 2011).

Finally, in spite of being very rare, pure aldosterone-producing adrenocortical carcinomas and ectopic aldosterone-secreting tumors (e.g. neoplasms in the ovary or kidney) may also occur.

The screening of PA is done by the demonstration of an elevated aldosterone level (> 15 ng/dl) together with the suppression of Plasma Renin Activity (PRA), translated in an increased Aldosterone (*in ng/dl*)/PRA (*in ng/ml/h*) ratio above 20 or 40 (accordingly to the desired sensitivity).

Then a confirmatory test is needed and this can be done by one of the following tests:

- fludrocortisone suppression test
- oral salt load
- saline infusion test
- Captopril test

Since these tumors are generally very small, CT scan has a low sensitivity to localize them, and the fact that in people above 40 to 50 years of age, the prevalence of incidentalomas is high makes its specificity also decrease. Therefore the gold standard for a correct diagnosis of APA is Adrenal Venous Sampling in spite of the fact that it is an invasive method with a good success rate only in the hands of experienced radiologists.

During the past two decades it has become increasingly recognized that primary aldosteronism is much more common than previously thought. It is currently acknowledged that primary aldosteronism accounts for up to 5–10% of hypertensive patients, correlating with the severity of hypertension and going up to 20% in cases of resistant hypertension (i.e one that does not respond to 3-drug-regimen).

The clinical features of PA are mostly determined by the renal actions of aldosterone. Its diagnosis is more frequently made in patients who are in the third to sixth decades of life, with resistant hypertension, accompanied by marked hypokalemia, possibly muscle weakness and cramping, headaches, palpitations, polydipsia, polyuria, nocturia, or a combination of these. There is, however, generally a characteristic lack of edema!

Hypokalemia, once the most important "screening" method for PA is observed less and less frequently both due to the sodium restriction that most doctors recommend to their patients with high blood pressure and also to the higher prevalence of BAH *vs* APA observed in the more recent series.

Patients' elevated blood pressure is a major clinical finding in PA (Mattsson & Young, 2006; Young, 2007a). However, PA is rarely associated with malignant hypertension (Zarifis et al., 1996). In a study of Blumenfeld and colleagues, the mean blood pressure was 184/112 mmHg in patients with an adrenal adenoma and 161/105 mmHg in patients diagnosed with bilateral hyperplasia (Blumenfeld et al., 1994). One important and special feature associated with PA hypertension is the failure to achieve the goal blood pressure (BP) despite a complete adherence to a multi-drug regimen of treatment.

It was also clearly demonstrated that aldosterone excess has direct adverse cardiovascular consequences that go well beyond the risks associated with this type of hypertension (Stowasser, 2009). Aldosterone is responsible for the development of myocardial fibrosis aggravating the prognosis post myocardial infarct (MI) and in congestive heart failure (CHF).

Cardiovascular risk factors seem to be more severe with PA, since when matched for age, blood pressure and the duration of hypertension, these patients have greater left ventricular mass measurements when compared to patients with other types of hypertension, including essential hypertension, pheochromocytoma, and Cushing's syndrome (Milliez et al., 2005; Tanabe et al., 1997). Also, in a case–control study of 124 patients with PA and 465 patients with essential hypertension, matched for age, sex, and systolic and diastolic blood pressure, it was found that patients presenting with either APA or bilateral hyperplasia had a significantly higher rate of cardiovascular events (e.g. stroke, atrial fibrillation and myocardial infarction) than the matched essential hypertension patients (Milliez et al., 2005).

Furthermore, some particular renal effects may be also experienced by PA patients, independently of their systemic hypertension. Several reports have shown that glomerular filtration rate (GFR) and urinary albumin excretion may be increased in these patients; however these changes appear to be largely reversible after appropriate treatment. Adrenalectomy increased the serum creatinine and decreased the mean GFR. Treatment with spironolactone resulted in a similar decline in GFR. Thus, surgical cure or mineralocorticoid receptor blockade reverse the hyperfiltration state and unmask the underlying renal insufficiency (Stowasser, 2009).

One final point to be stressed in relation to PA is that generally APA should be treated surgically while bilateral adrenal hyperplasias are better treated medically with mineralocorticoid inhibition by means of spironolactone, eplerenone or amiloride. Nevertheless, even APAs, specially the small ones, may also be treated appropriately with these drugs and hence, the choice should always be given to the patients.

4. Androgen-secreting adrenal cortex tumors

Androgen-secreting adrenal cortex tumors are rare tumors, accounting for only 0.2% of the causes of androgen excess (Azziz et al., 2004; Carmina et al., 2006). Androgen over-secretion results in the development of androgenic features in affected women, with the development of hirsutism, androgenic alopecia, acne, ovulatory dysfunction, and, if the oversecretion is extreme or prolonged, even virilization may ensue (Wajchenberg et al., 2000; Azziz et al., 2004).

Despite the fact that benign androgen-secreting adrenal tumors have been described, the finding of androgen secretion by an ACT is considered to be highly suggestive of malignancy. The presence of a virilizing adrenocortical carcinoma can be suggested by very high testosterone levels and the failure of androgen suppression in response to glucocorticoid administration (Kaltsas et al., 2003; Waggoner et al., 1999; Derksen et al., 1994). In a report of 21 women with androgen-secreting tumors, serum testosterone levels were 2.6-fold higher in the women with malignant tumors (n=10) than in women with benign tumors (n=11) (Moreno et al., 2004).

Benign cortisol-secreting adenomas can also produce small amounts of androgens, but the serum androgen levels are usually not elevated (Kamenicky et al., 2007).

Considering its elevated probability of malignancy it is of great importance to identify patients with this type of rare carcinomas among women with androgen excess, due to its life-threatening potential (Wajchenberg et al., 2000). Despite several authors having considered that a clinical presentation with rapidly progressive virilization was sufficient to identify patients requiring a more extensive investigation (Kettel, 1989), it is consensual that some androgen-secreting adrenocortical tumors may produce only moderate levels of androgens and have a rather indolent presentation (Rosenfield , 2005; Kaltsas et al., 2003).

It should also be noticed that androgen-secreting tumors in men same as estrogen secreting tumors in women, may not result in clinically significant syndromes, and both can be erroneously considered as non-functioning, delaying their treatment. If one doesn't apply an extensive analytical protocol to nonfunctioning adrenocortical tumors, only the development of mass effects or the occurrence of metastases would lead to their recognition as malignant.

5. Estrogen-secreting adrenal cortex tumors

Estrogen-secreting adrenal cortex tumors correspond to a very rare type of tumors characterized by the over-production of estrogens (estrone or estradiol). The over- secretion of these hormones may cause precocious puberty with very early menarche in girls and more often sex-reversal characteristics in men (feminizing symptoms) (Advani et al., 2010). The feminizing symptoms, such as the characteristic gynecomastia, are associated with the expression of the cytochrome P450 aromatase (aromatase) in adrenocortical cells. Normally, aromatase catalyses the conversion of C19 steroids into estrogens in tissues such as the ovarian follicles' granulosa layer and the adipose tissue, whereas normal adrenal tissues have no detectable aromatase activity (Watanabe & Nakajin, 2004).

6. Cushing's syndrome

The Cushing's syndrome was first described by Harvey Cushing in 1932, and can be caused by several mechanisms associated with increased levels of cortisol in the blood. The diagnosis of Cushing's syndrome is determined through biochemical tests, since the presence of suggestive symptoms and signs are not enough to sustain it. In fact none of its symptoms is pathognomonic and most of them are non-specific such as obesity, hypertension and increased cardiovascular risk, menstrual irregularity and infertility, osteoporosis and glucose intolerance. It can also cause some form of psychological distress, going from impaired quality of life to depression and even psychosis. It should always be borne in mind, however, that if left untreated, Cushing's syndrome has a 5 fold excess mortality.

The high levels of cortisol in the blood can be caused not only by adrenocortical tumors but also by adrenocorticotropic hormone (ACTH) or corticotropin-releasing hormone (CRH) hyperproduction, as well as by the excessive intake of glucocorticoid drugs. This is even one of the most frequent causes of Cushing's syndrome (Iatrogenic Cushing's). In the study of a Cushing's syndrome case these situations need to be excluded (Weber SL., 1997; Hughes et al., 1996; Quddusi et al., 1998). Moreover, special attention is also required for other disorders causing hypercortisolism-related symptoms and sometimes also exhibiting mild to moderate elevations of plasma cortisol, known as pseudo-Cushing's syndrome. The pseudo-Cushing's syndromes may include:

- Patients who are physically stressed (e.g. severe bacterial infections) (Liddle, 1960);
- Patients with severe obesity, especially visceral obesity or polycystic ovary syndrome (Liddle, 1960);
- Patients with psychological stress (major depressive disorder and severe melancholic syndromes) (Gold et al., 1986);
- Rarely, also patients with chronic alcoholism (Kirkman & Nelson, 1988).

The difficulties normally met in Cushing's syndrome diagnostic process are well translated by the fact that patients normally express some signs and symptoms of the syndrome, 2 years before a confirmation of diagnosis can be reached. After raising the suspicion by the observation of a patient with central (truncal) obesity plus hypertension, in many cases accompanied by a typical cushingoid facies (round, plethoric face), the most specific signs are the presence of thin skin, easy bruising and proximal myopathy. However, to avoid mistakes in diagnosing Cushing's syndrome due to all of the different conditions that might imitate its signs and symptoms, initial diagnostic tests for hypercortisolism must be highly sensitive. According to the evidence-based 2008 Endocrine Society Clinical Guidelines the *first-line tests* for this syndrome should be the late night salivary cortisol, the 24h urinary cortisol, or the low-dose dexamethasone suppression test (either the 1 mg, overnight or the 2mg/day, 48h dexamethasone suppression tests). To establish the diagnosis of Cushing's syndrome the following criteria should be met (Nieman et al., 2008):

- At least two of the first-line tests must be abnormal and conservative criteria should be used to interpret it to maximize sensitivity; for instance, in a patient with a symptomatic Cushing's syndrome, the cortisol cutoff level to be considered as un-suppressed after the Dexamethasone test should be >1.8 μg/dl (while in the case of incidentalomas studied to exclude subclinical Cushing's syndrome, specificity should be the main criterion and so the cutoff level should be >5 μg /dl).
- Urinary and salivary cortisol measurements should be obtained at least twice;
- The urinary cortisol excretion should be unequivocally increased (threefold above the upper limit of normal for the assay), or the diagnosis of Cushing's syndrome is uncertain and other tests should be performed;
- The patient should undergo additional evaluation if the test results are discordant or only slightly abnormal;
- If test results are normal, the patient does not have Cushing's syndrome unless it is extremely mild or cyclic. Additional evaluations are not suggested unless symptoms progress or cyclic Cushing's syndrome is suspected.

Cushing's syndrome is rare (it has an incidence of up to 3:1.000.000 persons per year) (Lindholm et al., 2001). It's also an intriguing condition both because of its complex diagnostic protocol and the demand for a correct treatment to avoid its devastating complications that can even conduct to death if left untreated. After diagnosing the hypercortisolism, it is important to determine its cause (Table 3) to better chose the appropriate treatment. It is a disease whose patients should be sent to a major hospital where multidisciplinary and well experienced teams will be available.

Diagnosis	Percentage of Patients (%)
ACTH-dependent Cushing's syndrome	
Cushing's disease	68
Ectopic ACTH syndrome	12
Ectopic CRH syndrome	< 1
ACTH-independent Cushing's syndrome	
Adrenal adenoma	10
Adrenal carcinoma	8
Micronodular hyperplasia	1
Macronodular hyperplasia	< 1
Pseudo-Cushing's syndrome	
Major depressive disorder	1
Alcoholism	< 1

Table 3. Frequency of causes of Cushing's syndrome

One of the most important, and therefore the initial, phase of determining Cushing's syndrome's etiology is to determine if the hypercortisolism is ACTH-dependent or ACTH independent. The ACTH-dependent hypercortisolism is normally due to a pituitary (or less frequently non-pituitary) ACTH secreting tumor, while ACTH-independent hypercortisolism is usually due to an adrenal tumor or hyperplasia. The preferred test is naturally the measurement of plasma ACTH. Usually a low plasma ACTH concentration of <5 pg/mL (1.1 pmol/L) in a hypercortisolemic patient is evidence of ACTH-independent disease (Invitti et al., 1999), while if the plasma ACTH concentration is above 15 pg/mL (3.3 pmol/L) it can be assumed that cortisol secretion is ACTH-dependent. Despite values between 5 and 15 pg/mL (1.1 to 3.3 pmol/L) being less definitive they normally indicate the hypercortisolism is ACTH-dependent. However, it is recommendable to perform a CRH stimulation test in these patients to confirm that hypothesis.

In the presence of an ACTH-independent Cushing's syndrome, it is important to proceed with a thin-section CT imaging of the adrenal glands, to determine its cause. When CT imaging suggests a suspicious lesion (for instance with large size) further investigation will be required to distinguish between the malignant ACC and benign ACT. The presence of bilateral disease on the other hand implies the distinction between, for instance, a bilateral tumor and bilateral macronodular adrenal hyperplasia.

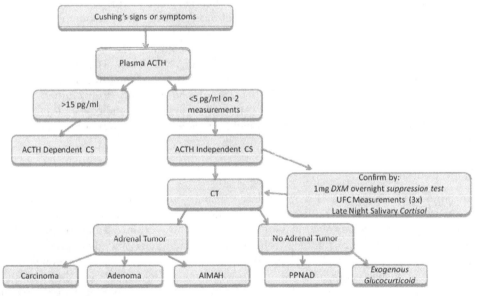

Fig. 2. Cushing syndrome

Unilateral adenomas causing Cushing's syndrome should be surgically removed as they imply a very significant increase in morbidity and mortality, which is due to cardiovascular diseases or infections.

For the great majority of ACTH-dependent Cushing's syndrome patients, the cause of the hypercortisolism is a pituitary corticotroph adenoma (Cushing's disease). Even so, patients with ACTH-dependent disease should undergo non-invasive tests such as the high-dose dexamethasone suppression test and the CRH stimulation test, to confirm the presence of Cushing's disease. It is also important to exclude extrapituitary (ectopic) sources of ACTH.

7. Subclinical Cushing's syndrome

The "subclinical" Cushing's syndrome (SCS) refers to autonomous cortisol production that is insufficient to generate the typical, clinically recognizable, combination of symptoms. The prevalence of overt Cushing's syndrome caused by an adrenal adenoma in the general population is lower than the prevalence of subclinical Cushing's syndrome in patients with clinically non-functioning adrenal adenoma (Ross, 1994).

Patients with SCS have an adrenal mass usually detected incidentally (an incidentaloma) and normally do not show any of the clinical manifestation of the Cushing's syndrome (Terzolo et al., 2005a). Still, they have some endocrine alterations that allows their recognition (Urinary free cortisol > 70 µg /24h; serum cortisol levels after a dexamethasone suppression   test >5 µg/dl; morning ACTH levels < 10 pg/ml). According to the Italian National survey on 1,004 adrenal incidentalomas (Mantero et al., 2000), of which 92 were classified as SCS, the hormonal evaluation showed low baseline secretion of ACTH in 79% of the SCS patients, lack of suppressibility of cortisol secretion after 1 mg dexamethasone in 73%, supra-normal 24-hour urinary cortisol excretion in 75% or disturbed cortisol circadian rhythm in 43%. Subclinical Cushing's syndrome is the most commonly detected abnormality in patients with adrenal incidentalomas.

Most patients with SCS may show one or more of the clinical manifestation of cortisol over-secretion, such as arterial hypertension, obesity or diabetes (Terzolo et al., 2000; Angeli & Terzolo, 2002). The association between a clinically silent adrenal adenoma and some of clinical manifestations of the metabolic syndrome has been studied and is considered well proven. In a retrospective study done by Terzolo and colleagues (Terzolo et al., 2005b), of 210 such patients, 53.8% had hypertension, 21.4% were obese and 22.4% had hyperglycemia.

8. Incidentalomas

An adrenal incidentaloma is a mass lesion, usually with 1cm or more in diameter, discovered incidentally by radiologic examination (Young, 2007b). In recent years these incidentally discovered adrenal masses have been found with increasing frequency due to the widespread use of imaging techniques of the abdomen and their prevalence is estimated to be around 4% in the general population (Bovio et al., 2006). Several studies have been published concerning the prevalence of adrenal incidentalomas. In a series of 739 autopsies, Hedeland and colleagues (Hedeland et al., 1968) reported the presence of adrenal masses in 9% of normotensive patients versus 12% in patients with hypertension. In another review including 25 studies (Kloos et al., 1995), the calculated prevalence of adrenal incidentaloma was of 6%. The prevalence of adrenal adenomas increases with age from 0.2%in a patient between 20 and 29 years of age to 7% in a patient over 70 years of age (Young, 2007; Kloos et al., 1995). It is noteworthy that they are rare under the age of 40.

Despite the fact that the majority of adrenal incidentalomas are clinically non-hypersecreting and benign adrenocortical adenomas (Mansmann et al., 2004), frequently, incidentalomas' series include cases that are cortisol secreting adrenocortical adenomas (5 to 9%) (Mantero et al., 2000; Young 2007) or pheochromocytomas (3 to 5%) (Young, 2007; Cawood et al., 2009). Of these pheochromocytomas, 50% are normotensive (Motta Ramirez et al., 2005). Incidentalomas can also be adrenocortical carcinomas and metastatic carcinomas. In a group of 2005 patients with adrenal incidentalomas, almost 5% were adrenocortical carcinomas and 2.5% corresponded to other primary carcinomas'metastases (Young, 2000).

The approach to the evaluation and management of adrenal incidentalomas usually begins with taking patients' clinical history and performing a physical examination, testing for signs or symptoms of adrenal hyperfunction or malignant disease, and performing a complete hormonal evaluation (Young, 2007; Kudva et al., 2003; Terzolo et al., 2005).

The probability to find a primary adrenal carcinoma in these cases has to be considered as rare, in spite of being dependant on the size of the tumor (above 4 cm the probability of an incidentaloma being malignant is 24% (Angeli et al., 1997); however, due to the importance of such a situation the initial major concern in evaluating an adrenal incidentaloma is the possibility of malignancy, followed by the evaluation of the possibility of metastatic cancer. In fact, one should also remember that several types of carcinomas may metastasize to the adrenal glands (e.g. lung, kidney, colon, breast, pancreas, liver and stomach).

Adrenal incidentalomas are bilateral in 10-to 15% of the cases. In these cases the etiology will be one of the following: metastases; congenital adrenal hyperplasia; bilateral adenomas, bilateral adrenocortical macronodular hyperplasia; bilateral pheochromocytomas; hemorrhage, lymphoma; infectious or infiltrative diseases.

As a main conclusion we would like to stress that it is of crucial importance to evaluate all patients with adrenal incidentalomas for the possibility of either subclinical hormonal hyper-function, including SCS and pheochromocytoma, as well as cancer. Table 4 describes major evaluations and clinical features for differential diagnosis of adrenal incidentalomas.

9. Pediatric adrenal cortex tumors

The presence and diagnosis of adrenal cortex tumors in children is rare and may occur sporadically or as a component of certain hereditary tumour syndromes, such as the Li-Fraumeni syndrome, the multiple endocrine neoplasia-1 (MEN1), the Beckwith-Wiedemann syndrome, the Carney complex, and even in some rare cases of congenital adrenal hyperplasia. Its incidence is around 1 to 3 in 10.000.000 except in the southern regions of Brazil where it reaches 1 to 3 :1.000.000 (Agrons et al., 1999; Ribeiro et al., 2000, Wasserman et al., 2011).).

In southern Brazil, these carcinomas are frequently associated with a particular mutation of TP53 (namely Arg337His) (Ribeiro et al., 1990).

Clinical and biological characteristics of adrenocortical tumours are different from those observed in other paediatric carcinomas. About 65% of them are diagnosed in children younger than 5 years of age (Ribeiro et al., 1990). This age distribution has been demonstrated in several reports, including a study of Zerbini and colleagues, with 32 pediatric patients with adrenocortical neoplasms, in which the age at diagnosis ranged from 6 months to 19 years (median age, 5 years), with a predominant number of patients being 5 years of age and younger (Zerbini et al., 1992). In another study of Lefebvre and colleagues, with 42 children with adrenocortical neoplasms, two-thirds were younger than 5 years of age (Lefevre et al., 1983).

Diagnosis	Suggestive Clinical Features	Imaging Characteristics
Adrenocortical Adenoma	May have symptoms related to excess glucocorticoid, mineralocorticoid, androgen, or estrogen secretion	• Round or oval, with smooth margins • Homogeneous • Rare tumor calcification, necrosis or hemorrhage • Small, usually ≤ 3 cm in diameter • Usually solitary, unilateral • CT unenhanced attenuation values ≤10 HU (25% may have low lipid content and hence have attenuation values >10%) • Not highly vascular • Isointense in relation to liver onT1- and T2-weighted images in MRI • No delay in contrast medium washout (ten minutes after administration of contrast, an absolute contrast medium washout of 50 % or more)
Adrenocortical carcinoma	Mass effect symptoms, symptoms related to excess glucocorticoid, mineralocorticoid, androgen, or estrogen secretion. The size (>4/6 cm) and the evolution are the most important signs to raise the suspicion	• Irregular shape • Inhomogeneous density because of central areas of low attenuation due to tumor necrosis • Common tumor calcification • Diameter usually >4 cm • Unilateral location • High unenhanced CT attenuation values (>20 HU) • Inhomogeneous enhancement on CT with intravenous contrast • Delay in contrast medium washout (ten minutes after administration of contrast, an absolute contrast medium washout of less than 50 %) • Hypo-intensity compared with liver on T-1 weighted MRI and high to intermediate signal intensity on T-2 weighted MRI • High standardized uptake value (SUV) on FDG-PET-CT study • Evidence of local invasion or metastases.

Diagnosis	Suggestive Clinical Features	Imaging Characteristics
Pheochromocytoma	Hypertension, Paroxysmal Symptoms (e.g. palpitation, diaphoresis, headache, pallor, tremor). Half of the cases will remain undiagnosed! Plasma metanephrines and 24h urine metanephrines are the initial screening tests	• Round or oval, with clear margins • Heterogeneous, with cystic areas • Usually large • Usually solitary, unilateral • High unenhanced CT attenuation values (>10 HU) (usually >25) • Usually vascular • Delay in contrast medium washout (ten minutes after administration of contrast, an absolute contrast medium washout of less than 50 percent) but may be normal, mimicking the adenomas • Markedly hyper intense in relation to the liver on T2-weighted images, in MRI • Chemical-shift imaging: Pheos and ACC don't loose signal intensity on out-of phase images in comparison with in-phase ones, whereas adenomas do • Hemorrhage and cystic areas common
Metastatic Cancer	Cancer-specific signs. The identification of a primary extra-adrenal cancer favors this possibility	• Irregular shape and inhomogeneous nature • Tendency to be bilateral • High unenhanced CT attenuation values (>20 HU) and enhancement with intravenous contrast on CT • Delay in contrast medium washout (ten minutes after administration of contrast, an absolute contrast medium washout of less than 50 percent) • Isointense or slightly less intense than the liver on T-1 weighted MRI and high to intermediate signal intensity on T-2 weighted MRI (representing an increased water content)

Adapted from Young WF, Jr. Clinical practice. The incidentally discovered adrenal mass. N Engl J Med 2007a; 356: 601-10

Table 4. Clinical features and imaging characteristics of adrenal incidentalomas

About half of the adrenocortical tumours in children have predisposing constitutional genetic factors, and are usually associated with the Li-Fraumeni syndrome or the Beckwith-Wiedemann syndrome (Li & Fraumeni, 1969a; Wiedemann, 1983; Lynch et al., 1978).

The Li-Fraumeni syndrome is a cancer-predisposing syndrome that includes breast cancer, brain carcinoma, sarcomas, leukaemia and adrenocortical carcinoma (Li & Fraumeni, 1969a; Lynch et al., 1978). This syndrome is a rare autosomal dominant condition associated with germline mutations of the tumour suppressor gene TP53 on the chromosome 17 (17p13) (Li & Fraumeni, 1969b; Li et al., 1998;). The patient and the affected family members may develop different types of tumours (Birch, 1994; Srivastava et al., 1990; Sandrini et al., 1997; Hisada et al., 1998).

On the other side the Beckwith-Wiedemann syndrome, associated with abnormalities involving chromosome 11p15, and defined as a growth disorder is sometimes referred to as the EMG [exomphalos-macroglossia-gigantism] syndrome. This syndrome is associated with an increased risk of benign and malignant tumors of multiple organs (Fraumeni & Miller et al., 1967; Wiedemann, 1983), particularly the Wilms tumor of the kidneys and adrenocortical carcinoma (Lack, 1997).

The incidence of adrenocortical carcinomas in children is higher in girls. These pediatric carcinomas are hormone secreting tumors more frequently than in adults (90% vs 50%) (Michalkiewicz et al., 2004; Patil et al., 2002; Bonfig et al., 2003). The classic endocrine syndromes (namely the virilising and the Cushing's syndromes) represent the most common presentations of adrenocortical carcinomas in this age group (Wilkins, 1948 and Ribeiro et al., 2000).

However in spite of being pathologically malignant these carcinomas have a much better prognosis, with many of them becoming cured by the first surgical intervention (Michalkiewicz et al., 2004; Sutter et al., 2006; Wieneke et al., 2003; 27: Sabbaga et al., 1993)

10. ACTH-independent adrenal cortex hyperplasias

ACTH-independent hypercortisolism is always of adrenocortical origin and an adrenocortical adenoma or carcinoma are by far its most common aetiologies (in up to 95% of patients). The remaining cases will be adrenocortical hyperplasias.

Even in these cases it's important to distinguish adrenocorticotropin (ACTH)–dependent forms like Cushing's disease or CAH (due to 21-hydroxylase deficiency) from ACTH-independent ones as a primary step in the differential diagnosis of Cushing's syndrome due to adrenocortical bilateral hyperplasias (Doppman et al., 2000).

Among the adrenal causes of Cushing's syndrome about 10-15% are due to bilateral adrenal lesions that include micronodular (particularly its most common variant the *Primary Pigmented Nodular Adrenocortical Disease – PPNAD*) and macronodular adrenal hyperplasias (*ACTH-Independent Macronodular Adrenocortical Hyperplasia - AIMAH*) and, more rarely, bilateral adenomas or carcinomas (Christopoulos et al., 2005; Stratakis & Boikos, 2007).

The hyperplasias can be sporadic or familial as is the case of PPNAD that can occur isolated or as part of an autosomal dominant disease including other tumors, endocrine and non-endocrine, called the Carney Complex.

Many adrenal cortex hyperplasia cases are thought to be the consequence of genetic changes in several key components of the cyclic AMP (cAMP) pathway (Libé & Betherat, 2005; Groussin et al., 2002a; Stratakis et al., 2007). Activating germline mutations of the ACTH receptor (MC2R) gene, making it display high levels of basal activity, have been reported

(Swords et al., 2002). The same occurred with GNAS activating mutations resulting in constitutive activation of the cAMP pathway that were shown to cause ACTH-independent macronodular adrenocortical hyperplasia (AIMAH) in McCune-Albright syndrome (Weinstein, 1991). On the other hand PRKAR1A-inactivating mutations resulting in a permanent activation of PKA may be associated to the development of PPNAD either isolated or as part of the Carney complex (Kirschner et al., 2000; Groussin et al., 2002b). More recently, inactivating mutations of the phosphodiesterase 11A gene, a gene coding for an enzyme that normally regulates cyclic nucleotide levels was reported both in cases of PPNAD and other bilateral hyperplasias (e.g. macronodular) (Libé et al., 2008).

11. ACTH-independent macronodular hyperplasias

The ACTH-independent macronodular adrenocortical hyperplasias (AIMAH) constitute a rare condition that consists of multiple bilateral adrenocortical macronodules causing a striking enlargement of the adrenal glands (Doppman et al., 1991; Malchoff et al., 1989; Swain et al., 1998). The great majority of AIMAH cases is sporadic. AIMAH is responsible for less than 1% of all the endogenous cases of Cushing's syndrome (Christopoulos et al., 2005). Usually patients present in the fifth and sixth decades of life, a significantly latter age of onset compared to other cortisol producing adenomas (Swain et al., 1998).

11.1 AIMAH pathogenesis
Increased cortisol levels in AIMAH result from the fact that hormones other than ACTH become able to activate cortisol secretion through receptors aberrantly located in the adrenal cortex cells and coupled to cAMP activation. Hormones like GIP, catecholamines, vasopressin, serotonin, LH among others can activate PKA signaling, via cAMP production, leading to a situation of Cushing's syndrome.
In fact a great number of patients with AIMAH have that ectopic expression of and/or increased responsiveness to one of several possible receptors like the gastric inhibitory polypeptide (GIP) receptors (food-dependent hypercortisolism) (Resnik et al., 1992; N'diaye et al., 1998), vasopressin receptors (Horiba et al., 1995), the β-adrenergic receptors (Lacroix et al., 1997), the LH receptors, the serotonin receptors, the leptin receptors and angiotensin II receptors (Lacroix et al., 1997; Lacroix et al., 2001; Lacroix et al., 1992).
In the example of GIP-activated-cortisol-production, k cells from the duodenum and small intestine release, after food ingestion, a gastro-intestinal hormone named GIP (Gastric Inhibiting Peptide or Glucose-dependent Insulinotropic Peptide) in physiological concentrations (Lacroix et al., 2001). The expression of GIP receptors in the cells of the *zona fasciculata*, where they normally don't exist, can then be activated by the GIP secreted in response to meals, causing what is known as "food-dependent" cortisol production. The presence of this receptor can be confirmed *in vivo* by clinical testing or by adrenal imaging following the injection of [^{123}I]-GIP (Lacroix et al., 1992).
To date, more than 30 cases were reported where the adrenal hormonal hypersecretion was associated to GIP stimulation. In the majority of cases patients presented with AIMAH (Lacroix et al., 2004; Groussin et al., 2002c). Besides that, other receptors were identified, some ectopically expressed and some being eutopic but showing an over-expression in the adrenocortical cells, as being the cause of cases of AIMAH and recently also demonstrated in cases of unilateral adenomas (Lacroix, 2009).
The majority of cases of AIMAH is sporadic. Some cases however are familial and in most an autosomal dominant hereditarity has been described (Lacroix, 2009). Nevertheless, the

genetic cause for these cases hasn't yet been identified. In addition to those familiar reports, AIMAH has been described in MEN-1 with a frequency between 6% (Burgess et al., 1996) and 21% (Skogseid et al., 1992), and in rare cases of Gs alpha subunit mutations (Weinstein et al., 1991; Fragoso et al., 2003) or activating mutations of the ACTH receptor (MC2R) (Swords et al., 2002):

- **Gs alpha-subunit mutations** — an activating mutation in the gene of the Gsa subunit of G-protein coupled receptors (stimulatory guanine nucleotide-binding protein, Gs) leads to constitutive activation of cAMP. These mutations may be responsible not only for increased production of cortisol but also for increased proliferation and consequently the formation of adrenal nodules (Weinstein et al., 1991; Fragoso et al., 2003).
- **MEN1** – In patients with multiple endocrine neoplasia syndrome type 1 (MEN1) caused by mutations in the the tumor suppressor gene *menin*, together with the more frequent endocrine tumors that are characteristic of the syndrome, adrenocortical adenomas or macronodular bilateral hyperplasias may also occur (Burgess et al., 1996; Skogseid et al., 1992).
- **Other genes** – There were some rare reports of activating mutations of the ACTH receptor (MC2R) gene in adrenal tumors and AIMAH (Swords et al., 2002). Moreover, AIMAH has also been reported in patients with: familial polyposis coli and a mutation in the adenomatous polyposis coli (APC) gene (Kartheuser et al., 1999); in patients with mutations in the fumarate hydratase gene (FH) (Matyakhina et al., 2005) on chromosome 1 (1q42.3-43); and in patients with germline mutations in phosphodiesterase 11A isoform 4 gene (PDE11A) (Libé et al., 2008) located on chromosome 2 (2q31-35).

11.2 AIMAH diagnosis and clinical presentation

Usually AIMAH cases can be discovered after an incidental radiological finding or following the investigation of an adrenal hypersecretion syndrome and can be distinguished from ACTH-dependent macronodular hyperplasia by a suppressed plasma ACTH (<5 pg/mL *vs.* ≥15 pg/mL).

The most common laboratory findings associated with AIMAH are the following:

- Increased serum and urinary cortisol and undetectable plasma ACTH in the basal state (Doppman et al., 2000; Swain et al., 1998; Kirschner et al., 1964; Bourdeau et al., 2001; Lieberman et al., 1994).
- As in any cause of adrenal cortisol hypersecretion, dexamethasone suppression test fails to suppress cortisol production (Christopoulos et al., 2005).

An exception to this general pattern occurs in patients with GIP-dependent Cushing's syndrome in whom cortisol hypersecretion occurs in response to meals and serum cortisol may be low in the fasting state (Resnik et al., 1992; Lacroix et al., 1992).

- Steroid hormone synthesis is relatively inefficient in AIMAH as a consequence of decreased steroidogenic enzymatic activity resulting frequently in elevated 17-hydroxyprogesterone levels after stimulation with ACTH (Bourdeau et al., 2001).
- Serum 18-hydroxycorticosterone, corticosterone and estrone may cause hypertension or feminization in the patients in whom they are increased (Wada et al., 2002).

The diagnosis of AIMAH is usually suspected after typical imaging studies, which can be variable. At the computed tomography (CT) the adrenal glands in patients with AIMAH are greatly enlarged with multiple macronodules up to 5 cm in diameter. These adrenals' weight may vary between 24 to 500g (Doppman et al., 2000; Malchoff et al., 1989).

The asymmetric appearance of the adrenal macronodules in AIMAH has been described (Liebermann et al., 1994; Lacroix et al., 2001) and also, according to a study including patients with surgically proven AIMAH, adrenal masses measuring up to 5 cm of soft tissue density can distort and obscure the adrenal glands (Doppman et al., 1991). This may conduct to the erroneous diagnosis of a unilateral adenoma.

Therefore, other clinical and molecular features must be used in diagnosing AIMAH.

One important suggestion consist of evaluating all patients with AIMAH and clinical and sub-clinical Cushing's syndrome for the presence of aberrant receptors, that are very frequently present in AIMAH (Lacroix et al., 2001; Mircescu et al., 2000).

In this scenario, tests that modulate the levels of ligands for those receptors may be useful determining cortisol and other steroid changes. These tests include physiological tests, such as upright posture and mixed meals, and pharmacological tests including gonadotropin-releasing hormone, thyrotropin-releasing hormone, vasopressin, glucagon and metoclopramide (Lacroix et al., 2001; Mircescu et al., 2000). Cortisol increases ≥25% are considered as significant, provided there is no increase in ACTH. If necessary, these tests should be carried out under Dexamethasone suppression. Responses between 25% and 49% are considered partial responses and if ≥50% complete responses. Any positive change should prompt the continuation of the study to identify all the receptors that may be involved (Lacroix et al., 2001)

The importance of identifying these aberrant receptors is the possibility to have specific therapeutical weapons that may permit avoiding bilateral adrenalectomy:

RECEPTOR	IN VIVO SCREENING	MEDICAL TREATMENT
GIP	Mixed meal (Food-dependent Cushing) Stimulation by GIP infusion	Octreotide GIPR antagonist
Vasopressin	Upright posture Inhibition by water load Stimulation by saline infusion Administration of Arginine Vasopressin Administration of DDAVP (- =V1R; + =V2R)	Vasopressin receptor antagonist DDAVP antagonist (V2)
B-adrenergic	Upright posture Stimulation by insulin-induced hypoglycemia Isoproterenol infusion Propranolol suppression	B-blocker (Propranolol)
LH / βHCG	GnRH test hCG Recombinant LH Pregnancy or Menopausal related cortisol elevation Sometimes also androgen secreting	Long acting GnRH agonist GnRH antagonist
5HT-4	Administration of 5HT-4 agonists Metoclopramide/Cisapride/Tegaserod test	5HT-4 receptor antagonist
Angiotensin	Upright posture Angiotensin infusion (?) Angiotensin antagonist	Angiotensin receptor antagonist

(Adapted from Lacroix et al., 2009 ACTH independent macronodular hyperplasia. Best Practice and Research Clinical Endocrinology and Metabolism. Vol 23. Pp 245-259)

Table 5. Receptors involved in AIMAH, in vivo screening tests and possible medical treatments

12. ACTH-independent micronodular hyperplasias

ACTH-independent micronodular hyperplasias are characterized by the presence of multiple cortical micronodules, with less than 1 cm in diameter (Louiset et al., 2010). These micronodular hyperplasias can be divided in two different subtypes, depending on the presence or absence of nodular pigment and internodular atrophy. The most common and predominant type of ACTH-independent micronodular adrenal hyperplasia is the primary pigmented nodular adrenocortical disease (PPNAD), characterized by multiple pigmented micronodules usually surrounded by internodular cortical atrophy. The pigmented nodules are observed in the zone between the cortex and the medulla and the cells have hybrid characteristics between cortical and medullar (for instance the high expression of synaptophysin). The pigment has been identified as lipofuscin (Louiset et al., 2010).

PPNAD is one of the possible causes of Cushing's syndrome. However, it must be stressed that it is a rare disease representing less than 1% of the cases of Cushing's syndrome. It may be sporadic or familial, and in this case it's one of the components of the Carney complex (Carney & Young, 1992; Stratakis et al., 2001).

12.1 ACTH-independent micronodular hyperplasia- pathogenesis

A few genes were already identified as causal for the development of ACTH-independent micronodular hyperplasia:

- **PRKAR1A** - Most patients with PPNAD, especially when the disease is a component of Carney complex, have germline-inactivating mutations of the PRKAR1A [protein kinase A (PKA) regulatory subunit type 1α] gene (Kirschner et al., 2000; Groussin et al., 2002a; Groussin et al., 2002b). These mutations code for a truncated protein that is not produced, and the loss of this protein leads to an increased activation of protein kinase A (PKA) by cyclic AMP (Nadella & Kirschner, 2005). In several different studies of patients with PPNAD associated with Carney complex, 65-82% had PRKAR1A mutations (Groussin et al., 2002; Veugelers et al., 2004; Bertherat et al 2009).

- **Phosphodiesterase 11A (PDE11A)** - PDE11A is a dual-specificity PDE with affinity both to cAMP and cGMP, expressed in several endocrine tissues (D'Andrea et al., 2005). Decreased expression of PDE11A has been correlated to increased adrenocortical levels of cAMP and cAMP-responsive element (CREB) phosphorylation presumably being the cause of adrenal hyperplasia. Besides having been identified in PPNAD and non-pigmented micronodular bilateral adrenocortical hyperplasias, in a study of Libé and colleagues, the PDE11A missense germline variants were also found in 18.8% of adrenocortical tumors (adrenocortical carcinomas, adenomas and bilateral macronodular adrenal hyperplasias) (Libé et al., 2008).

- **Other genes** - PDE8B gene mutations have also been described in patients with PPNAD or nonpigmented variants of the disease (Horvath et al., 2008).

Moreover, in addition to germline PRKAR1A mutations, somatic beta-catenin mutations have been found in the larger nodules of patients with PPNAD, suggesting that secondary events in the Wnt/beta-catenin signaling pathway can contribute to tumorigenesis in PPNAD (Tadjine et al., 2008; Gaujoux et al., 2008).

12.2 ACTH-independent micronodular hyperplasia – Diagnosis and clinical presentation

Most commonly patients with PPNAD present signs and symptoms of hypercortisolism such as weight gain, obesity, hypertension, and menstrual cycle disorders. However, in many of them these symptoms are subtle and slowly progressive. Besides, sometimes the cortisol hypersecretion can be cyclical rendering these cases difficult to diagnose. On the other hand, there are several characteristics that are unique to this type of micronodular hyperplasia (Carney & Young, 1992; Larsen et al., 1986; Stratakis et al., 2001).

- The majority of patients with PPNAD are diagnosed at a young age, usually before turning 30 years, and many cases occur in patients under 15 years of age.
- Another hallmark is the paradoxical cortisol response to Dexamethasone suppression test, meaning that cortisol raises in response to dexamethasone instead of being reduced (Stratakis et al., 1999).
- At surgery the characteristic pigmentation can be observed.
- Most of the nodules found in these patients are less than 4 mm, and reasonably well demarcated from the adjacent atrophic cortex.

As already mentioned, in some patients with this pathology the development of hypercortisolism symptoms can be cyclic and irregular what causes some typical Cushing's syndrome symptoms to be variable or discrete, therefore complicating its diagnosis. On the other hand, in patients with PPNAD, due to the presence of elevated cortisol levels, osteoporosis and avascular hip necrosis have been reported (Ruder et al., 1974; Carney & Young, 1992).

12.3 Carney complex

PPNAD occurs as part of Carney complex in more than 60% of the cases (Bertherat et al., 2009).

This syndrome is an autosomal dominant form of multiple neoplasia. The main signs that characterize this condition are the presence of spotty skin pigmentation (lentiginosis), the presence of endocrine tumors, including PPNAD (the most common endocrine finding in Carney's complex), testicular large cell calcifying Sertoli cells tumors, GH secreting pituitary adenomas and thyroid adenomas and carcinomas, and non-endocrine tumors, including atrial myxomas, cutaneous myxomas, breast ductal adenomas, psammomatous melanotic schwannomas, and osteochondromyxomas (Stratakis et al., 2001; Carney et al., 1985; Stratakis et al., 1997). Cushing's syndrome caused by PPNAD occurs in many of the cases of Carney Complex. However, if one considers also the subclinical cases of Cushing's syndrome, the percentage will surely be higher (Bertherat et al., 2009; Stratakis et al., 2001).

Three genetic loci were associated with the Carney Complex: 2p16, 17q22-24 and 17p12-13. More than 70% Carney Complex cases have a PRKAR1A mutation (Bertherat et al., 2009).

For being a heterogeneous disease that can present with different signs and symptoms, its diagnosis is usually difficult (Carson et al., 1988; Gunther et al., 2004), especially if it shows unusual clinical manifestations and if it is not present in other family members.

The most important steps for its diagnosis can be the same as for the diagnosis of Cushing's syndrome. Therefore initial phases must include confirming hypercortisolism, determining whether the hypercortisolism is ACTH-dependent or ACTH-independent, and whether there is paradoxical response to Dexamethasone suppression test. Then it will be necessary to identify the cause of that hypercortisolism. When investigating family members of patients affected by PPNAD or other forms of micronodular disease, the dexamethasone suppression tests should be used to identify subclinical adrenal disease, since for these patients, even subtle changes of cortisol secretion should be considered abnormal (plasma cortisol >1.8 µg/dL [50 nmol/L] following Liddle's test). ACTH suppression is also significant in this context. After that, the computerized tomography of the adrenals will help to distinguish unilateral from bilateral nodular disease or hyperplasia and so it must be performed next (Rockal et al., 2004). It must be stressed however that the adrenals are not very enlarged and so the interpretation of the images can be difficult (Bertherat et al., 2009). Treatment of PPNAD is often bilateral adrenalectomy, sometimes in two surgical timings years-apart, related to the fact that the development of this bilateral disease is frequently asymmetrical.

13. References

Abiven, G., Coste, J., Groussin, L., Anract, P., Tissier, F., Legmann, P., Dousset, B., Bertagna, X. & Bertherat, J. (2006). Clinical and biological features in the prognosis of adrenocortical cancer: poor outcome of cortisol-secreting tumors in a series of 202 consecutive patients. *J Clin Endocrinol Metab*, Vol. 91, pp. (2650-5), ISSN.

Abraham, J., Bakke, S., Rutt, A., Meadows, B., Merino, M., Alexander, R., Schrump, D., Bartlett, D., Choyke, P., Robey, R., Hung, E., Steinberg, SM., Bates, S. & Fojo, T. (2002). A phase II trial of combination chemotherapy and surgical resection for the treatment of metastatic adrenocortical carcinoma: continuous infusion doxorubicin, vincristine, and etoposide with daily mitotane as a P-glycoprotein antagonist. *Cancer*, Vol. 94, pp. (2333-43), ISSN.

Adam, R., Chiche, L., Aloia, T., Elias, D., Salmon, R., Rivoire, M., Jaeck, D., Saric, J., Le Treut, YP., Belghiti, J., Mantion, G. & Mentha, G., Association Française de Chirurgie. (2006). Hepatic resection for noncolorectal nonendocrine liver metastases: analysis of 1,452 patients and development of a prognostic model. *Ann Surg*, Vol. 244, No. 4, pp. (524-35), ISSN.

Advani, A., Johnson, SJ., Nicol, MR., Papacleovoulou, G., Evans, DB., Vaikkakara, S., Mason, JI. & Quinton, R. (2010). Adult-onset hypogonadotropic hypogonadism caused by aberrant expression of aromatase in an adrenocortical adenocarcinoma. *Endocr J*, Vol. 57, No. 7, pp. (651-6), ISSN.

Agrons, GA., Lonergan, GJ., Dickey, GE. & Perez-Monte, JE. (1999). Adrenocortical neoplasms in children: radiologic-pathologic correlation. *Radiographics*, Vol. 19, No. 4, pp. (989-1008), ISSN.

Allolio, B. & Fassnacht, M. (2006). Clinical review: Adrenocortical carcinoma: clinical update. *J Clin Endocrinol Metab*, Vol. 91, pp. (2027-37), ISSN.

Allolio, B., Hahner, S., Weismann, D. & Fassnacht, M. (2004). Management of adrenocortical carcinoma. *Clin Endocrinol (Oxf)*, Vol. 60, pp. (273-87), ISSN.

Angeli, A., Osella, G., Alì, A. & Terzolo, M. (1997). Adrenal incidentaloma: an overview of clinical and epidemiological data from the National Italian Study Group. *Horm Res*, Vol. 47, pp. (279-83), ISSN.

Angeli, A. & Terzolo, M. (2002). Adrenal incidentaloma − a modern disease with old complications. *J Clin Endocrinol Metab*, Vol. 87, pp. (4869-71), ISSN.

Aubert, S., Buob, D., Leroy, X., Devos, P., Carnaille, B., Do Cao, C., Wemeau, JL. & Leteurtre, E. (2005). Weiss system: a still in-use diagnostic tool for the assessment of adrenocortical malignancy. *Ann Pathol*, Vol. 25, No. 6, pp. (545-54), ISSN.

Azziz, R., Sanchez, LA., Knochenhauer, ES., Moran, C., Lazenby, J., Stephens, KC., Taylor, K. & Boots, LR. (2004). Androgen excess in women: experience with over 1000 consecutive patients. *J Clin Endocrinol Metab*, Vol. 89, pp. (453-62), ISSN.

Barzon, L., Chilosi, M., Fallo, F., Martignoni, G., Montagna, L., Palù, G. & Boscaro, M. (2001). Molecular analysis of CDKN1C and TP53 in sporadic adrenal tumors. *Eur J Endocrinol*, Vol. 145, pp. (207–12), ISSN.

Barzon, L., Sonino, N., Fallo, F., Palu, G. & Boscarom M. (2003). Prevalence and natural history of adrenal incidentalomas. *Eur J Endocrinol*, Vol. 149, pp. (273–85), ISSN.

Baudin, E., Pellegriti, G., Bonnay, M., Penfornis, A., Laplanche, A., Vassal, G. & Schlumberger, M. (2001). Impact of monitoring plasma 1,1-dichlorodiphenildichloroethane (o,p'DDD) levels on the treatment of patients with adrenocortical carcinoma. *Cancer*, Vol. 92, pp. (1385-92), ISSN.

Bernard, MH., Sidhu, S., Berger, N., Peix, JL., Marsh, DJ., Robinson, BG., Gaston, V., Le Bouc, Y. & Gicquel, C. (2003). A case report in favor of a multistep adrenocortical tumorigenesis. *J Clin Endocrinol Metab*, Vol. 88, pp. (998-1001), ISSN.

Bernini, GP., Moretti, A., Oriandini, C., Bardini, M., Taurino, C. & Salvetti. A. (2005). Long-term morphological and hormonal follow-up in a single unit on 115 patients with adrenal incidentalomas. *Br J Cancer*, Vol. 92, pp. (1104 – 9), ISSN.

Berruti, A., Terzolo, M., Sperone, P., Pia, A., Casa, SD., Gross, DJ., Carnaghi, C., Casali, P., Porpiglia, F., Mantero, F., Reimondo, G., Angeli, A. & Dogliotti, L. (2005). Etoposide, doxorubicin and cisplatin plus mitotane in the treatment of advanced adrenocortical carcinoma: a large prospective phase II trial. *Endocr Relat Cancer*, Vol. 12, pp. (657-66), ISSN.

Bertherat, J., Horvath, A., Groussin, L., Grabar, S., Boikos, S., Cazabat, L., Libe, R., René-Corail, F., Stergiopoulos, S., Bourdeau, I., Bei, T., Clauser, E., Calender, A., Kirschner, LS., Bertagna, X., Carney, JA. & Stratakis, CA. (2009). Mutations in regulatory subunit type 1A of cyclic adenosine 5'-monophosphate-dependent protein kinase (PRKAR1A): phenotype analysis in 353 patients and 80 different genotypes. *J Clin Endocrinol Metab*, Vol. 94, No. 6, pp. (2085-91), ISSN.

Beuschlein, F., Reincke, M., Karl, M., Travis, WD., Jaursch-Hancke, C., Abdelhamid, S., Chrousos, GP. & Allolio, B. (1944). Clonal composition of human adrenocortical neoplasms. *Cancer Research*, Vol. 54, pp. (4927–32), ISSN.

Birch, JM. (1994). Li-Fraumeni syndrome. *Eur J Cancer*, Vol. 30A, pp. (1935-41), ISSN.

Blumenfeld, JD., Sealey, JE., Schlussel, Y., Vaughan, ED., Sos, TA., Atlas, SA., Muller, FB., Acevedo, R., Ulick, S. & Laragh, JH. (1994). Diagnosis and treatment of primary hyperaldosteronism. *Ann Intern Med*, Vol. 121, pp. (877-85), ISSN.

Boland, GW., Lee, MJ., Gazelle, GS., Halpern, EF., McNicholas, MM. & Mueller, PR. (1998). Characterization of adrenal masses using unenhanced CT: an analysis of the CT literature. *AJR Am J Roentgenol*, Vol.171, pp. (201–4), ISSN.

Bonacci, R., Gigliotti, A., Baudin, E., Wion-Barbot, N., Emy, P., Bonnay, M., Cailleux, AF., Nakib, I. & Schlumberger, M. Réseau Comète. (1998). Cytotoxic therapy with etoposide and cisplatin in advanced adrenocortical carcinoma. *Br J Cancer*, Vol. 78, pp. (546-9), ISSN.

Bonfig, W., Bittmann, I., Bechtold, S., Kammer, B., Noelle, V., Arleth, S., Raile, K. & Schwarz, HP. (2003). Virilising adrenocortical tumours in children. *Eur J Pediatr*, Vol. 162, No. 9, pp. (623-8), ISSN.

Boulle, N., Logié, A., Gicquel, C., Perin, L. & Le Bouc, Y. (1998). Increased levels of insulin-like growth factor II (IGF-II) and IGF-binding protein-2 are associated with malignancy in sporadic adrenocortical tumors. *J Clin Endocrinol Metab*, Vol. 83, No. 5, pp. (1713-20), ISSN.

Bourdeau, I., D'Amour, P., Hamet, P., Boutin, JM. & Lacroix, A. (2001). Aberrant membrane hormone receptors in incidentally discovered bilateral macronodular adrenal hyperplasia with subclinical Cushing's syndrome. *J Clin Endocrinol Metab*, Vol. 86, pp. (5534-40), ISSN.

Bovio, S., Cataldi, A., Reimondo, G., Sperone, P., Novello, S., Berruti, A., Borasio, P., Fava, C., Dogliotti, L., Scagliotti, GV., Angeli, A. & Terzolo, M. (2006). Prevalence of adrenal incidentaloma in a contemporary computerized tomography series. *J Endocrinol Invest*, Vol. 29, pp. (298–302), ISSN.

Brembeck, FH., Rosário, M. & Birchmeier, W. (2006). Balancing cell adhesion and Wnt signaling, the key role of beta-catenin. *Curr Opin Genet Dev*, Vol. 16, No. 1, pp. (51-9), ISSN.

Bukowski, RM., Wolfe, M., Levine, HS., Crawford, DE., Stephens, RL., Gaynor, E. & Harker, WG. (1993). Phase II trial of mitotane and cisplatin in patients with adrenal carcinoma: a Southwest Oncology Group study. *J Clin Oncol*, Vol. 11, No. 1, pp. (161-5), ISSN.

Burgess, JR., Harle, RA., Tucker, P., Parameswaran, V., Davies, P., Greenaway, TM. & Shepherd, JJ. (1996). Adrenal lesions in a large kindred with multiple endocrine neoplasia type 1. *Arch Surg*, Vol. 131, No. 7, pp. (699-702), ISSN.

Caoili, EM., Korobkin, M., Brown, RK., Mackie, G. & Shulkin, BL. (2007). Differentiating adrenal adenomas from nonadenomas using (18)F-FDG PET/CT: quantitative and qualitative evaluation. *Acad Radiol*, Vol. 14, No. 4, pp. (468-75), ISSN.

Caoili, EM., Korobkin, M., Francis, IR., Cohan, RH., Platt, JF., Dunnick, NR. & Raghupathi, KI. (2002). Adrenal masses: characterization with combined unenhanced and delayed enhanced CT. *Radiology*, Vol. 222, No. 3, pp. (629–33), ISSN.

Carmina, E., Rosato, F., Janni, A., Rizzo, M. & Longo, RA. (2006). Extensive clinical experience: relative prevalence of different androgen excess disorders in 950 women referred because of clinical hyperandrogenism. *J Clin Endocrinol Metab*, Vol. 9, pp. (12-6), ISSN.

Carney, JA., Gordon, H., Carpenter, PC., Shenoy, BV. & Go, VL.. (1985). The complex of myxomas, spotty pigmentation, and endocrine overactivity. *Medicine (Baltimore)*, Vol. 64, No. 4, pp. (270-83), ISSN.

Carney, JA. & Young, WF Jr. (1992). Primary pigmented nodular adrenocortical disease and its associated conditions. *Endocrinologist*, Vol. 2, pp. (6), ISSN.

Carson, DJ., Sloan, JM., Cleland, J., Russell, CF., Atkinson, AB. & Sheridan, B. (1988). Cyclical Cushing's syndrome presenting as short stature in a boy with recurrent atrial myxomas and freckled skin pigmentation. *Clin Endocrinol (Oxf)*, Vol. 28, No. 2, pp. (173-80), ISSN.

Cawood, TJ., Hunt, PJ., O'Shea, D., Cole, D. & Soule, S. (2009). Recommended evaluation of adrenal incidentalomas is costly, has high false-positive rates and confers a risk of fatal cancer that is similar to the risk of the adrenal lesion becoming malignant; time for a rethink? *Eur J Endocrinol*, Vol. 161, No. 4, pp. (513-27), ISSN.

Choi, M., Scholl, UI., Yue, P., Björklund, P., Zhao, B., Nelson-Williams, C., Ji, W., Cho, Y., Patel, A., Men, CJ., Lolis, E., Wisgerhof, MV., Geller, DS., Mane, S., Hellman, P., Westin, G., Åkerström, G., Wang, W., Carling, T. & Lifton, RP. (2011). K+ channel mutations in adrenal aldosterone-producing adenomas and hereditary hypertension. *Science*, Vol. 331, No. 6018, pp. (768-72), ISSN.

Christopoulos, S., Bourdeau, I. & Lacroix, A. (2005). Clinical and subclinical ACTH-independent macronodular adrenal hyperplasia and aberrant hormone receptors. *Horm Res*, Vol. 64, pp. (119-31), ISSN.

Cobb, WS., Kercher, KW., Sing, RF. & Heniford, BT. (2005). Laparoscopic adrenalectomy for malignancy. *Am J Surg*, Vol. 189, pp. (405-11), ISSN.

Conn JW. (1964). Plasma renin activity in primary aldosteronism. Importance in differential diagnosis and in research of essential hypertension. *J Am Med Ass*, Vol. 190, pp. (222-5), ISSN.

Conn, JW. (1955). Presidential address. Part I. Painting the background. Part II. Primary aldosteronism, a new clinical syndrome. *J Lab Clin Med*, Vol. 45, pp. (3-17), ISSN.

Dackiw, AP., Lee, JE., Gagel, RF. & Evans, DB. (2001). Adrenal cortical carcinoma. *World J Surg*, Vol. 25, pp. (914-26), ISSN.

Daffara, F., De Francia, S., Reimondo, G., Zaggia, B., Aroasio, E., Porpiglia, F., Volante, M., Termine, A., Di Carlo, F., Dogliotti, L., Angeli, A., Berruti, A. & Terzolo, M. (2008). Prospective evaluation of mitotane toxicity in adrenocortical cancer patients treated adjuvantly. *Endocr Relat Cancer*, Vol. 15, No. 4, pp. (1043-53), ISSN.

D'Andrea, MR., Qiu, Y., Haynes-Johnson, D., Bhattacharjee, S., Kraft, P. & Lundeen, S. (2005). Expression of PDE11A in normal and malignant human tissues. *J Histochem Cytochem*, Vol. 53, No. 7, pp. (895-903), ISSN.

DeChiara, TM., Robertson, EJ. & Efstratiadis A. (1991). Parental imprinting of the mouse insulin-like growth factor II gene. *Cell*, Vol. 64, pp. (849-59), ISSN.

Decker, RA., Elson, P., Hogan, TF., Citrin, DL., Westring, DW., Banerjee, TK., Gilchrist, KW. & Horton, J. (1991). Eastern Cooperative Oncology Group study 1879: mitotane and adriamycin in patients with advanced adrenocortical carcinoma. *Surgery*, Vol. 110, No. 6, pp. (1006-13), ISSN.

DeLellis, RA., Lloyd, RV., Heitz, PU. & Eng, C. (2004). *Pathology and Genetics of Tumours of Endocrine Organs*, World Health Organization, ISBN, Lyon, France.

Derksen, J., Nagesser, SK., Meinders, AE., Haak, HR. & van de Velde, CJ. (1994). Identification of virilizing adrenal tumors in hirsute women. *N Engl J Med*, Vol. 331, pp. (968-73), ISSN.

Doppman, JL., Chrousos, GP., Papanicolaou, DA., Stratakis, CA., Alexander, HR. & Nieman, LK. (2000). Adrenocorticotropin-independent macronodular adrenal hyperplasia: an uncommon cause of primary adrenal hypercortisolism. *Radiology*, Vol. 216, No. 3, pp. (797-802), ISSN.

Doppman, JL., Nieman, LK., Travis, WD., Miller, DL., Cutler, GB Jr., Chrousos, GP. & Norton, JA. (1991). CT and MR imaging of massive macronodular adrenocortical disease: a rare cause of autonomous primary adrenal hypercortisolism. *J Comput Assist Tomogr*, Vol. 15, No. 5, pp. (773-9), ISSN.

Dunnick, NR., Korobkin, M. & Francis, I. (1996). Adrenal radiology: distinguishing benign from malignant adrenal masses. *AJR Am J Roentgenol*, Vol. 167, pp. (861-7), ISSN.

Edge, SB., Byrd, DR., Compton, CC., Fritz, AG., Greene, FL., Trotti, A. (Eds.). (2010). AJCC Cancer Staging Manual, 7th Ed. Springer, Chicago.

Fassnacht, M. & Allolio, B. (2009). Clinical management of adrenocortical carcinoma. *Best Pract Res Clin Endocrinol Metab*, Vol. 23, No. 2, pp. (273-89); ISSN.

Fassnacht, M., Johanssen, S., Quinkler, M., Bucsky, P., Willenberg, HS., Beuschlein, F., Terzolo, M., Mueller, HH., Hahner, S. & Allolio, B., German Adrenocortical Carcinoma Registry Group, European Network for the Study of Adrenal Tumors. (2009). Limited prognostic value of the 2004 International Union Against Cancer staging classification for adrenocortical carcinoma: proposal for a Revised TNM Classification. *Cancer*, Vol. 115, No. 2, pp. (243-50), ISSN.

Fassnacht, M., Libé R, Kroiss M, Allolio B. (2011). Adrenocortical carcinoma: a clinician's update. Nat Rev Endocrinol. Vol. 7, No 6, pp. (323-35).

Feige, JJ., Cochet, C., Savona, C., Shi, DL., Keramidas, M., Defaye, G. & Chambaz, EM. (1991). Transforming growth factor beta 1: an autocrine regulator of adrenocortical steroid genesis. *Endocr Res*, Vol. 17, pp. (267–79), ISSN.

Fottner, C., Hoeflich, A., Wolf, E. & Weber, MM. (2004). Role of the insulin-like growth factor system in adrenocortical growth control and carcinogenesis. *Horm Metab Res*, Vol. 36, pp. (397–405), ISSN.

Fragoso, MC., Domenice, S., Latronico, AC., Martin, RM., Pereira, MA., Zerbini, MC., Lucon, AM. & Mendonca, BB. (2003). Cushing's syndrome secondary to adrenocorticotropin-independent macronodular adrenocortical hyperplasia due to activating mutations of GNAS1 gene. *J Clin Endocrinol Metab*, Vol. 88, No. 5, pp. (2147), ISSN.

Fraumeni, JF Jr. & Miller, RW. (1967). Adrenocortical neoplasms with hemihypertrophy, brain tumors, and other disorders. *J Pediatr*, Vol. 70, pp. (129-38) ISSN.

Fuhrman, SA., Lasky, LC. & Limas, C. (1982). Prognostic significance of morphologic parameters in renal cell carcinoma. *Am J Surg Patho*, Vol. 6, No. 7, pp. (655-63), ISSN.

Gaujoux, S., Tissier, F., Groussin, L., Libé, R., Ragazzon, B., Launay, P., Audebourg, A., Dousset, B., Bertagna, X. & Bertherat, J. (2008). Wnt/beta-catenin and 3',5'-cyclic adenosine 5'-monophosphate/protein kinase A signaling pathways alterations and somatic beta-catenin gene mutations in the progression of adrenocortical tumors. *J Clin Endocrinol Metab*, Vol. 93, No. 10, pp. (4135-40), ISSN.

Gicquel, C., Bertagna, X., Gaston, V., Coste, J., Louvel, A., Baudin, E., Bertherat, J., Chapuis, Y., Duclos, JM., Schlumberger, M., Plouin, PF., Luton, JP. & Le Bouc, Y. (2001). Molecular markers and long-term recurrences in a large cohort of patients with sporadic adrenocortical tumors. *Cancer Res*, Vol. 61, No. 18, pp. (6762-7), ISSN.

Gicquel, C., Bertagna, X., Schneid, H., Francillard-Leblond, M., Luton, JP., Girard, F. & Le Bouc, Y. (1994). Rearrangements at the 11p15 locus and overexpression of insulin-like growth factor-II gene in sporadic adrenocortical tumors. *J Clin Endocrinol Metab*, Vol. 78, No. 6, pp. (1444–53), ISSN.

Gicquel, C., Raffin-Sanson, ML., Gaston, V., Bertagna, X., Plouin, PF., Schlumberger, M., Louvel, A., Luton, JP. & Le Bouc, Y. (1997). Structural and functional abnormalities at 11p15 are associated with the malignant phenotype in sporadic adrenocortical tumors: Study on a series of 82 tumors. *J Clin Endocrinol Metab*, Vol. 82, No. 8, pp. (2559–65), ISSN.

Giordano, TJ., Kuick, R., Else, T., Gauger, PG., Vinco, M., Bauersfeld, J., Sanders, D., Thomas, DG., Doherty, G. & Hammer, G. (2009). Molecular classification and prognostication of adrenocortical tumors by transcriptome profiling. *Clin Cancer Res*, Vol. 15, No. 2, pp. (668-76), ISSN.

Gittler, RD. & Fajans, SS. (1995). Primary aldosteronism (Conn's syndrome). *J Clin Endocrinol Metab*, Vol. 80, pp. (3438–41), ISSN.

Gold, PW., Loriaux, DL., Roy, A., Kling, MA., Calabrese, JR., Kellner, CH., Nieman, LK., Post, RM., Pickar, D. & Gallucci, W. (1986). Responses to corticotropin-releasing hormone in the hypercortisolism of depression and Cushing's disease. Pathophysiologic and diagnostic implications. *N Engl J Med*, Vol. 314, No. 21, pp. (1329-35), ISSN.

Gonzalez, RJ., Shapiro, S., Sarlis, N., Vassilopoulou-Sellin, R., Perrier, ND., Evans, DB. & Lee, JE. (2005). Laparoscopic resection of adrenal cortical carcinoma: a cautionary note. *Surgery*, Vol. 138, No. 6, pp. (1078–85), ISSN.

Gordon, MD. & Nusse, R (2006). Wnt signaling: Multiple pathways, multiple receptors, and multiple transcription factors. *J Biol Chem*, Vol. 281, pp. (22429–33), ISSN.

Groussin, L., Jullian, E., Perlemoine, K., Louvel, A., Leheup, B., Luton, JP., Bertagna, X. & Bertherat, J. (2002a). Mutations of the PRKAR1A gene in Cushing's syndrome due to sporadic primary pigmented nodular adrenocortical disease. *J Clin Endocrinol Metab*, Vol. 87, No. 9, pp. (4324-9), ISSN.

Groussin, L., Kirschner, LS., Vincent-Dejean, C., Perlemoine, K., Jullian, E., Delemer, B., Zacharieva, S., Pignatelli, D., Carney, JA., Luton, JP., Bertagna, X., Stratakis, CA. & Bertherat, J. (2002b). Molecular analysis of the cyclic AMP-dependent protein kinaseA (PKA) regulatory subunit1A (PRKAR1A) gene in patients with Carney complex and primary pigmented nodular adrenocortical disease (PPNAD) reveals novel mutations and clues for pathophysiology: augmented PKA signaling is associated with adrenal tumorigenesis in PPNAD. *Am J Hum Genet*, Vol. 71, No. 6, pp. (1433-42), ISSN.

Groussin, L., Perlemoine, K., Contesse, V., Lefebvre, H., Tabarin, A., Thieblot, P., Schlienger, JL., Luton, JP., Bertagna, X. & Bertherat, J. (2002c). The ectopic expression of the gastric inhibitory polypeptide receptor is frequent in adrenocorticotropin-independent bilateral macronodular adrenal hyperplasia, but rare in unilateral tumors. *J Clin Endocrinol Metab*, Vol. 87, No. 5, pp. (1980-5), ISSN.

Groussin, L., Bonardel, G., Silvéra, S., Tissier, F., Coste, J., Abiven, G., Libé, R., Bienvenu, M., Alberini, JL., Salenave, S., Bouchard, P., Bertherat, J., Dousset, B., Legmann, P., Richard, B., Foehrenbach, H., Bertagna, X. & Tenenbaum, F. (2009). 18F-Fluorodeoxyglucose positron emission tomography for the diagnosis of adrenocortical tumors: a prospective study in 77 operated patients. *J Clin Endocrinol Metab*, Vol. 94, No. 5, pp. (1713-22), ISSN.

Grumbach, MM., Biller, BM., Braunstein, GD., Campbell, KK., Carney, JA., Godley, PA., Harris, EL., Lee, JK., Oertel, YC., Posner, MC., Schlechte, JA. & Wieand, HS. (2003). Management of the clinically inapparent adrenal mass ("incidentaloma"). *Ann Intern Med*, Vol. 138, No. 5, pp. (424–9), ISSN.

Gunther, DF., Bourdeau, I., Matyakhina, L., Cassarino, D., Kleiner, DE., Griffin, K., Courkoutsakis, N., Abu-Asab, M., Tsokos, M., Keil, M., Carney, JA. & Stratakis, CA. (2004). Cyclical Cushing syndrome presenting in infancy: an early form of primary pigmented nodular adrenocortical disease, or a new entity? *J Clin Endocrinol Metab*, Vol. 89, no. 7, pp. (3173-82), ISSN.

Haak HR, Hermans J, van de Velde CJ, Lentjes EG, Goslings BM, Fleuren GJ, Krans HM. Optimal treatment of adrenocortical carcinoma with mitotane: results in a consecutive series of 96 patients. Br J Cancer. 1994 May;69(5):947-51

Hahner, S. & Fassnacht, M. (2005). Mitotane for adrenocortical carcinoma treatment. *Curr Opin Investig Drugs*, Vol. 6, pp. (386–94), ISSN.

Hamrahian, AH., Ioachimescu, AG., Remer, EM., Motta-Ramirez, G., Bogabathina, H., Levin, HS., Reddy, S., Gill, IS., Siperstein, A. & Bravo, EL. (2005). Clinical utility of noncontrast computed tomography attenuation value (hounsfield units) to differentiate adrenal adenomas/hyperplasias from nonadenomas: Cleveland Clinic experience. *J Clin Endocrinol Metab*, Vol. 90, No. 2, pp. (871-7), ISSN.

Harrison, LE., Gaudin, PB. & Brennan, MF. (1999). Pathologic features of prognostic significance for adrenocortical carcinoma after curative resection. *Arch Surg*, Vol. 134, pp. (181-5), ISSN.

Hedeland, H., Ostberg, G. & Hökfelt, B. (1968). On the prevalence of adrenocortical adenomas in an autopsy material in relation to hypertension and diabetes. *Acta Med Scand*, Vol. 184, pp. (211-4), ISSN.

Henley, DJ., van Heerden, JA., Grant, CS., Carney, JA. & Carpenter, PC. (1983). Adrenal cortical carcinoma--a continuing challenge. *Surgery*, Vol. 94, No. 6, pp. (926-31), ISSN.

Heppner, C., Reincke, M., Agarwal, SK., Mora, P., Allolio, B., Burns, AL., Spiegel, AM. & Marx, SJ. (1999). MEN1 gene analysis in sporadic adrenocortical neoplasms. *J Clin Endocrinol Metab*, Vol. 84, No. 1, pp. (216-9), ISSN.

Herrera, MF., Grant, CS., van Heerden, JA., Sheedy, PF. & Ilstrup, DM. (1991). Incidentally discovered adrenal tumors: an institutional perspective. *Surgery*, Vol. 110, No. 6, pp. (1014-21), ISSN.

Hisada, M., Garber, JE., Fung, CY., Fraumeni, Jr JF. & Li, FP. (1998). Multiple primary cancers in families with Li-Fraumeni syndrome. *J Natl Cancer Inst*, Vol. 90, pp. (606-11), ISSN.

Holland, OB. & Carr, B. (1993). Modulation of aldosterone synthase messenger ribonucleic acid levels by dietary sodium and potassium and by adrenocorticotropin. *Endocrinology*, Vol. 132, pp. (2666-73), ISSN.

Hollstein, M., Sidransky, D., Vogelstein, B. & Harris, CC. (1991). p53 mutations in human cancers. *Science*, Vol. 253, No. 5015, pp. (49–53), ISSN.

Horiba, N., Suda, T., Aiba, M., Naruse, M., Nomura, K., Imamura, M. & Demura, H. (1995). Lysine vasopressin stimulation of cortisol secretion in patients with adrenocorticotropinindependent macronodular adrenal hyperplasia. *J Clin Endocrinol Metab*, Vol. 80, No. 8, pp. (2336–41), ISSN.

Horvath, A., Mericq, V. & Stratakis, CA. (2008). Mutation in PDE8B, a cyclic AMP-specific phosphodiesterase in adrenal hyperplasia. *N Engl J Med*, Vol. 358, pp. (750-2), ISSN.

Hughes, JM., Hichens, M., Booze, GW. & Thorner, MO. (1986). Cushing's syndrome from the therapeutic use of intramuscular dexamethasone acetate. *Arch Intern Med*, Vol. 146, pp. (1848-9), ISSN.

Ilvesmaki, V., Kahri, AI., Miettinen, PJ. & Voutilainen, R. (1993). Insulin-like growth factors (IGFs) and their receptors in adrenal tumors: high IGF-II expression in functional adrenocortical carcinomas. *J Clin Endocrinol Metab*, Vol. 77, No. 3, pp. (852-8), ISSN.

Invitti, C., Pecori Giraldi, F., de Martin, M. & Cavagnini, F. (1999). Diagnosis and management of Cushing's syndrome: results of an Italian multicentre study. Study Group of the Italian Society of Endocrinology on the Pathophysiology of the Hypothalamic-Pituitary-Adrenal Axis. *J Clin Endocrinol Metab*, Vol. 84, pp. (440-8), ISSN.

Jhala, NC., Jhala, D., Eloubeidi, MA., Chhieng, DC., Crowe, DR., Roberson, J. & Eltoum, I. (2004). Endoscopic ultrasound-guided fine-needle aspiration biopsy of the adrenal glands: analysis of 24 patients. *Cancer*, Vol. 102, No. 5, pp. (308-14), ISSN.

Kaltsas, GA., Isidori, AM., Kola, BP., Skelly, RH., Chew, SL., Jenkins, PJ., Monson, JP., Grossman, AB. & Besser, GM. (2003). The value of the low-dose dexamethasone suppression test in the differential diagnosis of hyperandrogenism in women. *J Clin Endocrinol Metab*, Vol. 88, No. 6, pp. (2634–43), ISSN.

Kamenicky, P., Houdoin, L., Ferlicot, S., Salenave, S., Brailly, S., Droupy, S., Meduri, G., Sasano, H., Suzuki, T., Young, J. & Chanson, P. (2007). Benign cortisol-secreting adrenocortical adenomas produce small amounts of androgens. *Clin Endocrinol (Oxf)*, Vol. 66, No. 6, pp. (778-88), ISSN.

Kartheuser, A., Walon, C., West, S., Breukel, C., Detry, R., Gribomont, AC., Hamzehloei, T., Hoang, P., Maiter, D., Pringot, J., Rahier, J., Khan, PM., Curtis, A., Burn, J., Fodde, R. & Verellen-Dumoulin, C. (1999). Familial adenomatous polyposis associated with multiple adrenal adenomas in a patient with a rare 3' APC mutation. *J Med Genet*, Vol. 36, No. 1, pp. (65-7), ISSN.

Kebebew, E., Reiff, E., Duh, QY., Clark, OH. & McMillan, A. (2006) Extent of disease at presentation and outcome, for adrenocortical carcinoma: have we made progress? *World J Surgery*, Vol. 30, No. 5, pp. (872-8), ISSN.

Kendrick, ML., Lloyd, R., Erickson, L., Farley, DR., Grant, CS., Thompson, GB., Rowland, C., Young, WF Jr. & van Heerden, JA. (2001). Adrenocortical carcinoma: surgical progress or status quo? *Arch Surg*, Vol. 136, No. 5, pp. (543-9), ISSN.

Kettel, LM. (1989). Management of hirsutism. *Drug Ther Bull*, Vol. 27, pp. (49–51), ISSN.

Khan, TS., Imam, H., Juhlin, C., Skogseid, B., Gröndal, S., Tibblin, S., Wilander, E., Oberg, K. & Eriksson, B. (2000). Streptozocin and o,p'DDD in the treatment of adrenocortical cancer patients: long-term survival in its adjuvant use. *Ann Oncol*, Vol. 11, No. 10, pp. (1281-7), ISSN.

Khan, TS., Sundin, A., Juhlin, C., Wilander, E., Oberg, K. & Eriksson, B. (2004). Vincristine, cisplatin, teniposide, and cyclophosphamide combination in the treatment of recurrent or metastatic adrenocortical cancer. *Med Oncol*, Vol. 21, No. 2, pp. (167-77), ISSN.

Kirkman, S. & Nelson, DH. (1988). Alcohol-induced pseudo-Cushing's disease: a study of prevalence with review of the literature. *Metabolism*, Vol. 37, pp. (390-4), ISSN.

Kirschner, LS., Carney, JA., Pack, SD., Taymans, SE., Giatzakis, C., Cho, YS., Cho-Chung, YS. & Stratakis, CA. (2000). Mutations of the gene encoding the protein kinaseA type Ia regulatory subunit in patients with the Carney complex. *Nat Genet*, Vol. 26, No. 1, pp. (89-92), ISSN.

Kirschner MA, Powell RD Jr, Lipsett MB (1964). Cushing's syndrome: nodular cortical hyperplasia of adrenal glands with clinical and pathological features suggesting adrenocortical tumor. J Clin Endocrinol Metab. Vol.24, pp (947-55).

Kjellman, M., Roshani, L., Teh, BT., Kallioniemi, OP., Höög, A., Gray, S., Farnebo, LO., Holst, M., Bäckdahl, M. & Larsson, C. (1999). Genotyping of adrenocortical tumors: very frequent deletions of the MEN1 locus in 11q13 and of a 1-centimorgan region in 2p16. *J Clin Endocrinol Metab*, Vol. 84. No. 2, pp. (730-5), ISSN.

Kloos, RT., Gross, MD., Francis, IR., Korobkin, M. & Shapiro, B. (1995). Incidentally discovered adrenal masses. *Endocr Rev*, Vol. 16, pp. (460-484), ISSN.

Koch, CA., Pacak, K. & Chrousos, GP. (2002). The molecular pathogenesis of hereditary and sporadic adrenocortical and adrenomedullary tumors. *J Clin Endocrinol Metab*, Vol. 87, pp. (5367-84), ISSN.

Kocijancic, K., Kocijancic, I. & Guna, F. (2004). Role of sonographically guided fine-needle aspiration biopsy of adrenal masses in patients with lung cancer. *J Clin Ultrasound*, Vol. 32, pp. (12-6), ISSN.

Kopf, D., Goretzki, PE. & Lehnert, H. (2001). Clinical management of malignant adrenal tumors. *J Cancer Res Clin Oncol*, Vol. 127, pp. (143-55), ISSN.

Korobkin, M., Francis, IR., Kloos, RT. & Dunnick, NR. (1996). The incidental adrenal mass. *Radiol Clin North Am*, Vol. 34, pp. (1037-54), ISSN.

Kudva, YC., Sawka, AM. & Young, WF. (2003). The laboratory diagnosis of adrenal pheochromocytoma: the Mayo Clinic experience. *J Clin Endocrinol Metab*, Vol. 88, pp. (4533-9), ISSN.

Lack, LEE. (1997). *Atlas of tumor pathology*, Armed Forces Institute of Pathology, ISBN, Washington, DC.

Lacroix, A., Bolte, E., Tremblay, J., Dupré, J., Poitras, P., Fournier, H., Garon, J., Garrel, D., Bayard, F., Taillefer, R., Flanagan & RJ. & Hamet, P.(1992). Gastric inhibitory polypeptide-dependent cortisol hypersecretion – a new cause of Cushing's syndrome. *N Engl J Med*, Vol. 327, No. 14, pp. (974-80), ISSN.

Lacroix, A., Tremblay, J., Rousseau, G., Bouvier, M. & Hamet, P. (1997). Propranolol therapy for ectopic b-adrenergic receptors in adrenal Cushing's syndrome. *N Engl J Med*, Vol. 337, pp. (429–34), ISSN.

Lacroix, A., N'diaye, N., Tremblay, J. & Hamet, P. (2001). Ectopic and abnormal hormone receptors in adrenal Cushing's syndrome. *Endocr Rev*, Vol. 22, pp. (75-110), ISSN.

Lacroix, A., Baldacchino, V., Bourdeau, I., Hamet, P. & Tremblay, J. (2004). Cushing's syndrome variants secondary to aberrant hormone receptors. *Trends Endocrinol Metab*, Vol. 15, pp. (375-82), ISSN.

Lacroix A. (2009). ACTH-independent macronodular hyperplasia. *Best Practice and Research Clinical Endocrinology and Metabolism*, Vol. 23, pp. (245-259), ISSN.

Larsen, JL., Cathey, WJ. & Odell, WD. (1986). Primary adrenocortical nodular dysplasia, a distinct subtype of Cushing's syndrome. Case report and review of the literature. *Am J Med*, Vol. 80, pp. (976-84), ISSN.

Latronico, AC., Pinto, EM., Domenice, S., Fragoso, MC., Martin, RM., Zerbini, MC., Lucon, AM. & Mendonca, BB. (2001). An inherited mutation outside the highly conserved DNA-binding domain of the p53 tumor suppressor protein in children and adults with sporadic adrenocortical tumors. *J Clin Endocrinol Metab*, Vol. 86, No. 10, pp. (4970-3), ISSN.

Lau, SK. & Weiss, LM. (2009). The Weiss system for evaluating adrenocortical neoplasms: 25 years later. *Hum Pathol*, Vol. 40, No. 6, pp. (757-68), ISSN.

Lee, MH., Reynisdottir, I. & Massague, J. (1995). Cloning of p57kip2, a cyclindependent kinase inhibitor with unique domain structure and tissue distribution. *Genes Dev*, Vol. 9, pp. (639–49), ISSN.

Lefevre, M., Gerard-Marchant, R., Gubler, JP., Chaussain, JL. & Lemerle, J. (1983). *Adrenal and endocrine tumors in children*, Nijhoff, ISBN, Boston.

Li, FP. & Fraumeni, JF Jr. (1969a). Soft-tissue sarcomas, breast cancer, and other neoplasms: a familial syndrome? *Ann Intern Med*, Vol. 71, pp. (747-52), ISSN.

Li, FP. & Fraumeni, Jr JF. (1969b). Rhabdomyosarcoma in children: epidemiologic study and identification of a familial cancer syndrome. *J Natl Cancer Inst*, Vol. 43, pp. (1365-73), ISSN.

Li, FP., Fraumeni, Jr JF., Mulvihil, JJ., Blattner, WA., Dreyfus, MG., Tucker, MA. & Miller, RW. (1998). A cancer family syndrome in twenty-four kindreds. *Cancer Res*, Vol. 48, pp. (5358-62), ISSN.

Libé, R. & Bertherat, J. (2005). Molecular genetics of adrenocortical tumours, from familial to sporadic diseases. *Eur J Endocrinol*, Vol. 153, pp. (477-87), ISSN.

Libé, R., Fratticci, A. & Bertherat, J. (2007). Adrenocortical cancer: pathophysiology and Clinical management. *Endocr Relat Cancer*, Vol. 14, pp. (13–28), ISSN.

Libé, R., Fratticci, A., Coste, J., Tissier, F., Horvath, A., Ragazzon, B., Rene-Corail, F., Groussin, L., Bertagna, X., Raffin-Sanson, ML., Stratakis, CA. & Bertherat, J. (2008). Phosphodiesterase 11A (PDE11A) and genetic predisposition to adrenocortical tumors. *Clin Cancer Res*, Vol. 14, No. 12, pp. (4016-24), ISSN.

Liddle, GW. (1960). Tests of pituitary-adrenal suppressibility in the diagnosis of Cushing's syndrome. *J Clin Endocrinol Metab*, Vol. 20, pp. (1539-60), ISSN.

Lieberman, SA., Eccleshall, TR. & Feldman, D. (1994). ACTH-independent massive bilateral adrenal disease (AIMBAD): A subtype of Cushing's syndrome with major diagnostic and therapeutic implications. *Eur J Endocrinol*, Vol. 131, pp. (67–73), ISSN.

Lin, SR., Lee, YJ. & Tsai, JH. (1994). Mutations of the p53 gene in human functional adrenal neoplasms. *J Clin Endocrinol Metab*, Vol. 78, No. 2, pp. (483-91), ISSN.

Lindholm J, Juul S, Jorgensen JO, Astrup J, Bjerre P, Feldt-Rasmussen U, Hagen C, Jorgensen J, Kosteljanetz M, Kristensen L, Laurberg P, Schmidt K, Weeke J. (2001). Incidence and late prognosis of Cushing's syndrome: a population based study. *J Clin Endocrinol Metab* 86: 117-123

Logie, A., Boulle, N., Gaston, V., Perin, L., Boudou, P., Le Bouc, Y. & Gicquel, C. (1999). Autocrine role of IGF-II in proliferation of human adrenocortical carcinoma NCI H295R cell line. *J Mol Endocrinol*, Vol. 23, pp. (23–32), ISSN.

Louiset, E., Gobet, F., Libé, R., Horvath, A., Renouf, S., Cariou, J., Rothenbuhler, A., Bertherat, J., Clauser, E., Grise, P., Stratakis, CA., Kuhn, JM. & Lefebvre, H. (2010). ACTH-independent Cushing's syndrome with bilateral micronodular adrenal hyperplasia and ectopic adrenocortical adenoma. *J Clin Endocrinol Metab*, Vol. 95, No. 1, pp. (18-24), ISSN

Luton, JP., Cerdas, S., Billaud, L., Thomas, G., Guilhaume, B., Bertagna, X., Laudat, MH., Louvel, A., Chapuis, Y., Blondeau, P., Bonnin, A. & Bricaire, H. (1990). Clinical features of adrenocortical carcinoma, prognostic factors, and the effect of mitotane therapy. *N Engl J Med*, Vol. 322, No. 17, pp. (1195-201), ISSN.

Lynch, HT., Mulcahy, GM., Harris, RE., Guirgis, HA. & Lynch, JF. (1978). Genetic and pathologic findings in kindred with hereditary sarcoma, breast cancer, brain tumors, leukemia, lung, laryngeal, and adrenal cortical carcinoma. *Cancer*, Vol. 41, pp. (2055-64), ISSN.

Magee, BJ., Gattamaneni, HR. & Pearson, D. (1987). Adrenal cortical carcinoma: survival after radiotherapy. *Clin Radiol*, Vol. 38, pp. (587-8), ISSN.

Malchoff, CD., Rosa, J., DeBold, CR., Kozol, RA., Ramsby, GR., Page, DL., Malchoff, DM. & Orth, DN. (1989). Adrenocorticotropin-independent bilateral macronodular adrenal hyperplasia: an unusual cause of Cushing syndrome. *J Clin Endocrinol Metab*, Vol. 68, No. 4, pp. (855-60), ISSN.

Mansmann, G., Lau, J., Balk, E., Rothberg, M., Miyachi, Y. & Bornstein, SR. (2004). The clinically inapparent adrenal mass: update in diagnosis and management. *Endocr Rev*, Vol. 25, pp. (309-40), ISSN.

Mantero, F., Terzolo, M., Arnaldi, G., Osella, G., Masini, AM., Alì, A., Giovagnetti, M., Opocher, G. & Angeli, A. (2000). A survey on adrenal incidentaloma in Italy. Study Group on Adrenal Tumors of the Italian Society of Endocrinology. *J Clin Endocrinol Metab*, Vol. 85, No. 2, pp. (637-44), ISSN.

Matsuoka, S., Edwards, MC., Bai, C., Parker, S., Zhang, P., Baldini, A., Harper, JW. & Elledge, SJ. (1995). P57kip2, a structurally distinct member of the p21CIP1 Cdk inhibitor family, is a candidate tumor suppressor gene. *Genes Dev*, Vol. 9, No. 6, pp. (650-62), ISSN.

Mattsson, C. & Young, WF Jr. (2006). Primary aldosteronism: diagnostic and treatment strategies. *Nat Clin Pract Nephrol*, Vol. 2, pp. (198), ISSN.

Matyakhina, L., Freedman, RJ., Bourdeau, I., Wei, MH., Stergiopoulos, SG., Chidakel, A., Walther, M., Abu-Asab, M., Tsokos, M., Keil, M., Toro, J., Linehan, WM. & Stratakis, CA. (2005). Hereditary leiomyomatosis associated with bilateral, massive, macronodular adrenocortical disease and atypical cushing syndrome: a clinical and molecular genetic investigation. *J Clin Endocrinol Metab*, Vol. 90, No. 6, pp. (3773-9), ISSN.

Maurea, S., Klain, M., Mainolfi, C., Ziviello, M. & Salvatore, M. (2001). The diagnostic role of radionuclide imaging in evaluation of patients with nonhypersecreting adrenal masses. *J Nucl Med*, Vol. 42, No. 6, pp. (884-92), ISSN.

Mayo-Smith, WW. & Dupuy, DE. (2004). Adrenal neoplasms: CT-guided radiofrequency ablation--preliminary results. *Radiology*, Vol. 231, pp. (225-30), ISSN.

Mesiano, S., Mellon, SH., Gospodarowicz, D., Di Blasio, AM. & Jaffe, RB. (1991). Basic fibroblast growth factor expression is regulated by corticotropin in the human fetal adrenal: a model for adrenal growth regulation. *PNAS*, Vol. 88, pp. (5428-32), ISSN.

Mesiano, S., Mellon, SH. & Jaffe, RB. (1993). Mitogenic action, regulation, and localization of insulin-like growth factors in the human fetal adrenal gland. *J Clin Endocrinol Metab*, Vol. 76, pp. (968-76), ISSN.

Metser, U., Miller, E., Lerman, H., Lievshitz, G., Avital, S. & Even-Sapir, E. (2006). 18F-FDG PET/CT in the evaluation of adrenal masses. *J Nucl Med*, Vol. 47, No. 1, pp. (32-7), ISSN.

Meyer, A., Niemann, U. & Behrend, M. (2004). Experience with the surgical treatment of adrenal cortical carcinoma. *Eur J Surg Oncol*, Vol. 30, pp. (444-9), ISSN.

Michalkiewicz, E., Sandrini, R., Figueiredo, B., Miranda, EC., Caran, E., Oliveira-Filho, AG., Marques, R., Pianovski, MA., Lacerda, L., Cristofani, LM., Jenkins, J., Rodriguez-Galindo, C. & Ribeiro, RC. (2004). Clinical and outcome characteristics of children with adrenocortical tumors: a report from the International Pediatric Adrenocortical Tumor Registry. *J Clin Oncol*, Vol. 22, No. 5, pp. (838-45), ISSN.

Milliez, P., Girerd, X., Plouin, PF., Blacher, J., Safar, ME. & Mourad, JJ. (2005). Evidence for an increased rate of cardiovascular events in patients with primary aldosteronism. *J Am Coll Cardiol*, Vol. 45, pp. (1243-8), ISSN.

Minn, H., Salonen, A., Friberg, J., Roivainen, A., Viljanen, T., Långsjö, J., Salmi, J., Välimäki, M., Någren, K. & Nuutila, P. (2004). Imaging of adrenal incidentalomas with PET using (11)C-metomidate and (18)F-FDG. *J Nucl Med*, Vol. 45, No. 6, pp. (972-9), ISSN.

Mircescu, H., Jilwan, J., N'Diaye, N., Bourdeau, I., Tremblay, J., Hamet, P. & Lacroix, A. (2000). Are ectopic or abnormal membrane hormone receptors frequently present in adrenal Cushing's syndrome? *J Clin Endocrinol Metab*, Vol. 85, No. 10, pp. (3531-6), ISSN.

Moreno, S., Montoya, G., Armstrong, J., Leteurtre, E., Aubert, S., Vantyghem, MC., Dewailly, D., Wemeau, JL. & Proye, C. (2004). Profile and outcome of pure androgen-secreting adrenal tumors in women: experience of 21 cases. *Surgery*, Vol. 136, No. 6, pp. (1192-8), ISSN.

Motta Ramirez, G., Remer, E., Herts, B., Gill, I. & Hamrahian, A. (2005). Comparison of CT findings in symptomatic and incidentally discovered pheochromocytomas. *Am J Roentgenol*, Vol. 185, pp. (684-688), ISSN.

N'diaye, N., Tremblay, J., Hamet, P., de Herder, WW. & Lacroix, A. (1998). Adrenocortical overexpression of gastric inhibitory polypeptide receptor underlies food-dependent Cushing's syndrome. *J Clin Endocrinol Metab*, Vol. 83, pp. (2781-5), ISSN.

Nadella, KS. & Kirschner, LS. (2005). Disruption of Protein Kinase A regulation causes immortalization and dysregulation of D-type cyclins. *Cancer Res*, Vol. 65, pp. (10307-15), ISSN.

National Institutes of Health. (2002). NIH state-of-the-science statement on management of the clinically inapparent adrenal mass ("incidentaloma"). *NIH Consensus State-of-the-Science Statements*, Vol. 19, pp. (1-25), ISSN.

Ng, L. & Libertino, JM. (2003). Adrenocortical carcinoma: diagnosis, evaluation and treatment. *J Urol*, Vol. 169, pp. (5-11), ISSN.

Nieman, L., Biller, B., Findling, J., Newell-Price, J., Savage, M., Stewart, P. & Montori, VM. (2008). The diagnosis of Cushing's syndrome: an Endocrine Society Clinical Practice guideline. *J Clin Endocrinol Metab*, Vol. 93, No. 5, pp. (1526-40), ISSN

Ohgaki, H., Kleihues, P. & Heitz, PU. (1993). P53 mutations in sporadic adrenocortical tumors. *Intern J Cancer*, Vol. 54, pp. (408-10), ISSN.

Patil, KK., Ransley, PG., McCullagh, M., Malone, M. & Spitz, L. (2002). Functioning adrenocortical neoplasms in children. *BJU Int*, Vol. 89, No. 6, pp. (562-5), ISSN.

Polakis, P. Wnt signaling and cancer. *Genes Dev*, Vol. 14, No. 15, pp. (1837-51), ISSN.

Polat, B., Fassnacht, M., Pfreundner, L., Guckenberger, M., Bratengeier, K., Johanssen, S., Kenn, W., Hahner, S., Allolio, B. & Flentje, M. (2009). Radiotherapy in adrenocortical carcinoma. *Cancer*, Vol. 115, No. 13, pp. (2816-23), ISSN.

Quddusi, S., Browne, P., Toivola, B. & Hirsch, IB. Cushing syndrome due to surreptitious glucocorticoid administration. *Arch Intern Med*, Vol. 158, pp. (294-6), ISSN.

Quinkler, M., Hahner, S., Wortmann, S., Johanssen, S., Adam, P., Ritter, C., Strasburger, C., Allolio, B. & Fassnacht, M. (2008). Treatment of advanced adrenocortical carcinoma with erlotinib plus gemcitabine. *J Clin Endocrinol Metab*, Vol. 93, No. 6, pp. (2057-62), ISSN.

Reincke, M., Karl, M., Travis, WH., Mastorakos, G., Allolio, B., Linehan, HM. & Chrousos, GP. (1994). P53 mutations in human adrenocortical neoplasms: Immunohistochemical and molecular studies. *J Clin Endocrinol Metab*, Vol. 78, No. 3, pp. (790 –4), ISSN.

Resnik, Y., Allali Zerah, V., Chayvilalle, JA., Leroyer, R., Leymarie, P., Travert, G., Lebrethon, MC., Budi, I., Balliere, AM. & Mahoudeau, J. (1992). Food-dependent Cushing's syndrome mediated by aberrant adrenal sensitivity to gastric inhibitory polypeptide. *N Engl J Med*, Vol. 327, No. 14, pp. (981–6), ISSN.

Ribeiro, RC., Sandrini Neto, RS., Schell, MJ., Lacerda, L., Sambaio, GA. & Cat, I. (1990). Adrenocortical carcinoma in children: A study of 40 cases. *J Clin Oncol*, Vol. 8, pp. (67-74), ISSN.

Ribeiro, RC., Michalkiewicz, EL., Figueiredo, BC., DeLacerda, L., Sandrini, F., Pianovsky, MD., Sampaio, G. & Sandrini, R. (2000). Adrenocortical tumors in children. *Braz J Med Biol Res*, Vol. 33, No. 10, pp. (1225-34), ISSN.

Ribeiro, RC., Sandrini, F., Figueiredo, B., Zambetti, GP., Michalkiewicz, E., Lafferty, AR., DeLacerda, L., Rabin, M., Cadwell, C., Sampaio, G., Cat, I., Stratakis, CA. & Sandrini, R. (2001). An inherited p53 mutation that contributes in a tissue-specific manner to pediatric adrenal cortical carcinoma. *Proc Natl Acad Sci U S A*, Vol. 98, No. 16, pp. (9330-5), ISSN.

Rockall, AG., Babar, SA., Sohaib, SA., Isidori, AM., Diaz-Cano, S., Monson, JP., Grossman, AB. & Reznek, RH. (2004). CT and MR imaging of the adrenal glands in ACTH-independent cushing syndrome. *Radiographics*, Vol. 24, No. 2, pp. (435-52), ISSN.

Rosenfield, RL. Clinical practice. Hirsutism. *N Engl J Med*, Vol. 353, pp. (2578–88), ISSN.

Ross, NS. (1994). Epidemiology of Cushing's syndrome and subclinical disease. *Endocrinol Metab Clin North Am*, Vol. 23, pp (539-46), ISSN.

Ruder, HJ., Loriaux, DL. & Lipsett, MB. (1974). Severe osteopenia in young adults associated with Cushing's syndrome due to micronodular adrenal disease. *J Clin Endocrinol Metab*, Vol. 39, pp. (1138-47), ISSN.

Sabbaga, CC., Avilla, SG., Schulz, C., Garbers, JC. & Blucher, D. (1993). Adrenocortical carcinoma in children: clinical aspects and prognosis. *J Pediatr Surg*, Vol. 28, No. 6, pp. (841-3), ISSN.

Sandrini, R., Ribeiro, R. & DeLacerda, L. (1997). Extensive personal experience: childhood adrenocortical tumors. *J Clin Endocrinol Metab*, Vol. 82, pp. (2027-31), ISSN.

Sbiera S, Schmull S, Assie G, Voelker HU, Kraus L, Beyer M, Ragazzon B, Beuschlein F, Willenberg HS, Hahner S, Saeger W, Bertherat J, Allolio B, Fassnacht M. (2010).

High diagnostic and prognostic value of steroidogenic factor-1 expression in adrenal tumors. J Clin Endocrinol Metab. Vol. 95, No. 10, pp. (161-71).

Schlumberger, M., Ostronoff, M., Bellaiche, M., Rougier, P., Droz, JP. & Parmentier, C. (1988). 5-Fluorouracil, doxorubicin, and cisplatin regimen in adrenal cortical carcinoma. *Cancer*, Vol. 61, No. 8, pp. (1492-4), ISSN.

Schteingart, DE., Motazedi, A., Noonan, RA. & Thompson, NW. (1982). Treatment of adrenal carcinomas. *Arch Surg*, Vol. 117, pp. (1142-6), ISSN.

Schteingart, DE., Doherty, GM., Gauger, PG., Giordano, TJ., Hammer, GD., Korobkin, M. & Worden, FP. (2005). Management of patients with adrenal cancer: recommendations of an international consensus conference. *Endocr Relat Cancer*, Vol. 12, No. 3, pp. (667–80), ISSN.

Schulte, KM., Mengel, M., Heinze, M., Simon, D., Scheuring, S., Köhrer, K. & Röher, HD. (2000). Complete sequencing and messenger ribonucleic acid expression analysis of the MEN I gene in adrenal cancer. *J Clin Endocrinol Metab*, Vol. 85, No. 1, pp. (441-8), ISSN.

Sidhu, S., Marsh, DJ., Theodosopoulos, G., Philips, J., Bambach, CP., Campbell, P., Magarey, CJ., Russell, CF., Schulte, KM., Röher, HD., Delbridge, L. & Robinson, BG. (2002). Comparative genomic hybridization analysis of adrenocortical tumors. *J Clin Endocrinol Metab*, Vol. 87, No. 7, pp. (3467-74), ISSN.

Sidhu, S., Sywak, M., Robinson, B. & Delbridge, L. (2004). Adrenocortical cancer: recent clinical and molecular advances. *Curr Opin Oncol*, Vol. 16, pp. (13-8), ISSN.

Skogseid, B., Larsson, C., Lindgren, PG., Kvanta, E., Rastad, J., Theodorsson, E., Wide, L., Wilander, E. & Oberg, K. (1992). Clinical and genetic features of adrenocortical lesions in multiple endocrine neoplasia type 1. *J Clin Endocrinol Metab*, Vol. 75, No. 1, pp. (76-81), ISSN.

Soon, P., MsDonald, K., Robinson, B. & Sidhu, S. (2008). Molecular markers and the pathogenesis of adrenocortical cancer. *Oncologist*, Vol. 13, pp. (548-61), ISSN.

Srivastava, S., Zou, ZQ., Pirollo, K., Blattner, W. & Chang, EH. (1990). Germ-line transmission of a mutated p53 gene in a cancerprone family with Li-Fraumeni syndrome. *Nature*, Vol. 348, pp. (747-9), ISSN.

Stojadinovic, A., Ghossein, RA., Hoos, A., Nissan, A., Marshall, D., Dudas, M., Cordon-Cardo, C., Jaques, DP. & Brennan, MF. (2002). Adrenocortical carcinoma: clinical, morphologic, and molecular characterization. *J Clin Oncol* , Vol. 20, No. 4, pp. (941-50), ISSN.

Stowasser, M. (2009). Update in primary aldosteronism. *J Clin Endocrinol Metab*, Vol 94, No. 10, pp. (3623-30), ISSN.

Stratakis, CA., Courcoutsakis, NA., Abati, A., Filie, A., Doppman, JL., Carney, JA. & Shawker, T. (1997). Thyroid gland abnormalities in patients with the syndrome of spotty skin pigmentation, myxomas, endocrine overactivity, and schwannomas (Carney complex). *J Clin Endocrinol Metab*, Vol. 82, No. 7, pp. (2037-43), ISSN.

Stratakis CA, Sarlis N, Kirschner LS, Carney JA, Doppman JL, Nieman LK, Chrousos GP, Papanicolaou DA. (1999) Paradoxical response to dexamethasone in the diagnosis of primary pigmented nodular adrenocortical disease. Ann Intern Med. Vol. 131(8), pp (585-91).

Stratakis, CA., Kirschner, LS. & Carney, JA. (2001). Clinical and molecular features of the Carney complex: diagnostic criteria and recommendations for patient evaluation. *J Clin Endocrinol Metab*, Vol. 86, pp. (4041-6), ISSN.

Stratakis, CA. & Boikos, SA. (2007). Genetics of adrenal tumors associated with Cushing's syndrome: a new classification for bilateral adrenocortical hyperplasias. *Nat Clin Pract Endocrinol Metab*, Vol. 3, pp. (748–57), ISSN.

Sturgeon C, Shen WT, Clark OH, Duh QY, Kebebew E. (2006). Risk assessment in 457 adrenal cortical carcinomas: how much does tumor size predict the likelihood of malignancy? J Am Coll Surg. Vol. 202(3), pp (423-30).

Sullivan, M., Boileau, M. & Hodges, CV. (1978). Adrenal cortical carcinoma. *J Urol*, Vol. 120, pp. (660–5), ISSN.

Sutter, JA. & Grimberg, A. (2006). Adrenocortical tumors and hyperplasias in childhood: etiology, genetics, clinical presentation and therapy. *Pediatr Endocrinol Rev*, Vol. 4, No. 1, pp. (32-9), ISSN.

Swain, JM., Grant, CS., Schlinkert, RT., Thompson, GB., vanHeerden, JA., Lloyd, RV. & Young, WF. (1998). Corticotropin-independent macronodular adrenal hyperplasia: a clinicopathologic correlation. *Arch Surg*, Vol. 133, No. 5, pp. (541–6), ISSN.

Swords, FM., Baig, A., Malchoff, DM., Malchoff, CD., Thorner, MO., King, PJ., Hunyady, L. & Clark, AJ. (2002). Impaired desensitization of a mutant adrenocorticotropin receptor associated with apparent constitutive activity. *Mol Endocrinol*, Vol. 16, No. 12, pp. (2746-53), ISSN.

Szolar, DH., Korobkin, M., Reittner, P., Berghold, A., Bauernhofer, T., Trummer, H., Schoellnast, H., Preidler, KW. & Samonigg, H. (2005). Adrenocortical carcinomas and adrenal pheochromocytomas: mass and enhancement loss evaluation at delayed contrast-enhanced CT. *Radiology*, Vol. 234, No. 2, pp. (479–85), ISSN.

Tadjine, M., Lampron, A., Ouadi, L., Horvath, A., Stratakis, CA. & Bourdeau, I. (2008). Detection of somatic beta-catenin mutations in primary pigmented nodular adrenocortical disease (PPNAD). *Clin Endocrinol (Oxf)*, Vol. 69, No. 3, pp. (367-73), ISSN.

Tanabe, A., Naruse, M., Naruse, K., Hase, M., Yoshimoto, T., Tanaka, M., Seki, T., Demura, R. & Demura, H. (1997). Left ventricular hypertrophy is more prominent in patients with primary aldosteronism than in patients with other types of secondary hypertension. *Hypertens Res*, Vol. 20, No. 2, pp. (85–90), ISSN.

Terzolo, M., Osella, G., Alì, A. & Angeli, A. (2000). Adrenal incidentalomas. *In*: De Herder WW (ed). Functional and Morphological Imaging of the Endocrine System. *Boston: Kluwer Academic Publishers*, Vol. 7, pp. (191-211), ISSN.

Terzolo M, Boccuzzi A, Bovio S, Cappia S, De Giuli P, Alì A, Paccotti P, Porpiglia F, Fontana D, Angeli A. (2001). Immunohistochemical assessment of Ki-67 in the differential diagnosis of adrenocortical tumors. Urology. Vol. 57(1), pp (176-82).

Terzolo, M., Bovio, S., Reimondo, G., Pia, A., Osella, G., Borretta, G. & Angeli, A. (2005a). Subclinical Cushing's syndrome in adrenal incidentalomas. *Endocrinol Metab Clin North Am*, Vol. 34, No. 2, pp. (423-39), ISSN.

Terzolo, M., Bovio, S., Pia, A., Conton, PA., Reimondo, G., Dall'Asta, C., Bemporad, D., Angeli, A., Opocher, G., Mannelli, M., Ambrosi, B. & Mantero, F. (2005b). Midnight serum cortisol as a marker of increased cardiovascular risk in patients with a clinically inapparent adrenal adenoma. *Eur J Endocrinol*, Vol. 153, No. 2, pp. (307-15), ISSN.

Terzolo, M., Angeli, A., Fassnacht, M., Daffara, F., Tauchmanova, L., Conton, PA., Rossetto, R., Buci, L., Sperone, P., Grossrubatscher, E., Reimondo, G., Bollito, E., Papotti, M., Saeger, W., Hahner, S., Koschker, AC., Arvat, E., Ambrosi, B., Loli, P., Lombardi, G., Mannelli, M., Bruzzi, P., Mantero, F., Allolio, B., Dogliotti, L. & Berruti, A. (2007). Adjuvant mitotane treatment for adrenocortical carcinoma. *N Engl J Med*, Vol. 356, No. 23, pp. (2372-80), ISSN.

Tissier, F., Cavard, C., Groussin, L., Perlemoine, K., Fumey, G., Hagneré, AM., René-Corail, F., Jullian, E., Gicquel, C., Bertagna, X., Vacher-Lavenu, MC., Perret, C. & Bertherat, J. (2005). Mutations of beta-catenin in adrenocortical tumors: Activation of the Wnt signaling pathway is a frequent event in both benign and malignant adrenocortical tumors. *Cancer Res*, Vol. 65, No. 17, pp. (7622-7), ISSN.

Tissier, F. (2010). Classification of adrenal cortical tumors: what limits for the pathological approach? *Best Pract Res Clin Endocrinol Metab*, Vol. 24, No. 6, pp. (877-85), ISSN.

Ulick, S., Wang, JZ. & Morton, DH. (1992). The biochemical phenotypes of two inborn errors in the biosynthesis of aldosterone. *J Clin Endocrinol Metab*, Vol. 74, pp. (1415-20), ISSN.

van Ditzhuijsen, CI., van de Weijer, R. & Haak, HR. (2007). Adrenocortical carcinoma. *Neth J Med*, Vol. 65, No. 2, pp. (55-60), ISSN.

Varley, JM., McGown, G., Thorncroft, M., James, LA., Margison, GP., Forster, G., Evans, DG., Harris, M., Kelsey, AM. & Birch, JM. (1999). Are there low-penetrance TP53 Alleles? Evidence from childhood adrenocortical tumors. *Am J Hum Genet*, Vol. 65, No. 4, pp. (995-1006), ISSN.

Veugelers, M., Wilkes, D., Burton, K., McDermott, DA., Song, Y., Goldstein, MM., La Perle, K., Vaughan, CJ., O'Hagan, A., Bennett, KR., Meyer, BJ., Legius, E., Karttunen, M., Norio, R., Kaariainen, H., Lavyne, M., Neau, JP., Richter, G., Kirali, K., Farnsworth, A., Stapleton, K., Morelli, P., Takanashi, Y., Bamforth, JS., Eitelberger, F., Noszian, I., Manfroi, W., Powers, J., Mochizuki, Y., Imai, T., Ko, GT., Driscoll, DA., Goldmuntz, E., Edelberg, JM., Collins, A., Eccles, D., Irvine, AD., McKnight, GS. & Basson, CT. (2004). Comparative PRKAR1A genotype-phenotype analyses in humans with Carney complex and PRKAR1a haploinsufficient mice. *Proc Natl Acad Sci U S A*, Vol. 101, No.39, pp. (14222-7), ISSN.

Volante, M., Buttigliero, C., Greco, E., Berruti, A. & Papotti, M. (2008). Pathological and molecular features of adrenocortical carcinoma: an update. *J Clin Pathol*, Vol. 61, No. 7, pp. (787-93), ISSN.

Wada, S., Kitahama, S., Togashi, A., Inoue, K., Iitaka, M. & Katayama, S. (2002). Preclinical Cushing's syndrome due to ACTH-independent bilateral macronodular adrenocortical hyperplasia with excessive secretion of 18-hydroxydeoxycorticosterone and corticosterone. *Intern Med*, Vol. 41, No. 4, pp. (304-8), ISSN.

Waggoner, W., Boots, LR. & Azziz, R. (1999). Total testosterone and DHEAS levels as predictors of androgen-secreting neoplasms: a populational study. *Gynecological Endocrinology*, Vol. 13, pp. (394-400), ISSN.

Wagner, J., Portwine, C., Rabin, K., Leclerc, JM., Narod, SA. & Malkin, D. (1994). High frequency of germline p53 mutations in childhood adrenocortical cancer. *J Natl Cancer Inst*, Vol. 86, No. 22, pp. (1707-10), ISSN.

Wajchenberg, BL., Albergaria Pereira, MA., Medonca, BB., Latronico, AC., Campos Carneiro, P., Alves, VA., Zerbini, MC., Liberman, B., Carlos Gomes, G. & Kirschner,

MA. (2000). Adrenocortical carcinoma: clinical and laboratory observations. *Cancer*, Vol. 88, No. 4, pp. (711-36), ISSN.

Wasserman JD, Zambetti GP, Malkin D. (2011) Towards an understanding of the role of p53 in adrenocortical carcinogenesis. *Mol Cell Endocrinol*. Sep 10. [Epub ahead of print]

Watanabe, M. & Nakajin, S. (2004). Forskolin up-regulates aromatase (CYP19) activity and gene transcripts in the human adrenocortical carcinoma cell line H295R. *J Endocrinol*, Vol. 180, No. 1, pp. (125-33), ISSN.

Weber MM., Auernhammer CJ., Kiess W., and Engelhardt D. (1997) Insulin-like growth factor receptors in normal and timorous adult human adrenocortical glands. European Journal of Endocrinology Vol. 136 pp. (296-303).

Weber, SL. (1997). Cushing's syndrome attributable to topical use of lotrisone. *Endocr Pract*, Vol. 3, pp. (140-4), ISSN.

Weinstein, LS., Shenker, A., Gejman, PV., Merino, MJ., Friedman, E. & Spiegel, AM. (1991). Activating mutations of the stimulatory G protein in the McCune-Albright syndrome. *N Engl J Med*, Vol. 325, pp. (1688-95), ISSN.

Weiss, LM. (1984). Comparative histologic study of 43 metastasizing and nonmetastasizing adrenocortical tumors. *Am J Surg Pathol*, Vol. 8, pp. (163-9), ISSN.

White, PC., New, MI. & Dupont, B. (1987). Congenital adrenal hyperplasia. *N Engl J Med*, Vol. 316, pp. (1519-24), ISSN.

White, PC. (1994). Disorders of aldosterone biosynthesis and action. *N Engl J Med*, Vol. 331, pp. (250-8), ISSN.

Wiedemann, HR. (1983). Tumours and hemihypertrophy associated with Wiedemann-Beckwith syndrome. *Eur J Pediatr*, Vol. 141, pp. (29), ISSN.

Wieneke, JA., Thompson, LD. & Heffess, CS. (2003). Adrenocortical neoplasms in the pediatric population: a clinicopathologic and immunophenotypic analysis of 83 patients. *Am J Surg Pathol*, Vol. 27, No. 7, pp. (867-81), ISSN.

Wilkins, L. (1948). A feminizing adrenal tumor causing gynecomastia in a boy of five years contrasted with a virilizing tumor in a five-year-old girl: classification of seventy cases of adrenal tumor in children according to their hormonal manifestations and a review of eleven cases of feminizing adrenal tumor in adults. *J Clin Endocrinol Metab*, Vol. 8, pp. (111-32), ISSN.

Wood, BJ., Abraham, J., Hvizda, JL., Alexander, HR. & Fojo, T. (2003). Radiofrequency ablation of adrenal tumors and adrenocortical carcinoma metastases. *Cancer*, Vol. 97, pp. (554-60), ISSN.

Young, WF. (2000). Management approaches to adrenal incidentalomas: a view from Rochester, Minnesota. Endocrinol Metab Clin North Am. Vol. 29, pp (159-85).

Young, WF. (2007a). Primary aldosteronism: renaissance of a syndrome. *Clin Endocrinol (Oxf)*, Vol. 66, No. 5, pp. (607-18), ISSN.

Young, WF. (2007b). The incidentally discovered adrenal mass. *N Engl J Med*, Vol. 356, pp. (601-10), ISSN.

Zarifis, J., Lip, GY., Leatherdale, B. & Beevers, G. (1996). Malignant hypertension in association with primary aldosteronism. *Blood Press*, Vol. 5, pp. (250-4), ISSN.

Zerbini, CA., Kozakewich, HP., Weinberg, DS., Mundt, DJ., Edwards, JAI. & Lack, EE. (1992). Adrenocortical neoplasms in childhood and adolescence: analysis of prognostic factors including DNA content. *Endocr Pathol*, Vol. 3, pp. (116-28), ISSN.

2

Adrenal Incidentaloma and Adrenocortical Carcinoma: A Clinical Guideline on Treating the Unexpected and a Plea for Specialized Care

S.H.A. Brouns, T.M.A. Kerkhofs, I.G.C. Hermsen and H.R. Haak
Máxima Medical Center, Eindhoven
The Netherlands

1. Introduction

An adrenal incidentaloma is an important clinical finding that is often considered harmless, but can be the tip of the iceberg. The term incidentaloma indicates an adrenal mass larger than 1 cm, incidentally discovered during imaging studies performed for reasons other than suspicion of adrenal pathology. Lesions identified during staging procedure or work-up for patients with a known extra-adrenal malignancy are not considered to be an incidentaloma (Young, Jr. 2000; Grumbach et al. 2003; Young, Jr. 2007; Singh & Buch 2008; Terzolo et al. 2009; Androulakis et al. 2011).

The entity incidentaloma is not a new finding and has been reported for many years (Grumbach et al. 2003; Young, Jr. 2007; Singh & Buch 2008; Terzolo et al. 2009; Androulakis et al. 2011). Because of the increased use of imaging techniques and improvement in abdominal imaging, the frequency of incidentaloma findings is increasing as well. Recent studies using high-resolution computed tomography (CT) have reported an estimated prevalence of 4% (Young, Jr. 2007; Singh & Buch 2008). In autopsy studies the prevalence ranged 0.2%-8.7%, depending on definitions used and age group, as there is an age-dependent occurrence of adrenal incidentalomas (Young, Jr. 2000; Grumbach et al. 2003; Young, Jr. 2007; Singh & Buch 2008; Terzolo et al. 2009; Androulakis et al. 2011). The estimated prevalence in patients younger than 30 years is < 1%, in contrast to a 7% frequency in patients 70 years of age or older (Young, Jr. 2007). With an aging population and advanced radiological techniques becoming more widely available, the increasing frequency of adrenal incidentalomas is of growing importance.

When an incidentaloma is found, it is of vital importance to make an early and reliable differentiation between benign and (potentially) malignant lesions, but also to assess tumor functionality. The mass can originate from either the adrenal medulla or cortex (Androulakis et al. 2011). Consequently, a spectrum of different pathological conditions may underlie an incidentaloma, all requiring a different therapeutic approach. As much as 38 different diagnoses have been reported in patients with a serendipitous discovered adrenal tumor (Young, Jr. 2000). Most adrenal incidentalomas are clinically nonhypersecretory benign adenomas, with an estimated frequency of 70-80%, which cause no health problems. However, in 5-20% of patients who have no endocrinological signs or symptoms, analysis reveals subclinical hypercortisolism (Grumbach et al. 2003; Young, Jr. 2007; Singh & Buch

2008; Terzolo et al. 2009). Other frequently reported diagnoses besides a nonfunctioning adenoma include adrenocortical carcinoma (ACC), pheochromocytoma, metastasis and aldosterone-producing adenoma. Although malignancy is rare, it is of great clinical concern because of the poor prognosis (Grumbach et al. 2003; Terzolo et al. 2009).

After recognition of an incidentaloma both patient and physician are faced with uncertainties regarding the course, likelihood of a malignancy and treatment of the adrenal mass. Unfortunately, no diagnostic or therapeutic strategy has been validated in prospective clinical trials. Thus, the diagnostic work-up as well as management of an incidentaloma is a growing public health challenge (Young, Jr. 2007; Singh & Buch 2008; Terzolo et al. 2009).

The goal of this chapter is to provide a diagnostic guideline, which contains information about clinical presentation, biochemical work-up and radiological imaging. In addition, this chapter offers practical recommendations for the management of adrenal incidentaloma, including surgery and follow-up. Also, therapeutic options for adrenal carcinoma are discussed. Furthermore, we present organisational recommendations concerning the management of adrenal incidentaloma and emphasize the need for centralization of adrenal disease-research and patient care. This will provide patients with an opportunity to receive optimal care, as the beneficial effects of specialization have been proven multiple times in other rare diseases.

2. Diagnostics of incidentaloma

The first step in the evaluation of adrenal incidentalomas is establishing the definition of the tumor type, beginning with a thorough history taking and extensive physical examination, with attention to signs or symptoms of hormonal overproduction, a malignancy or pheochromocytoma. Furthermore, hormonal work-up and radiological imaging is required in the diagnostic evaluation of the adrenal mass.

2.1 History and physical examination
2.1.1 History
Signs suggestive of hormonal overproduction may include Cushing's characteristics, symptoms of hyperaldosteronism or sex hormone excess. Cushing's syndrome may be asymptomatic in the event of subclinical disease or present with weight gain and central obesity, flushes, proximal muscle weakness, and polydipsia. Furthermore, cognitive changes, such as irritability, depression or restlessness, may also be present. Hirsutism, acne, gynaecomastia and oligomenorrhoe may be symptoms of hypercortisolism or sex hormone overproduction. Features of primary hyperaldosteronism are nocturia, muscle cramps and polyuria in case of hypokalaemia and palpitations (Young, Jr. 2007; Singh & Buch 2008; Androulakis et al. 2011).

The classic triad of symptoms associated with a pheochromocytoma includes episodic headaches of variable duration, tachycardia and generalized sweating. However, this combination of symptoms is present in only a small percentage of patients (10%) (Nieman 2010). Characteristics less commonly present are pallor, dyspnea and anxiety and secondary, complaints of hyperglycemia, unintentional weight loss, arrhythmias and cardiomyopathy (Young, Jr. 2007; Androulakis et al. 2011).

An adrenocortical carcinoma may either present with signs of adrenal hypersecretion as mentioned above or symptoms related to mass effect, such as abdominal fullness or abdominal pain. Cancer-related signs (e.g. fever, unintentional weight loss) are less frequently present (Young, Jr. 2007; Singh & Buch 2008; Terzolo et al. 2009; Androulakis et al. 2011).

2.1.2 Physical examination

Clinical features of Cushing's syndrome detected during physical examination are hypertension, central obesity, striae, facial rounding ('moon face'), supraclavicular and dorsocervical fat pads ('buffalo hump'), proximal muscle weakness, clitoris hypertrophy, acne and hirsutism. Primary aldosteronism is characterized by hypertension. In rare cases, female patients can present with signs of virilization (e.g. acne, hirsutism) as a result of testosterone excess. In contrast, an estrogen secreting adrenal lesion can produce signs of feminization, such as gynaecomasty in the male patient. A pheochromocytoma may present with hypertension (paroxysmal or sustained), orthostatic hypotension, pallor and sweating on physical examination. Adrenocortical carcinoma may as well present signs of hormonal overproduction mentioned above. In addition, a palpable mass may be present at abdominal examination (Young, Jr. 2007; Singh & Buch 2008; Terzolo et al. 2009; Androulakis et al. 2011).

Causes	Estimated prevalence	Clinical presentation
Adenoma		
Subclinical Cushing's Syndrome	9 %	Weight gain with central obesity, flushes, proximal muscle weakness, polydipsia, cognitive changes
Primary aldosteronism	1.2 %	Nocturia, muscle cramps, polyuria, palpitations
Androgen overproduction	Rare	Hirsutism, acne, oligomenorrhoe
Nonfunctioning	73.9 %	-
Pheochromocytoma	4.7 %	Episodic headaches, tachycardia, generalized sweating, pallor, dyspnea, anxiety
Malignancy		
Adrenocortical carcinoma	4.8 %	Symptoms of functioning mass (see above), abdominal pain or fullness
Metastasis	2.3 %	Cancer-related symptoms (fever, unintentional weight loss)

Table 1. Prevalence and clinical presentation of the most frequent types of adrenal incidentaloma (Young, Jr. 2007, Singh and Buch 2008)

2.2 Hormonal evaluation

Additional hormonal work-up is necessary in the evaluation of tumor functionality. Although an adrenal mass may appear clinically nonhypersecretory, up to 20% of patients with an incidentaloma may have hormonal dysfunction, which might be associated with a higher risk of morbidity, such as metabolic disorders and cardiovascular disease (Singh & Buch 2008; Androulakis et al. 2011).

2.2.1 Subclinical Cushing's Syndrome

The most frequently diagnosed endocrine alteration in patients with an incidentaloma is Subclinical Cushing's Syndrome (SCS), which refers to autonomous and dysregulated cortisol secretion by the tumor, which may cause mild cortisol excess without typical signs and symptoms of hypercortisolism (Young, Jr. 2007; Singh & Buch 2008; Androulakis et al. 2011). It is also known as subclinical autonomous glucocorticoid hypersecretion (Grumbach et al. 2003). The average prevalence is 9% (range 1-29%, depending on criteria used)(Singh and Buch 2008). It is difficult to characterize, since clinical Cushing's syndrome is not present and patients may have normal 24-hour urinary free cortisol secretion (Terzolo et al. 2009). Therefore, late-night salivary cortisol and/or overnight dexamethasone (1 mg) suppression test is recommended to detect subclinical hypercortisolism (Grumbach et al. 2003; Nieman 2010). The optimal cut-off value is much discussed. A cortisol value greater than 138 nmol per liter (5 microg/dL) in response to 1mg dexamethasone overnight is associated with glucocorticoid overproduction and has an estimated sensitivity of 98% and specificity of 80-98% (Singh and Buch 2008). When a level between 50-70 nmol/L (1.8-2.5 microg/dL) is used as cut-off value, confirmatory testing is indicated, such as midnight plasma cortisol or serum ACTH level (Grumbach et al. 2003; Young, Jr. 2007; Singh & Buch 2008; Terzolo et al. 2009).

Recent studies and own observations identify urinary steroid profiling as a very promising screening instrument for early differentiation between benign and malignant tumors. A quantitative analysis of steroid precursors by gas chromatography and mass spectrometry reveals steroid patterns associated with particular clinical problems. A recently designed algorithm screens for nine metabolites in a 24-hour urine sample and has impressive test characteristics with high sensitivity and specificity (Taylor A & Arlt 2010).

2.2.2 Primary aldosteronism

Primary aldosteronism (Conn's syndrome) is present in approximately 1.2% of patients with an adrenal incidentaloma (Androulakis et al. 2011). The textbook presentation comprises hypertension and hypokalaemia, however almost 40% of patients are normokalaemic (Young, Jr. 2000; Singh & Buch 2008). Therefore, serum potassium level is not considered a reliable screening method. Hormonal work-up includes routine measurement of ambulatory morning plasma aldosterone concentration to plasma renin activity ratio (PAC/PRA ratio) in hypertensive patients. This can be performed during treatment with antihypertensive drugs with the exception of beta blockers and aldosterone antagonists. A PAC/PRA ratio ≥ 30 and plasma aldosterone concentration greater than 0.5 nmol/L is indicative of autonomous aldosterone secretion. Since the PAC/PRA ratio is influenced by time of sampling and posture of the patient, the diagnosis needs to be confirmed by additional measurement of mineralocorticoid secretory autonomy (e.g. saline infusion test) (Young, Jr. 2000; Grumbach et al. 2003; Young, Jr. 2007; Singh & Buch 2008; Nieman 2010).

2.2.3 Sex hormone overproduction

Sex hormone-secreting adrenal tumors rarely present as an incidentaloma, since they are usually symptomatic (e.g. hirsutism, virilization, gynaecomasty). Androgen overproduction

Adrenal Incidentaloma and Adrenocortical Carcinoma: A Clinical Guideline on Treating the Unexpected
and a Plea for Specialized Care

51

may be a feature of ACC, but measurement of androgens and their precursors in serum has a low diagnostic accuracy in differentiating malignant from benign adrenal masses. Routine measurement of androgen or estrogen production is not necessary in patients with an incidentaloma (Young, Jr. 2000; Young, Jr. 2007)

Nonclassical congenital adrenal hyperplasia may cause unilateral or bilateral adrenal lesions and is an uncommon cause (< 1%) of incidentalomas. Routine cosyntropin-stimulation testing with measurement of cortisol precursors is not warranted, unless the diagnosis is suspected based on clinical manifestation (hirsutism, acne, menstrual irregularities) or the presence of bilateral adrenal masses (Young, Jr. 2000; Young, Jr. 2007; Nieman 2010).

2.2.4 Silent pheochromocytoma

The estimated prevalence of a pheochromocytoma among patients with an adrenal incidentaloma is 4-7% Although it is mostly a benign condition, it may cause significant morbidity and mortality. Hypertension is constantly present in only half of the patients and paroxysmal in approximately 30%. It is essential to diagnose a catecholamine-secreting pheochromocytoma, since it has the potential to cause cardiac arrhythmias and hemodynamic instability even in asymptomatic patients. Therefore, routine measurement of fractionated metanephrines and catecholamines in 24-hour urine specimen is indicated in all patients presenting with an incidentaloma. Recent research reported the superiority of determination of fractionated plasma free metanaphrines, with a diagnostic sensitivity of 99% and specificity of 89%. However, this method is not widely available (Grumbach et al. 2003; Young, Jr. 2007; Singh & Buch 2008; Terzolo et al. 2009; Nieman 2010; Androulakis et al. 2011).

2.3 Radiologic evaluation

Imaging studies that brought the incidentaloma to light should be reviewed with a focus on the adrenal glands, but will often be insufficient. The goal is to distinguish adenomas from malignant masses. Several imaging characteristics are used to assess the malignant potential and to provide information concerning appropriate management.

2.3.1 Computed Tomography

It is advised to perform an unenhanced CT-scan to help distinguish adenomas from nonadenomas, followed by a delayed contrast-enhanced sequence and computed wash-out percentage (Hamrahian et al. 2005). Attenuation of adrenal masses is measured in Hounsfield Units. A low attenuation on CT before contrast administration indicates high lipid content and is found in adenomas. However, around 30% (range 10-40%) of adenomas do not have a large lipid content and consequently may be difficult to discriminate from nonadenomas.

Furthermore, size and appearance of the adrenal lesion may as well help to differentiate between benign and malignant tumors. The probability of an incidentaloma being an ACC is directly related to size of the lesion. A diameter greater than 4 cm is reported to have 90% sensitivity for identifying ACC, but a low specificity, since only approximately 25% of lesions greater than 4 cm are malignant. In addition, calcifications, necrosis and hemorrhage are indicative of a malignancy (Young, Jr. 2000; Terzolo et al. 2009; Nieman 2010).

CT-characteristic	Adenoma	Pheochromocytoma	Adrenocortical carcinoma	Metastasis
Size	Usually < 4 cm	Large, usually > 3 cm	Large, usually > 3 cm	Variable, usually < 3 cm
Shape	Round, smooth margins	Round, smooth margins	Irregular, unclear margins	Oval, irregular margins
Attenuation on unenhanced CT	< 10 HU	> 10 HU	> 10 HU	> 10 HU
Washout (in 10 minutes)	Rapid, > 50%	Delayed, < 50%	Delayed, < 50%	Delayed, < 50%
Growth rate	Stable	Slow (usually)	Rapid (usually)	Variable
Other features	Rarely necrosis, hemorrhage or calcification	Hemorrhage, cystic necrotic areas	Necrosis, hemorrhage, calcification	Hemorrhage, cystic necrotic areas

HU = Hounsfield Units

Table 2. CT characteristics of the most frequent types of an incidentaloma (Young, Jr. 2000; Young, Jr. 2007; Terzolo et al. 2009)

2.3.2 Magnetic Resonance Imaging
Magnetic Resonance Imaging (MRI) is equally effective as CT in differentiating benign from malignant adrenal masses (Grumbach et al. 2003). A normal adrenal gland is characterized by an equal or slightly lower intensity than that of the liver on T1 and T2. In contrast, malignant lesions are hyperintense on T2-weighted images (Young, Jr. 2000; Androulakis et al. 2011).

2.3.3 Positron Emission Tomography
Additional advanced radiological testing is generally not indicated. 18-Fluoro-2-deoxy-D-glucose positron emission tomography (PET) is highly sensitive in identifying malignant lesions. However, it is of limited use regarding the evaluation of adrenal incidentaloma (in patients without a prior history of malignancy) (Young, Jr. 2007; Singh & Buch 2008; Boland 2011)

2.4 Fine-Needle Aspiration
There is no evidence to support the routine use of computed tomography-guided fine-needle aspiration (FNA) in the diagnostic evaluation of an incidentaloma. It is rarely informative, since it has a high-false negative rate, and there is a risk of complications, such as hemorrhage, abdominal pain, pancreatitis and pneumothorax. Moreover, its added value over radiological imaging has not been established. In case of a suspected pheochromocytoma FNA is contraindicated, since manipulation of the tumor can potentially cause a hypertensive crisis. Furthermore, biopsy of an adrenocortical carcinoma may lead to tumourspill and consequently tumor recurrence along the needle track. The only role of FNA in the evaluation of an incidentaloma is in confirming metastatic disease in patients with a known extra-adrenal malignancy without other signs of metastases (Young,

Adrenal Incidentaloma and Adrenocortical Carcinoma: A Clinical Guideline on Treating the Unexpected
and a Plea for Specialized Care

53

Jr. 2000; Grumbach et al. 2003; Young, Jr. 2007; Quayle et al. 2007; Singh & Buch 2008; Terzolo et al. 2009; Nieman 2010).

3. Diagnostic evaluation

The work-up leads to a preliminary conclusion which determines further management. The spectrum varies from benign adenoma to the presumption of malignancy or a pheochromocytoma.

3.1 Suspect adenoma

As noted before, the first step in evaluation of an adrenal incidentaloma is discrimination between a benign or malignant adrenal mass, in which radiological imaging by CT-scan has a fundamental role. Most adrenal incidentalomas exhibit characteristic features of adrenocortical adenoma (ACA). Adenomas typically present as small (< 4 cm) lesions, with clear margins and high lipid content, which is characterized by low attenuation (< 10 HU) on unenhanced CT. Furthermore, they display rapid washout of contrast medium (e.g. more than 50% after 10 minutes) (see figure 1) (Androulakis et al. 2011).

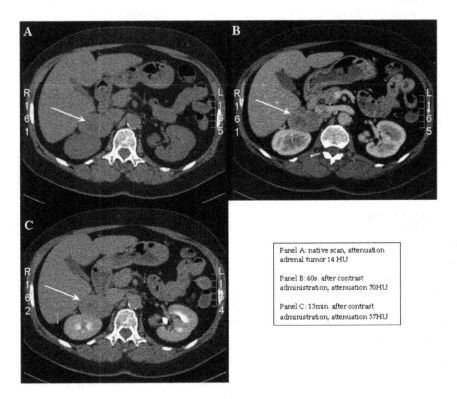

Panel A: native scan, attenuation adrenal tumor 14 HU

Panel B: 60s. after contrast administration, attenuation 70HU

Panel C: 15min. after contrast administration, attenuation 57HU

Fig. 1. Washout sequence of an adrenocortical adenoma

In patients with non-functioning ACA, size of the adrenal mass is the major determinant in choice of management (Nieman 2010; Androulakis et al. 2011). Over 60% of incidentalomas less than 4 cm in diameter are ACA, in contrast only 2% are malignant. For a small non-functioning adenoma surgical resection is not necessary, follow-up through CT-imaging and biochemical screening will suffice. In lesions larger than 6 cm the prevalence of ACC increases to approximately 25% and surgery is indicated (Singh & Buch 2008). Management of adrenal masses with a diameter between 4 to 6 cm is less well defined. Because of a higher risk of malignancy in this subgroup of patients, surgical approach is recommended in most cases.

In about 20% of adrenal adenomas hormonal work-up reveals overproduction of aldosterone (0.5-1%) or cortisol (5-20%), which may have a negative influence on patient's health. Primary hyperaldosteronism is associated with increased risk of cardiovascular events. Additionally, patients with SCS may be at risk for potential morbidity attributable to cortisol overproduction. However, progression to clinical overt Cushing's syndrome is uncommon. Surgical resection is considered the treatment of choice when biochemical overproduction is confirmed.

3.2 Suspect pheochromocytoma

It is essential to exclude a pheochromocytoma in patients presenting with an adrenal incidentaloma, because they are potentially lethal even when clinically asymptomatic (Young, Jr. 2007). Increased metanephrines and catecholamines in 24-hour urine specimen or fractionated plasma free metanephrines in combination with features on CT, such as increased attenuation on unenhanced CT (>10 HU), prominent vascularity of the mass and delayed washout of contrast (<50% after 10 minutes), are highly suggestive of a pheochromocytoma (Terzolo et al. 2009). Characteristics indicative of pheochromocytoma on MRI include hyperintensity on T2-weighted imaging, with approximately 92% sensitivity and 88% specificity (Androulakis et al. 2011). When a pheochromocytoma is suspected, surgical treatment is indicated. Patients should be adequately prepared pre-operatively by adrenergic blockade, to prevent a perioperative hypertensive crisis caused by manipulation of the tumor and subsequent catecholamine-release.

3.3 Suspect malignancy
3.3.1 Adrenocortical carcinoma

The risk of a malignancy is the main concern in patients with an incidentaloma. The prevalence of ACC in these patients without a history of malignancy is estimated at 4.8%, which makes it the most commonly identified adrenal malignancy (Terzolo et al. 2009). It is an aggressive malignancy with a median survival of 19 months (range 8-29 months), as calculated from data of 191 patients diagnosed between 2000 and 2010 in The Netherlands. Prognosis of ACC is still mainly dependent on stage at diagnosis (Fassnacht & Allolio 2009). For that reason it is vital to make accurate decisions regarding the necessary diagnostic and therapeutic measurements.

A smaller tumor size corresponds with a lower tumor stage and consequently better prognosis. The risk of ACC is, as mentioned, associated with mass size. However, because the prevalence of adrenal adenoma is age-dependent, the presence of small adrenal masses in young patients should raise major concern of a potential malignancy. A malignant adrenal lesion typically presents as a larger mass (> 6 cm) and is characterized by an irregular border,

Adrenal Incidentaloma and Adrenocortical Carcinoma: A Clinical Guideline on Treating the Unexpected
and a Plea for Specialized Care

55

high attenuation on unenhanced CT (> 10 HU) and slow washout after contrast administration (see figure 2) (Terzolo et al. 2009). Own observations from the authors show that although an ACC may appear clinically non-functioning, in about 80-95% additional hormonal work-up and urinary steroid profiling reveals presence of hormone excess.

When an adrenal malignancy is suspected, further investigation concerning cancer staging is warranted before directing the patient to surgery.

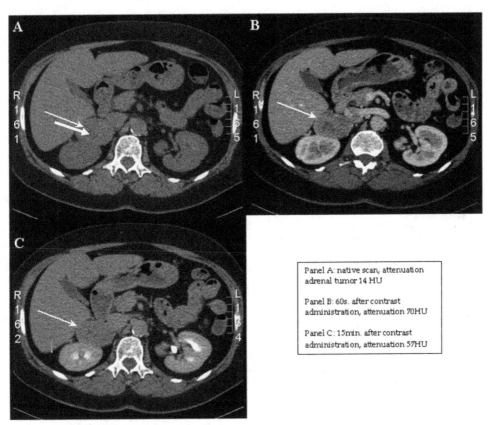

Panel A: native scan, attenuation adrenal tumor 14 HU

Panel B: 60s. after contrast administration, attenuation 70HU

Panel C: 15min. after contrast administration, attenuation 57HU

Fig. 2. Washout sequence of an adrenocortical carcinoma

3.3.2 Metastasis

Tumors that frequently metastasize to adrenal glands include carcinomas of lungs, esophagus, kidney, colon, breast, liver, pancreas and stomach (Young, Jr. 2007). Metastases frequently occur bilateral and are variable in size, mostly smaller than 3 cm. Abdominal imaging may also reveal the presence of necrosis, hemorrhage or calcifications (Young, Jr. 2000). Adrenal metastasis may cause beginning adrenal insufficiency. The suspicion of metastasis in an incidentaloma has clinical implications for prognosis and management and the search for a primary neoplasm is indicated. Resection of an isolated adrenal metastasis is associated with improved (disease-free and overall) survival. However, only in a limited number of cases adequate treatment of adrenal metastasis is possible (Terzolo et al. 2009).

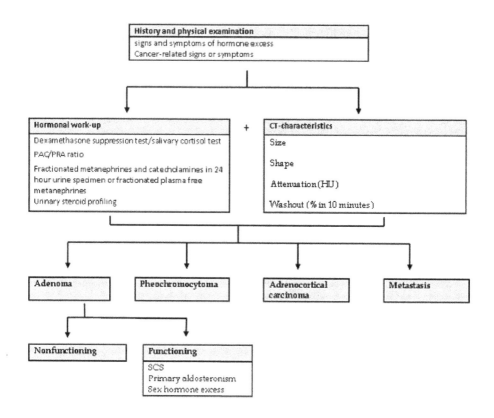

PPAC/PRA ratio = plasma aldosterone concentration to plasma renin activity ratio.
HU = Hounsfield Units. SCS = Subclinical Cushing's Syndrome.

Fig. 3. Algorithm for diagnostic evaluation of adrenal incidentaloma

Adrenal Incidentaloma and Adrenocortical Carcinoma: A Clinical Guideline on Treating the Unexpected
and a Plea for Specialized Care

57

4. Surgical treatment of incidentaloma

Based on results of the diagnostic evaluation of the adrenal incidentaloma, decisions are made regarding the required therapeutic approach. However, a prospective randomized comparison of laparoscopic versus open adrenalectomy has not yet been performed. Recommendations are made based on little known evidence and pragmatism.

4.1 Adenoma

When an adrenocortical adenoma is suspected, subsequent management is founded on size of the mass and functionality. As mentioned, in case of overproduction of cortisol, aldosterone or sex hormones, surgical resection of the mass is the treatment of choice. Mortality associated with adrenalectomy is estimated at less than 2% (Grumbach et al. 2003). Laparoscopic approach allows for a minimal invasive procedure associated with less morbidity in the patient and shorter period of hospitalization, while surgical results are comparable if performed by an experienced surgical team (Gill 2001). An important issue in resection of functioning adrenal masses is steroid suppletion peri- and postoperatively, because of the risk of adrenal insufficiency, hemodynamic crisis and death. In most cases this can be tapered over time.

It is common practice to perform a surgical resection of incidentalomas larger then 6 cm, even if they are non-functioning and there are no signs of malignancy. It is unclear whether this is a good indication for a surgical resection, as follow-up might be sufficient as well. In lesions smaller than 4 cm, surgical resection is deemed not necessary and follow-up is generally accepted as the correct management. For lesions between 4 cm and 6 cm in diameter, a clear recommendation is lacking. In this group, surgery might be the safest option regarding the increasing risk of malignancy, however the number needed to treat with respect to curing a carcinoma will be large. The other option is to repeat medical imaging on a shorter term, for example 3 months. We expect urinary steroid profiling to become a valuable instrument in differentiating between benign and malignant lesions in this particular subgroup.

4.2 Pheochromocytoma

In patients with an adrenal incidentaloma and suspicion of a pheochromocytoma, rapid surgical resection is the standard curative option, associated with an excellent prognosis (Terzolo et al. 2009). Due to potential perioperative catecholamine excess, removal of a pheochromocytoma is accompanied with unusual hemodynamic and technical conditions, which require thorough preoperative medical preparation and adrenergic blockade to minimize perioperative cardiovascular morbidity. Furthermore, close perioperative monitoring is mandatory (Gill 2001; Ichikawa et al. 2002). Catecholamine release is suggested to be lower during laparoscopy than open adrenalectomy. Therefore, and because of the other benefits of laparoscopic surgery mentioned earlier, a laparoscopic approach is recommended in patients with an incidentaloma suspected for a pheochromocytoma (Cheah et al. 2002; Matsuda et al. 2002).

4.3 Adrenocortical carcinoma

A radical surgical resection is the only chance of cure for patients with an adrenocortical carcinoma, so an aggressive surgical approach is warranted (Dackiw et al. 2001; Miller et al. 2010). A complete resection is possible in most cases when the diagnosis is suspected pre-operatively. Success rates drop significantly in cases where a carcinoma is not recognized before or during surgery, as follows from own observations from the authors. This emphasizes the need of a complete diagnostic work-up before the patient is directed for a surgical resection of an incidentaloma. The surgeon has to be prepared to perform an extensive resection and to keep the tumour capsule intact, as tumour spill is strongly associated with the occurrence of peritoneal carcinomatosis and a poor prognosis (Dackiw et al. 2001; Schteingart et al. 2005). Therefore, several authors recommend an open surgical approach instead of a laparoscopic technique, which is being used increasingly in adrenal surgery (Gonzalez et al. 2005; Zografos et al. 2009; Leboulleux et al. 2010; Miller et al. 2010). This topic is controversial, as prospective studies are lacking and retrospective studies show contradictory results. It is our belief that in general, a laparotomy is the safest option with respect to achieving a complete resection, although an expert surgeon in laparoscopic adrenalectomies might achieve better results than a less experienced surgeon can achieve performing a laparotomy.

We therefore recommend that these patients should be treated by a multidisciplinary team with at least an endocrinologist, a surgeon, an oncologist, a pathologist and an experienced radiologist. The team should evaluate all patients with a suspect adrenal incidentaloma and decide on which patients will be treated surgically. Peri-operative hydrocortisone suppletion is recommended in all patients. The surgical technique should be determined with respect to the preference and specific qualities of the surgeon. The pathological examination of the tumour requires special attention, as carcinomas might be difficult to recognize. Rating systems as the Weiss-score and the Van Slooten score should be applied to all adrenal tumours. Close follow-up using medical imaging is strongly recommended as the risk of recurrence is high, even after complete resection. The debate regarding adjuvant therapy with mitotane is still ongoing, but it is the opinion of the authors that this is recommended if the tumor has a ki-67 index >10% (Terzolo et al. 2007).

5. Follow-up of nonfunctioning adenoma

A much discussed matter in the management of patients with an non-functioning adrenal adenoma is the frequency and duration of follow-up evaluation. Recommendations regarding follow-up are aimed at identifying changes in size or functionality of the adrenal adenoma and to recognize lesions with malignant potential that have escaped detection on primary analysis. Research suggests that approximately 8% of non-functional adrenal incidentalomas increase in size by at least 1 cm during follow-up, whereas 3-4% decrease in size (Singh and Buch 2008, Young, Jr. 2000). The majority of adrenal adenomas remain stable. In contrast, adrenocortical carcinomas usually display rapid growth. It is recommended to repeat adrenal imaging by CT-scan in patients with nonfunctioning adenomas smaller than 4 cm within 6-12 months after the initial discovery to detect size changes (Grumbach et al. 2003).

Approximately 20% of adrenal adenomas which displayed no excess hormone secretion at time of discovery, become autonomous during subsequent period of 4 years. Lesions of at least 3 cm in diameter are more likely to develop subclinical hyperfunction in contrast to smaller tumors (Androulakis et al. 2011). It is reported that the risk seems to disappear after 3-4 years follow-up. Hyperaldosteronism or catecholamine hypersecretion occurs rarely during follow-up (Grumbach et al. 2003). Cortisol overproduction is more likely to occur. Hence, annual repetition of hormonal work-up, including late-night salivary cortisol and/or overnight dexamethasone (1 mg) suppression test is recommended during 4 years of follow-

Adrenal Incidentaloma and Adrenocortical Carcinoma: A Clinical Guideline on Treating the Unexpected
and a Plea for Specialized Care

59

up. Whether measurement of PAC/PRA ratio and determination of fractionated metanephrines and catecholamines in 24-hour urine specimen or fractionated plasma free metanephrines should be repeated, is left to the discretion of the clinician as the indication may vary per patient.

Further follow-up is not indicated in patients with an adrenal mass that remains stable on two imaging studies, done at least 6 months apart and do not demonstrate hormonal overproduction during 4 years of follow-up (Grumbach et al. 2003). Recommendations regarding follow-up of patients with a functional adenoma who are surgically treated, have not been developed.

Suspicion	Management	Considerations
Adenoma		
Functioning	Laparoscopic resection	Post-operative steroid hormone suppletion
Nonfunctioning		
< 4 cm	Follow-up - CT-scan within 6-12 months - Hormonal work-up annually during 4 years	
4-6 cm	Risk group: - Repeat CT-scan within 6 months - Consider surgical resection - Urinary steroid profiling - Consider referral to specialized centre	Suspicious imaging phenotype: open adrenalectomy
> 6 cm	Laparoscopic resection	
Pheochromocytoma	Laparoscopic resection	Pre-operative preparation
Adrenocortical carcinoma	Referral to specialized centre Open adrenalectomy by specialized surgical team	Post-operative steroid hormone suppletion Additional treatment depending on stage

Fig. 4. Recommendations for management of adrenal incidentaloma

6. Treatment in advanced stages

6.1 Introduction

The occurrence of metastatic disease in patients with adrenocortical carcinoma is not rare, as 35% of patients present with stage 4 disease. 50% of patients who initially have had a curative resection, ultimately suffer a recurrence (Pommier & Brennan 1992; Stojadinovic et al. 2002). Even in advanced stages, a surgical debulking should be considered as our own observations indicate this might give a survival benefit. The backbone of treatment in advanced stages is formed by drug therapy with mitotane. Cytotoxic chemotherapy may be added, but response percentages vary. The role of radiation therapy remains disputed. Current experimental treatments include IGF-R blockers (OSI-906) and sunitinib.

6.2 Surgery

In their recent review article, Fassnacht and Allolio provide a flowchart for management of ACC, which advocates at least consideration of surgery in every stage of disease (Fassnacht & Allolio 2009). Surgery including metastasectomy should at least be considered in stage IV patients and should be pursued if technically feasible and if the patient is motivated and in appropriate physical condition. On the other hand, the absolute survival gain might not weigh up against morbidity after surgery in certain (older) patients. This implies that the decision to perform surgery should be tailored to individual cases and should be discussed in a multidisciplinary team including an experienced surgeon. An additional benefit in cases of hormonal overproduction is that surgery might help controlling hormonal excess (Fassnacht & Allolio 2009).

Repeat surgery should be considered individually, results indicate that this could be beneficial with regard to survival, especially if the interval between the two operations is more than 6 months (Allolio & Fassnacht 2006; Veytsman et al. 2009).

6.3 Mitotane

Mitotane is the only adrenal-specific agent available for the treatment of ACC (Haak et al. 1994). The exact mechanism of action is not known, but it is proposed and generally accepted that mitotane is metabolized in adrenal mitochondria and causes cytotoxicity by oxidative damage through the production of free radicals (Veytsman et al. 2009). Whatever the exact pathway may be, the main effect is focal degeneration of the fascicular and (particularly) the reticular zone, which clinically leads to adrenal insufficiency for which glucocorticoid substitution is needed. (Hahner & Fassnacht 2005).

When describing results of mitotane, one should differentiate between antitumor- and antihormonal effects. Regarding antitumor activity, mitotane has been assessed in several clinical studies, with variable results. Most studies were retrospective and comprised only small numbers of patients. Results show that mitotane does have activity against ACC. Percentages vary, but most investigators report total or partial tumor responses in about 25% to 30% of cases.

Concerning hormone excess, therapy with mitotane is sufficient in the majority of patients. However, the onset of mitotane is slow due to its lipophilic properties and the resulting accumulation in adipose tissues. It can take up to three months before therapeutic levels are established, so in patients with severe hypercortisolism another agent must be used concurrently to treat this condition while mitotane levels are being built up. The recommended treatment in this situation would be ketoconazol, which is generally well tolerated. Other options, dependent on the case at hand, could be etomidate, mifeprestone or metyrapone (Igaz et al. 2008; Veytsman et al. 2009).

Mitotane treatment with a plasma concentration >14mg/L is associated with prolonged survival (Haak et al. 1994). Adverse effects occur in over 80% of patients and involve mainly the gastro-intestinal tract: anorexia, nausea, vomiting and diarrhea are frequently observed (Hahner & Fassnacht 2005). Reported symptoms caused by effects on the central nervous system are ataxia, speed disturbances, confusion and somnolence. Typically, all adverse effects are reversible after mitotane withdrawal (Lanser et al. 1992).

It is important to bear in mind that mitotane not only has adrenolytic effects, impairing adrenal steroidogenesis and thus inducing a need for replacement hydrocortisone, but also stimulates peripheral cortisol metabolism, so that hydrocortisone should be administered in higher doses. A second issue in managing patients on mitotane is monitoring thyroid

Adrenal Incidentaloma and Adrenocortical Carcinoma: A Clinical Guideline on Treating the Unexpected
and a Plea for Specialized Care

61

hormone and thyroid stimulating hormone levels, as mitotane can decrease thyroid hormone as well. A third and possibly favorable interaction is the supposedly increased efficacy of cytotoxic chemotherapy when combined with mitotane. However, evidence on this topic is not conclusive. The proposed mechanism for this synergistic effect is the possible negative effect of mitotane on multidrug resistance proteins, as investigated in vitro, which could decrease the resistance of adrenocortical cancer cells to cytotoxic agents (Hahner & Fassnacht 2005; Igaz et al. 2008).

Given the rarity of the indication and use of mitotane, it is recommended to leave treatment with mitotane to experienced doctors who are familiar with possible adverse events and are able to manage them.

6.4 Cytotoxic chemotherapy

Regarding cytotoxic chemotherapy, several combinations of agents have been tried so far. The highest response rates have been found in a trial with a treatment regimen combining mitotane with etoposide, doxorubicine and cisplatin (response rate 49%) and another trial with a treatment regimen combining mitotane and streptozotocine (response rate 36%) (Berruti et al. 2005), (Khan et al. 2000). Recently, these two regimens were compared in the First International Trial in Locally Advanced and Metastatic Adrenocortical Cancer (FIRM-ACT). Results of this trial are expected in 2011.

6.5 Radiation therapy

Whether there is a place for radiation therapy in the treatment of adrenocortical carcinoma, is not yet clear according to the literature. Some authors claim to have accomplished favorable results, like prevention of local recurrence and adequate pain relief in metastatic disease, whereas toxicity was low (Fassnacht et al. 2006; Polat et al. 2009; Hermsen et al. 2010).

Other investigators recommend a more conservative approach, seeing that re-operations in a post-radiation tumor bed would be more difficult and that the favorable results are not all too convincing, given the retrospective character of research so far (Veytsman et al. 2009). One could argue that radiation therapy can be of use in a palliative setting, especially in alleviating pain or neurologic complaints caused by metastatic disease in bone or brain and that a prospective trial is needed to determine the efficacy in an adjuvant setting.

6.6 Future therapeutic agents

The insulin-like growth factor receptor (IGF-R) in adrenocortical carcinoma is regarded as a possible target for treatment. Both antibody and tyrosine kinase inhibitor trials targeted against IGF-R are in progress. A trial using sunitinib as therapeutic agent produced disappointing results, but a better understanding of the metabolic complexity of the disease might lead to better trials in the future. Other areas of interest are VEGFR inhibitors and FGFR inhibitors, but these have not been translated into clinical trials yet.

7. Limitations

Due to limited evidence and guidelines, there are still multiple unresolved issues regarding management of incidentalomas, mainly concerning the duration of follow-up. The most important health risk in patients with an incidentaloma is related to several characteristics of the adrenal mass associated with a malignant mass or pheochromocytoma (Kievit & Haak 2000). The rate of growth of a benign adrenal lesion remains unclear. Besides this, the percentage of patients that will develop hormonal overproduction when initial analysis was negative is uncertain as well. Furthermore, there is some concern regarding the side effects of repeated CT imaging. One report estimated the risk of fatal cancer due to exposure to ionising radiation during CT-imaging to be one in 430-2170 (Androulakis et al. 2011). This is comparable to the chance of developing an adrenocortical carcinoma during 3-year follow-up of an incidentaloma. Additionally, a long follow-up period with repeated extensive hormonal work-up and radiological imaging is associated with high costs. Since the frequency of discovered adrenal incidentalomas is expected to increase and the use of abdominal imaging is also increasing, the cost-effectiveness of repeated hormonal work-up and imaging becomes an important issue in health care. However, in practice, choices of follow-up or treatment are also based on psychological or social mechanisms, such as anxiety, doubt and risk aversion as well as cost-effectiveness. To elucidate these uncertainties prospective trials are warranted to evaluate the optimal diagnostic approach and management of an incidentaloma and provide an answer for unresolved questions.

8. Organization of care

The rarity of a number of adrenal disorders, such as ACC or pheochromocytoma, and the dismal prognosis associated with an adrenal malignancy, requires a multidisciplinary approach of each patient. In the event of an ACC, physicians often are not familiar with the disorder and its few available treatment options, resulting in inferior patient care. Given that a large part of diagnostics and management is based on pragmatism and expert opinion instead of prospective trials, additional studies concerning treatment and follow-up of adrenal tumors are necessary. In order to improve care in patients with adrenal disorders and stimulate scientific research, national and international collaboration is vital. In a number of European countries (France, Germany, Italy, The Netherlands), national networks have been set up to coordinate adrenal diseases-research and - patient care. (Koschker et al. 2006; van Ditzhuijsen et al. 2007)

In the southern region of The Netherlands, our hospital acts as a tertiary referral center for patients with adrenal tumors. We have provided local hospitals with a guideline for diagnostics and patient referral similar to the procedure described in this chapter. The subsequent centralization of these patients facilitates reliable pre-operative diagnostics and specialized surgery, of which the importance cannot be overemphasized. Too many patients each year see their chance of survival be ruined because an adrenal malignancy is not recognized before, during or even after surgery. Irradical resection and/or rupture of the tumor capsule in adrenocortical carcinoma is fatal without exception, but can often be prevented if treated by experienced doctors.

Therefore, we strongly support initiatives of centralization being deployed in other regions and countries, as the beneficial effects of specialization have been proven multiple times in other rare diseases (Sosa et al. 1998; Kumar et al. 2001). Centralization and multidisciplinary approach is associated with more complete resections, improved survival and enhanced patient care. A secondary benefit is the facilitation of scientific research and participation in clinical trials in centralized populations of patients with a rare disease.

Adrenal Incidentaloma and Adrenocortical Carcinoma: A Clinical Guideline on Treating the Unexpected
and a Plea for Specialized Care

63

9. Conclusion

Due to the increasing discovery of adrenal incidentalomas, the diagnostic work-up as well as the management of incidentalomas is a growing public health challenge. Hormonal functionality and malignant potential of the lesion need to be evaluated. Incidentalomas are mostly benign nonhypersecretory adrenal adenomas, however important diagnoses to exclude are (subclinical) Cushing's Syndrome, primary aldosteronism, sex hormone overproduction, pheochromocytoma or malignancy (e.g. adrenocortical carcinoma, metastasis). Surgical treatment is recommended in all patients with a hormonally active tumor or a tumor larger than 6 cm. Furthermore, surgery may be indicated in individual cases depending on radiological characteristics. In patients with nonfunctioning adrenal adenomas smaller than 4 cm follow-up with CT-scan after 6-12 months and annual hormonal work-up for 4 years is recommended. An adrenocortical carcinoma is rare, but often lethal. Surgery is the cornerstone of initial treatment, whereas drug therapy with mitotane is inevitable in advanced stages. It is recommended that patients with adrenal disorders are treated in a multidisciplinary setting by experienced physicians. Centralization of care is strongly encouraged in order to improve patient outcome and to stimulate research and trial participation.

10. References

Allolio,B. & Fassnacht,M. 2006. Clinical review: Adrenocortical carcinoma: clinical update. J Clin Endocrinol. Metab, 91, 2027-2037.

Androulakis,I.I., Kaltsas,G., Piaditis,G. & Grossman,A.B. 2011. The clinical significance of adrenal incidentalomas. Eur J Clin Invest, 41, 552-560.

Berruti,A., Terzolo,M., Sperone,P., Pia,A., Casa,S.D., Gross,D.J., Carnaghi,C., Casali,P., Porpiglia,F., Mantero,F., Reimondo,G., Angeli,A. & Dogliotti,L. 2005. Etoposide, doxorubicin and cisplatin plus mitotane in the treatment of advanced adrenocortical carcinoma: a large prospective phase II trial. Endocr. Relat Cancer, 12, 657-666.

Boland,G.W. 2011. Adrenal imaging: why, when, what, and how? Part 3. The algorithmic approach to definitive characterization of the adrenal incidentaloma. AJR Am J Roentgenol., 196, W109-W111.

Cheah,W.K., Clark,O.H., Horn,J.K., Siperstein,A.E. & Duh,Q.Y. 2002. Laparoscopic adrenalectomy for pheochromocytoma. World J Surg, 26, 1048-1051.

Dackiw,A.P., Lee,J.E., Gagel,R.F. & Evans,D.B. 2001. Adrenal cortical carcinoma. World J Surg, 25, 914-926.

Fassnacht,M. & Allolio,B. 2009. Clinical management of adrenocortical carcinoma. Best. Pract. Res. Clin Endocrinol. Metab, 23, 273-289.

Fassnacht,M., Hahner,S., Polat,B., Koschker,A.C., Kenn,W., Flentje,M. & Allolio,B. 2006. Efficacy of adjuvant radiotherapy of the tumor bed on local recurrence of adrenocortical carcinoma. J Clin Endocrinol. Metab, 91, 4501-4504.

Gill,I.S. 2001. The case for laparoscopic adrenalectomy. J Urol., 166, 429-436.

Gonzalez,R.J., Shapiro,S., Sarlis,N., Vassilopoulou-Sellin,R., Perrier,N.D., Evans,D.B. & Lee,J.E. 2005. Laparoscopic resection of adrenal cortical carcinoma: a cautionary note. Surgery, 138, 1078-1085.

Grumbach,M.M., Biller,B.M., Braunstein,G.D., Campbell,K.K., Carney,J.A., Godley,P.A., Harris,E.L., Lee,J.K., Oertel,Y.C., Posner,M.C., Schlechte,J.A. & Wieand,H.S. 2003. Management of the clinically inapparent adrenal mass ("incidentaloma"). Ann Intern Med, 138, 424-429.

Haak,H.R., Hermans,J., van de Velde,C.J., Lentjes,E.G., Goslings,B.M., Fleuren,G.J. & Krans,H.M. 1994. Optimal treatment of adrenocortical carcinoma with mitotane: results in a consecutive series of 96 patients. Br J Cancer, 69, 947-951.

Hahner,S. & Fassnacht,M. 2005. Mitotane for adrenocortical carcinoma treatment. Curr. Opin. Investig. Drugs, 6, 386-394.

Hamrahian,A.H., Ioachimescu,A.G., Remer,E.M., Motta-Ramirez,G., Bogabathina,H., Levin,H.S., Reddy,S., Gill,I.S., Siperstein,A. & Bravo,E.L. 2005. Clinical utility of noncontrast computed tomography attenuation value (hounsfield units) to differentiate adrenal adenomas/hyperplasias from nonadenomas: Cleveland Clinic experience. J Clin Endocrinol. Metab, 90, 871-877.

Hermsen,I.G., Groenen,Y.E., Dercksen,M.W., Theuws,J. & Haak,H.R. 2010. Response to Radiation Therapy in Adrenocortical Carcinoma. J Endocrinol. Invest.

Ichikawa,T., Mikami,K., Suzuki,H., Imamoto,T., Yamazaki,T., Naya,Y., Ueda,T., Igarashi,T. & Ito,H. 2002. Laparoscopic adrenalectomy for pheochromocytoma. Biomed. Pharmacother., 56 Suppl 1, 149s-153s.

Igaz,P., Tombol,Z., Szabo,P.M., Liko,I. & Racz,K. 2008. Steroid biosynthesis inhibitors in the therapy of hypercortisolism: theory and practice. Curr Med Chem., 15, 2734-2747.

Khan,T.S., Imam,H., Juhlin,C., Skogseid,B., Grondal,S., Tibblin,S., Wilander,E., Oberg,K. & Eriksson,B. 2000. Streptozocin and o,p'DDD in the treatment of adrenocortical cancer patients: long-term survival in its adjuvant use. Ann Oncol, 11, 1281-1287.

Kievit,J. & Haak,H.R. 2000. Diagnosis and treatment of adrenal incidentaloma. A cost-effectiveness analysis. Endocrinol. Metab Clin North Am, 29, 69-ix.

Koschker,A.C., Fassnacht,M., Hahner,S., Weismann,D. & Allolio,B. 2006. Adrenocortical carcinoma -- improving patient care by establishing new structures. Exp. Clin Endocrinol. Diabetes, 114, 45-51.

Kumar,H., Daykin,J., Holder,R., Watkinson,J.C., Sheppard,M.C. & Franklyn,J.A. 2001. An audit of management of differentiated thyroid cancer in specialist and non-specialist clinic settings. Clin Endocrinol. (Oxf), 54, 719-723.

Lanser,J.B., van Seters,A.P., Moolenaar,A.J., Haak,H.R. & Bollen,E.L. 1992. Neuropsychologic and neurologic side effects of mitotane and reversibility of symptoms. J Clin Oncol, 10, 1504.

Leboulleux,S., Deandreis,D., Al,G.A., Auperin,A., Goere,D., Dromain,C., Elias,D., Caillou,B., Travagli,J.P., De,B.T., Lumbroso,J., Young,J., Schlumberger,M. & Baudin,E. 2010. Adrenocortical carcinoma: is the surgical approach a risk factor of peritoneal carcinomatosis? Eur J Endocrinol..

Matsuda,T., Murota,T., Oguchi,N., Kawa,G. & Muguruma,K. 2002. Laparoscopic adrenalectomy for pheochromocytoma: a literature review. Biomed. Pharmacother., 56 Suppl 1, 132s-138s.

Adrenal Incidentaloma and Adrenocortical Carcinoma: A Clinical Guideline on Treating the Unexpected
and a Plea for Specialized Care

65

Miller,B.S., Ammori,J.B., Gauger,P.G., Broome,J.T., Hammer,G.D. & Doherty,G.M. 2010. Laparoscopic Resection is Inappropriate in Patients with Known or Suspected Adrenocortical Carcinoma. World J Surg.

Nieman,L.K. 2010. Approach to the patient with an adrenal incidentaloma. J Clin Endocrinol. Metab, 95, 4106-4113.

Polat,B., Fassnacht,M., Pfreundner,L., Guckenberger,M., Bratengeier,K., Johanssen,S., Kenn,W., Hahner,S., Allolio,B. & Flentje,M. 2009. Radiotherapy in adrenocortical carcinoma. Cancer, 115, 2816-2823.

Pommier,R.F. & Brennan,M.F. 1992. An eleven-year experience with adrenocortical carcinoma. Surgery, 112, 963-970.

Quayle,F.J., Spitler,J.A., Pierce,R.A., Lairmore,T.C., Moley,J.F. & Brunt,L.M. 2007. Needle biopsy of incidentally discovered adrenal masses is rarely informative and potentially hazardous. Surgery, 142, 497-502.

Schteingart,D.E., Doherty,G.M., Gauger,P.G., Giordano,T.J., Hammer,G.D., Korobkin,M. & Worden,F.P. 2005. Management of patients with adrenal cancer: recommendations of an international consensus conference. Endocr. Relat Cancer, 12, 667-680.

Singh,P.K. & Buch,H.N. 2008. Adrenal incidentaloma: evaluation and management. J Clin Pathol, 61, 1168-1173.

Sosa,J.A., Bowman,H.M., Tielsch,J.M., Powe,N.R., Gordon,T.A. & Udelsman,R. 1998. The importance of surgeon experience for clinical and economic outcomes from thyroidectomy. Ann Surg, 228, 320-330.

Stojadinovic,A., Ghossein,R.A., Hoos,A., Nissan,A., Marshall,D., Dudas,M., Cordon-Cardo,C., Jaques,D.P. & Brennan,M.F. 2002. Adrenocortical carcinoma: clinical, morphologic, and molecular characterization. J Clin Oncol, 20, 941-950.

Taylor A & Arlt,W. Urinary Steroid Profiling as a High-Throughput Screening Tool for the Detection of Malignancy in Patients with Adrenal Tumors. Society for Endocrinology BES 2010 Abstract, 3-72. 2010.

Terzolo,M., Angeli,A., Fassnacht,M., Daffara,F., Tauchmanova,L., Conton,P.A., Rossetto,R., Buci,L., Sperone,P., Grossrubatscher,E., Reimondo,G., Bollito,E., Papotti,M., Saeger,W., Hahner,S., Koschker,A.C., Arvat,E., Ambrosi,B., Loli,P., Lombardi,G., Mannelli,M., Bruzzi,P., Mantero,F., Allolio,B., Dogliotti,L. & Berruti,A. 2007. Adjuvant mitotane treatment for adrenocortical carcinoma. N Engl J Med, 356, 2372-2380.

Terzolo,M., Bovio,S., Pia,A., Reimondo,G. & Angeli,A. 2009. Management of adrenal incidentaloma. Best. Pract. Res Clin Endocrinol. Metab, 23, 233-243.

van Ditzhuijsen,C.I., van de,W.R. & Haak,H.R. 2007. Adrenocortical carcinoma. Neth. J Med, 65, 55-60.

Veytsman,I., Nieman,L. & Fojo,T. 2009. Management of Endocrine Manifestations and the Use of Mitotane as a Chemotherapeutic Agent for Adrenocortical Carcinoma. J Clin Oncol.

Young,W.F., Jr. 2000. Management approaches to adrenal incidentalomas. A view from Rochester, Minnesota. Endocrinol. Metab Clin North Am., 29, 159-85, x.

Young,W.F., Jr. 2007. Clinical practice. The incidentally discovered adrenal mass. N. Engl. J Med, 356, 601-610.
Zografos,G.N., Vasiliadis,G., Farfaras,A.N., Aggeli,C. & Digalakis,M. 2009. Laparoscopic surgery for malignant adrenal tumors. JSLS., 13, 196-202.

3

Autoimmunity to Steroid-Producing Cells

Alberto Falorni and Stefania Marzotti
Department of Internal Medicine, Section of Internal Medicine and Endocrine and
Metabolic Sciences, University of Perugia
Italy

1. Introduction

Addison's disease, named after the English physician who provided its full description in 1855, is the result of the destruction or impaired function of adrenocortical cells. Of the 11 cases described by Addison, 10 were likely subsequent to an infiltrative disease (the most common being the secondary localization of *Mycobacterium tuberculosis* to the adrenal gland) and 1 was clinically idiopathic (likely of an autoimmune origin, on the basis of the current knowledge of disease mechanisms). In recent years the ethiologic spectrum of the disease has considerably expanded to include genetic causes not present in the 11 cases described by Thomas Addison. Accordingly, the definition of primary adrenal insufficiency (PAI) appears today more correct. Nevertheless, Autoimmune Addison's Disease (AAD) and post-tuberculosis Addison's disease are still adequate definitions according to the clinical characteristics of the cases described in 1855.

Prevalence of PAI is estimated at 120-160 cases per million in western countries, corresponding to 1 case every 7,000-7,500 individuals (Laureti *et al*, 1999; Løvås *et al*, 2002). The clinical manifestations of the disease result from the glucocorticoid, mineralcorticoid and androgen deficiency (Oelkers, 1996). In western countries and Japan, an autoimmune process is responsible for the destruction of the adrenocortical cells and for the clinical manifestations of PAI in around 70-90% of cases (Betterle *et al*, 2002; Nomura *et al*, 1994).

AAD occurs frequently in concomitance with other organ-specific and non-organ-specific autoimmune diseases in the so-called autoimmune polyendocrine syndromes (APS). Since at least two-thirds of patients with AAD have one or more other manifestations of an ongoing autoimmune process against other endocrine glands or different tissues, AAD can be considered a paradigmatic disease for the study of endocrine autoimmunity. On the basis of the type of diseases present in the same patient, different APSs are recognized. APS 1 is caused by mutations of the AIRE (AutoImmune REgulator) gene, which is located on chromosome 21 (The Finnish-German APECED Consortium, 1997). This syndrome is characterized by the concomitant presence of at least two of three diseases: chronic mucocutaneous candidiasis, hypoparathyroidism and AAD. In first-degree relatives of APS1 patients a single disease manifestation is sufficient to formulate the diagnosis. No general agreement exists for the classification of the remaining APSs. Some authors discriminate APS 2, APS 3 and APS 4 according to the different combination of autoimmune diseases present in the same patients. With this classification, APS 2 would identify the association of clinical or pre-clinical AAD with thyroid autoimmune diseases and/or type 1 diabetes mellitus (T1DM). APS 3 would be the association of thyroid autoimmune diseases with other endocrine and non-endocrine autoimmune manifestations (with the exception of AAD) and APS 4 would include all other possible combinations. No sound pathophysiological and/or genetic background, however, supports this classification, as the different endocrine autoimmune diseases tend to share a common genetic background and the same subject that might be initially be classified as APS 3 or APS 4 would be reclassified as APS2 if clinical or subclinical signs of adrenal or thyroid autoimmunity occur at a later stage. Throughout this chapter we will then refer to APS 2 to include all combinations of AAD with other immuno-mediated diseases, different from hypoparathyroidism or chronic mucocutaneous candidiasis.

Most frequently AAD is associated with Hashimoto's thyroiditis or Graves's disease, one or the other being present in over 50% of patients with autoimmune adrenal insufficiency (Betterle et al, 2002; Nerup, 1974; Kong et al, 1994; Irvine et al, 1967, 1979; McHardy-Young et al, 1974; De Rosa et al, 1987; Papadopoulos et al, 1990; Kasperlik-Zaluska et al, 1991; Zelissen et al, 1995; Söderbergh et al, 1996; Neufeld et al, 1981). Atrophic gastritis is present in 20-25% of AAD patients, while type 1 diabetes mellitus (T1DM) has been reported in 1-20% of addisonian patients (Betterle et al, 2002; Nerup, 1974; Kong et al, 1994; Irvine et al, 1967, 1979; McHardy-Young et al, 1974; De Rosa et al, 1987; Papadopoulos et al, 1990; Kasperlik-Zaluska et al, 1991; Zelissen et al, 1995; Söderbergh et al, 1996; Neufeld et al, 1981). Hypergonadotropic hypogonadism is present in 4.5-19% of AAD women. Other autoimmune diseases found associated with AAD at lower frequency include: vitiligo, alopecia, celiac disease, pernicious anemia, multiple sclerosis, inflammatory bowel disease, Sjögren's syndrome, chronic hepatitis and lymphocytic hypophysitis (Betterle et al, 2002; Nerup, 1974; Kong et al, 1994; Irvine et al, 1967, 1979; McHardy-Young et al, 1974; De Rosa et al, 1987; Papadopoulos et al, 1990; Kasperlik-Zaluska et al, 1991; Zelissen et al, 1995; Söderbergh et al, 1996; Neufeld et al, 1981).

2. Adrenal autoimmunity

The human adrenal autoimmune process is made evident by the apperance of circulating autoantibodies directed against the adrenal cortex or its components, which can be detected in the serum of affected individuals.

The first demonstration of adrenal cortex autoantibodies (ACA), detected by a complement-fixation test in the sera from patients with AAD, was provided in 1957 (Anderson et al, 1957). The use of the indirect immunofluorescence (IIF) approach, introduced by Blizzard and Kyle, 1963, has subsequently enabled the development of more sensitive assays for the detection of ACA (Blizzard et al, 1963, 1967; Goudie et al, 1966; Andrada et al, 1968; Wuepper et al, 1969; Nerup, 1974; Irvine & Barnes, 1974; Sotsiou et al, 1980; Elder et al, 1981; Papadopoulos et al, 1990). ACA have been detected in 40-75% patients with clinically idiopathic Addison's disease (Blizzard et al, 1963, 1967; Goudie et al, 1966; Andrada et al, 1968; Wuepper et al, 1969; Nerup, 1974; Irvine & Barnes, 1974; Sotsiou et al, 1980; Elder et al, 1981; Stechmesser et al, 1985; Kosowicz et al, 1986; Papadopoulos et al, 1990). Differences in the substrate used for detection of autoantibodies (human vs. animal adrenals), in disease duration and in selection of patients are responsible for the high variability in ACA frequency in patients with PAI.

In spite of the very well known technical limitations, because of the relative simplicity of the assay and the high diagnostic sensitivity, ACA-IIF have represented the gold standard for adrenal autoantibody determination until the middle of the '90s. ACA react with cytoplasm autoantigen(s) of cells located in all three layers of the adrenal cortex. More recent studies have detected ACA in approximately 80% of patients with AAD, representing over 90% of patients with recent-onset disease and 79% with long-standing disease (>2 years of disease duration) (Betterle *et al*, 1999). ACA are more frequent in patients with APS1 or APS2 than in patients with isolated Addison's disease (Betterle *et al*, 1999).

Attempts to identify the molecular targets of ACA started during the 1980's, which led to the initial identification of a 55-kDa autoantigen present in human adrenal microsomes (Furmaniak *et al*, 1988). Subsequent studies of the beginning of the 1990's have identified steroid-21-hydroxylase (21OH) as the main autoantigen target of ACA (Winqvist *et al*, 1992; Baumann-Antczak *et al*, 1992; Bednarek *et al*, 1992). Around the same time, steroid-17α-hydroxylase (17OH) (Krohn *et al*, 1992) and P450 side chain cleavage (P450scc) enzyme (Winqvist *et al*, 1993) were identified as additional autoantigens.

The discovery of the molecular targets of ACA led to development of radiobinding assays with radiolabelled human autoantigen. The use of either in vitro translated ^{35}S-21OH (Falorni *et al*, 1995, 1997; Colls *et al*, 1995) or 125 I-21OH (Tanaka *et al*, 1997) has enabled the demonstration that 21OH autoantibodies (21OHAb) have a high diagnostic sensitivity and specificity for AAD, being detected in over 95% of cases with clinically idiopathic adrenal insufficiency. The major epitopes recognised by human 21OHAb are located in the central and COOH-terminal domains of the enzyme. In addition, naturally occurring mutations, associated with the development of congenital adrenal hyperplasia, inhibit the binding of human autoantibodies to recombinant 21OH (Chen *et al*, 1998, Nikoshkov *et al*, 1999). *In vitro* studies (Furmaniak *et al*, 1994) have shown that 21OHAb may inhibit the enzymatic activity of the autoantigen, but this finding has not been confirmed *in vivo*, during the natural history of the disease (Boscaro *et al*, 1996; Laureti *et al*, 2002).

Similarly to other organ-specific autoantibodies, 21OHAb have no major pathogenic role in the development of adrenal insufficiency, as they can be detected in approximately 1/200 healthy subjects who do not necessarily progress towards clinical adrenal insufficiency. During pregnancy, 21OHAb cross the placental barrier, but do not determine any sign of clinical or pre-clinical adrenal insufficiency in the newborn (Betterle *et al*, 2004). Hence, 21OHAb are a highly senstive and specific immunological marker of the ongoing adrenal autoimmune process, but do not act as an effector of the destructive autoimmune process.

Our group has recently shown that 21OHAb are predominantly IgG1, with a minor expression of IgG2 and IgG4, which demonstrates a Th1-oriented type of immune response (Brozzetti *et al*, 2010a). However, approximately 10% of AAD patients express IgG4-21OHAb in the absence of IgG1 (Brozzetti *et al*, 2010a). This type of IgG subclass selection reveals a more Th2-oriented type of activation. At present, it is still unclear whether this distinct subgroup of patients with a more Th2-oriented type of immune response represents a different population of AAD subjects or is the expression of a different stage of the natural history of the disease.

Although 17OHAb and P450sccAb can be detected in a small fraction of patients with AAD, these markers are more frequently present in patients with APS 1 or in women with autoimmune oophoritis which causes autoimmune ovarian insufficiency (*see paragraph on Ovarian Autoimmunity*) (Betterle *et al*, 1999; Perniola *et al*, 2000; Falorni *et al*, 2002a).

Diagnosis of PAI is based on clinical ground and hormonal determination, but the ethiologic diagnosis of AAD requires detection of circulating 21OHAb, by using a radiobinding assay.

Autoantibody titer is also important, because the presence of low titre adrenal autoantibodies does not enable the unequivocal diagnosis of AAD in all cases (Falorni et al, 2004). ACA and 21OHAb have sporadically been found also in patients with unequivocal post-tuberculosis Addison's disease (Nomura et al, 1994; do Carmo Silva et al, 2000). A flow-chart for the etiological classification of PAI, that takes into consideration immunological, biochemical and imaging data, has been developed by the Italian Addison Network (Falorni et al, 2004). Published data indicate that the diagnostic accuracy of the 21OHAb assay is higher than that of the ACA-IIF (Falorni et al, 2004), and 21OHAb is currently the gold standard for detection of adrenal autoantibodies. In the case of a simultaneous presence of both ACA and 21OHAb, the probability of an accurate diagnosis of AAD is higher than 99% (Falorni et al, 2004). All patients with AAD should undergo additional autoantibody analyses, such as thyroid autoantibodies, GAD autoantibodies (GADA), steroid-cell autoantibodies (StCA), 17OHAb, P450sccAb or parietal cell autoantibodies, as approximately two thirds of AAD patients show clinical or pre-clinical signs of another autoimmune disease. Autoimmune AAD can be diagnosed also in the presence of medium-high levels of either 21OHAb or ACA (Falorni et al, 2004). In the case of patients positive only for 21OHAb or ACA at low levels, as well as in autoantibody-negative subjects, adrenal imaging should be performed to exclude an infiltrative form of adrenal insufficiency (such as post-tuberculosis, sarcoidosis, mycosis or metastatic localization of non-adrenal tumours) (Falorni et al, 2004). In male patients negative for both adrenal autoantibody measurement and adrenal imaging analysis, determination of plasmatic very long chain fatty acids (VLCFA) must be performed to exclude X-linked adrenoleukodystrophy (ALD).

At present, no clear and standardised cut-off is available to discriminate between low and medium-high level autoantibody titers and worskhops for the standardization of adrenal autoantibody assays are strongly needed. In a first international serum exchange to compare the results of 21OHAb determination in four independent laboratories, a good positive-negative concordance was observed, but major discrepancies emerged in quantitation of autoantibody titre (Falorni et al, 2011). A European program for the standardization of 21OHAb assay is currently being organised, and is expected to be completed within 2012.

Screening of subjects with endocrine autoimmune diseases for the presence of 21OHAb enables the identification of subjects with so-called *preclinical AAD*, which is characterised by the presence of adrenal autoantibodies in the absence of clinical signs of adrenal insufficiency and in the presence of normal basal cortisol concentrations. In patients with autoimmune diseases, 21OHAb can be detected in around 0.5-1.5% T1DM patients, 0.5-1.5% patients with autoimmune thyroid diseases, 0.5-1.0% patients with vitiligo and in 4-8% women with primary ovarian insufficiency (Betterle et al, 2002). 21OHAb-positive individuals exhibit a variable degree of adrenal dysfunction that can be classified in four different stages (Betterle et al, 1988).

Stage 0 indicates the apperance of adrenal autoantibodies, as a sign of the ongoing adrenal autoimmune process. 21OHAb appears before ACA, and lasts longer than ACA, during the natural history of the disease.

Often the first dysfunction observed as a consequence of the progression of the autoimmune process is an initial increase of plasmatic renin activity (PRA), at a time when normal ACTH-cortisol axis response is still present (*stage 1*). In *stage 2*, an impaired response to the ACTH stimulation test is documented, while the final *stage 3* represents the pre-clinical stage characterized by increased basal ACTH levels, along with the dysfunctions observed in stage 1 and 2.

No preventative therapy is yet available to delay or block the progressive destruction of adrenocortical cells in pre-clinical AAD. An Italian study has shown that an immunosuppressive therapy with high-dose corticosteroids for the treatment of Graves' ophthalmopathy had been able to revert a stage 2 pre-clinical AAD in a 21OHAb-positive individual (De Bellis et al, 1993). As a result of the treatment, disappearance of adrenal autoantibodies and normalization of both ACTH-cortisol and PRA-aldosterone axis function was observed and maintained for over 10 years at follow-up (De Bellis et al, 1993). However, the possibility to revert an advanced pre-clinical adrenal insufficiency by high-dose steroid immunosuppression has not yet been confirmed in other independent studies and it is not recommended for the sole purpose of preventing the progression towards clinical AAD.

Among the factors associated with progression towards clinical adrenal insufficiency are adrenal autoantibody levels that tend to increase during the progression of the adrenal dysfunction (Betterle et al, 1997).

Approximately 80% of patients with stage 0 and stage 1 do not progress to clinical AAD and may show a spontaneous remission of the pre-clinical dysfunction (Laureti et al, 1998). On the other hand, no such spontaneous remission seems to occur in patients with stage 2 and stage 3, in whom progression to clinical AAD is observed in over 95% of cases. A matematical formula that takes into consideration all known factors influencing risk of progression towards clinical AAD has been generated (Coco et al, 2006).

In subjects positive for 21OHAb and/or ACA, an ACTH stimulation test discriminates between a potentially reversible and an irreversible stage of the pre-clinical dysfunction. It has been shown that the high-dose 250 µg of synthetic ACTH used in the classical ACTH test (HDT) is supra-maximal and that as little as 1 µg of synthetic ACTH can determine a maximal stimulation of the adrenocortical cells (Arvat et al, 2000). The low-dose test with 1 µg of ACTH (LDT) has a high diagnostic sensitivity and specificity for pre-clinical adrenal dysfunction and can substitute the classical high-dose test (Laureti et al, 2000, 2002). An ongoing European multicenter study is currently testing the diagnostic accuracy and the predictive value of a 0.5 µg low-dose ACTH test.

Among the factors increasing significantly the risk of progression towards clinical adrenal insufficiency, in subjects with subclinical AAD, the most important are: male gender, presence of other concomitant autoimmune diseases, impaired response to the LDT and a high 21OHAb titer (Coco et al, 2006). HLA-DR3-DQ2, DR4-DQ8 and CTLA-4 gene polymorphism are significantly associated with appearance of 21OHAb, but do not influence the natural history of the disease and do not predict future clinical adrenal insufficiency (Coco et al, 2006; Falorni et al, unpublished data). Homozygosity for MICA5.1 was found to increase significantly the risk of progression towards clinical adrenal insufficiency (Barker et al, 2005), but larger, prospective studies are needed to confirm this finding. Because of the high predictive value of 21OHAb for future AAD, which is higher than 30% at 10 years of follow-up, screening of patients with ongoing endocrine autoimmune diseases with this marker is recommended to identify subjects with pre-clinical adrenal insufficiency.

3. Genetics of autoimmune adrenal insufficiency

Autoimmune Regulator (AIRE) is the causative gene for APS1 (The Finnish-German APECED Consortium, 1997). The AIRE gene product, Aire, acts as a strong activator of transcription (Pitkänen et al, 2000, 2001; Björses et al, 2000). Over 60 disease-associated mutations of the AIRE gene have been so far identified. Many mutations are located in the homogeneously staining region (HSR) in the N-terminal end of the protein. Other mutations, such as C311Y, P326Q, L397fsX478 are located in the plant homeodomain zinc finger 1 and 2, while only a few mutations, such as G228W or R257X have been identified in the DNA binding motif (Bottomley *et al*, 2001). It has been reported that a kindred carrying the G228W variant presented with an autosomal dominant autoimmune phenotype manifesting predominantly with thyroidits and distinct from APS1 (Cetani *et al*, 2001). The generation of a G228W-knocking mouse model showed that this AIRE variant acts in a dominant-negative manner causing a unique autoimmune syndrome (Su *et al*, 2008).

Disease-associated AIRE mutations are highly conserved within defined geographical areas. The R257X is the most frequently found mutation in Northern Italy and in Finland, while 964del13 is the most common mutation in the UK. In Sardinia, R139X is the typical AIRE mutation found in APS 1 patients.

Outside APS1, AAD shares many predisposing genetic factors with other endocrine autoimmune diseases that are components of APS2, such as thyroid autoimmune diseases and T1DM, the major genetic markers associated with the diseases beeing located in the HLA region on chromosome 6. The disease is strongly and positively associated with both HLA-DRB1*0301-DQA1*0501-DQB1*0201 (DR3-DQ2) and DRB1*04-DQA1*0301-DQB1*0302 (DR4-DQ8) (Falorni *et al*, 2008). The HLA-DRB1*01-DQA1*01-DQB1*0501 and DRB1*13-DQA1*0103-DQB1*0603 haplotypes are negatively associated with genetic risk for AAD. Several studies have shown that the association of HLA class II haplotypes is still highly significant in patients with isolated AAD and does not depend on the coexistence of other autoimmune disorders in the same patient. DRB1-*0404 was more frequent among DRB1*04-positive AAD patients from US (Yu *et al*, 1999) and Norway (Myhre *et al*, 2002) as compared to both DRB1*04-positive healthy control subjects and DRB1*04-positive T1DM patients. The DRB1*0401 subtype was strongly and positively associated with T1DM, but not with AAD (Yu *et al*, 1999; Myhre *et al*, 2002). However, an Italian study from our group (Gambelunghe *et al*, 2005) did not confirm this hypothesis. In that study (Gambelunghe *et al*, 2005), it was observed that no statistically different distribution of DRB1*0401 and DRB1*0404 was detectable among T1DM patients and AAD patients. On the other hand, it was observed that the DRB1*0403 subtype, which was already known to confer strong protection for T1DM, was absent among 56 DRB1*04-positive AAD patients, but present in 27 % DRB1*04-positive healthy control subjects, thus conferring protection also for the development of AAD.

Other HLA genes contribute to the risk for AAD, among which the MHC class I chain-related A (MICA) gene polymorphism. The MICA gene encodes for a ligand for an activating receptor (NKG2D) present on $\gamma\delta$ T cells, CD8+CD28- $\alpha\beta$ T cells, natural killer cells and CD4+CD28- $\alpha\beta$ T cells and is located within the HLA class III region. There are speculations that MICA gene polymorphism might influence affinity for the NKG2D receptor. AAD is strongly associated with the transmembrane MICA 5.1 allele, with odds ratio similar to those observed for HLA class II haplotypes (Gambelunghe *et al*, 1999; Park *et al*, 2002). MICA6 appears to be negatively associated with disease risk for AAD (Gambelunghe *et al*, 1999).

Though the association of MICA with AAD appears to be independent from that with HLA class II haplotypes, the strong *linkage disequilibrium* existing within the DRB1*03-DQA1*0501-DQB1*0201-MICA5.1-HLA-B extended haplotype has so far limited the possibility to discriminate the relative contribution of each gene marker and further studies on large populations are needed to provide an answer to this specific question.

Similarly to T1DM and other autoimmune diseases, the genetic background for AAD includes also other genes believed to modulate the function of the immune system. The CTLA-4 gene polymorphism and the PTPN22 gene polymorphism have been found to modulate genetic risk for AAD (Falorni *et al*, 2008; Skinningsrud *et al*, 2008a). A recent metanalysis of European studies has confirmed that the CTLA-4 Ala 17 polymorphism is strongly associated with genetic risk for AAD, independentenly from the well known association with the polymorphism of HLA class II genes (Brozzetti *et al*, 2010b).

Two independent European studies have shown the association of the class II transactivator (CIITA) (also denominated MHC2TA) gene with AAD (Ghaderi *et al*, 2006; Skinningsrud *et al*, 2008b). Modulation of the expression of HLA class II determinants in antigen-presenting cells may represent a critical factor in the activation and maintenance of the organ-specific autoimmune process and genetic factors that may influence such expression may have an important role on the pathogenesis of autoimmune diseases. The regulatory factor X complex (RFX) and CIITA are essential and specific for activation of class II promoters (Durand *et al*, 1997; Masternak *et al*, 1998; Reith & Mach, 2001; Nekrep *et al*, 2002). More specifically, the class II expression on antigen presenting cells is under the control of CIITA, that exhibits cell-specific, cytokine-inducible and differentiation-specific expression and is expressed in the same cells that express class II molecules, such as B cells, monocytes, dendritic cells and activated T cells. The genetic association of CIITA with AAD appears to be independent from that with HLA gene markers.

Other reported AAD genetic associations include the vitamin D receptor and the CYP27B1 (25-hydroxyvitamin D3-1α-hydroxylase) gene and the NACHT leucine-rich-repeat protein 1 (NALP1) gene (Magitta *et al*, 2009).

4. Pathophysiology of AAD

No model of spontaneous autoimmune primary adrenal insufficiency is yet available. Experimental autoimmune adrenalitis has been induced in mice, guinea pigs, rats and monkeys by injection of adrenal homogenates mixed with adjuvants (Betterle *et al*, 2002), with a resulting delayed type of hypersensitivity to adrenal antigens, rather than the induction of an adrenal autoimmune process. No conclusive data are yet available on the possibility of inducing an autoimmune reaction by injecting the major adrenal autoantigen 21-hydroxylase.

The current unavailability of a reliable animal model of spontaneous adrenal autoimmunity similar to the human disease, has so far limited the studies on the pathophysiology of AAD. Major efforts are being profused to develop an animal model of AAD that may prove useful for the understanding of the molecular mechanisms responsible for the human disease.

The effector cells of the autoimmune-mediated destruction of adrenocortical cells are thought to be T lymphocytes (Hayashi *et al*, 1989; Freeman & Weetman, 1992). Nerup *et al.*, 1969, 1970, showed that patients with autoimmune adrenal insufficiency have T cells reactive against fetal adrenal extracts or adrenal mitochondrial fraction. Subsequently, it was shown that patients with recent-onset AAD have an increased expression of circulating Ia-positive T cells when compared to healthy control subjects (Rabinowe *et al*, 1984). Freeman & Weetman, 1992 were able to demonstrate T cell proliferation in response to stimulation with adrenal proteins fractionated according to molecular weight. Patients with autoimmune polyendocrine syndrome type II, but not individuals with isolated Addison's disease, seem to have CD4+CD25+regulatory T cells with defective suppressive capacity (Kriegel *et al*, 2004; Coles *et al*, 2005).

Although several studies support the hypothesis of a major role of cellular immunity in the autoimmune destruction of the adrenocortical cells in Addison's disease, little is known of the individual antigens recognised by autoreactive T cells. Husebye et al. immunized BALB/c and SJL mice with recombinant 21OH and showed a selective significant proliferative response of T cells from lymph nodes against the peptide 342-361 of 21OH that corresponds to the substrate binding site of the enzyme (Husebye *et al*, 2006).

Among Th cell subtypes, two main subtypes, denominated Th1 and Th2, are recognized. AAD is thougth to result from an unbalance of Th1/Th2 responses with a predominance of Th1 activity. Chemokines produced at the site of inflammation participate by recruiting T cells and by sustaining the immune reaction (Rotondi *et al*, 2007). Th1 cells mainly express CXCR3 and are recruited at the site of inflammation by CXCL9, CXCL10 and CXCL11. Th2 cells express different chemokine receptors, such as CCR4 and CCR8, thus being recruited in target tissues by CCL17, CCL22 and CCL1. The existence of an important IFN-γ-mediated pathogenetic loop has been proposed for endocrine autoimmunity, as release of CXCR3-binding chemokines is stimulated by IFN-γ and, in turn, these chemokines recruit Th-1 cells that produce IFN-γ (Rotondi *et al*, 2007).

In one report concerning the role of serum CXCL10 in AAD, serum levels of CXCL10 were significantly increased in patients with either clinically evident or subclinical adrenal insufficiency, as compared to healthy control subjects (Rotondi *et al*, 2005). The absence of a gender-related effect in AAD, either isolated or occurring within APS-2, suggested that autoimmune adrenalitis by itself was responsible for the high circulating levels of CXCL10. In the same study (Rotondi *et al*, 2005), it was also shown that release of CXCL10 by primary cell cultures of human zona fasciculata cells (hZFC) was undetectable basally, but significantly induced by stimulation with IFN-γ or IFN-γ plus TNF-α, while stimulation of hZFC with TNF-α alone was not able to induce chemokine secretion. Interestingly, increasing concentrations of hydrocortisone progressively and significantly inhibited IFN-γ-induced and IFN-γ- plus TNF-α-induced CXCL10 secretion (Rotondi *et al*, 2005).

The inhibitory effect of glucocorticoids on chemokine production is in line with their antiinflammatory and immunosuppressive actions. Glucocorticoids are able to suppress the production of several cytokines and chemokines by inhibiting the nuclear factor-κB and by activating protein-1 transcription factor families (Karin, 1998).

More recently, increased serum levels of Th1-related chemokines CXCL10 and macrophage inflammatory proteins 1alpha (CCL3/MIP-1alpha) and of the Th2- related chemokine macrophage inflammatory proteins 1 beta (CCL4/MIP-1beta) were observed in patients with AAD, which confirms the role of these chemokines in the autoimmune pathology of adrenal gland through the recruitment in loco of Th1 and Th2 cells (Bellastella *et al*, 2011).

Based on the above described body of evidence, we can hypothesize that Th1 cells play a major pathogenetic role, while autoantibody production is a side effect with no pathogenic relevance. The decrease in Treg activity is probably one of the main mechanisms at the basis of the unbalanced activity of Th1 cells. The active role of the adrenocortical cells in modulating the autoimmune inflammation, by producing Th1-attracting chemokines and cortisol, should not be underestimated. Based on knowledge derived from studies on ovarian autoimmunity (Samy *et al*, 2005), it is likely that the continuous drainage of autoantigens to regional lymph nodes be essential to maintain an adequate activity of antiinflammatory Treg cells and that the reduced activity of Tregs and the unbalance Th1/Th2 ratio observed in human endocrine autoimmunity occur at the site of regional lymph nodes.

5. Ovarian autoimmunity

Although it has been proposed that up to 30% of cases of primary ovarian insufficiency (POI) would have an autoimmune origin (Meskhi *et al*, 2006; Calongos *et al*, 2009), a more accurate estimate indicates that a documented ovarian autoimmune reaction is present in not more than 4-5% of women with ovarian insufficiency (Hoek *et al*, 1997; Bakalov *et al*, 2005).

Similarly to the study of adrenal autoimmunity, the unavailability of an animal model of spontaneous autoimmune oophoritis has limited the possibility to define the molecular mechanisms of immune-mediated ovarian insufficiency. The animal model of neonatal thymectomy has proven instrumental to unravel the critical role of $CD4^+CD25^+$ regulatory T (Treg) cells (Samy *et al*, 2006) in suppressing autoimmune processes in regional lymph nodes, under a continuous stimulation by autologous antigens (Samy *et al*, 2005). The ovarian autoantigen identified in the animal model of neonatal thymectomy is the ooplasm-specific MATER (Maternal Antigen That Embryo Requires) protein.

Immunization of mice with a peptide of inhibin alpha chain induced an initial increase in fertility, mediated by high serum levels of inhibin alpha neutralizing antibodies, that prevented inhibin-mediated downregulation of activin-induced FSH release (Altuntas *et al*, 2006). In a second, delayed phase, the activation of CD4+ T-cells resulted in a lymphocytic infiltration of the ovary that occurred in parallel with a progressive decrease in fertility and ovarian function (Altuntas *et al*, 2006).

However, it is still unclear to what extent these animal models are similar to human autoimmune POI.

Several lines of evidence support the autoimmune origin of a fraction of POI cases. Some autoimmune diseases are more frequent in women with POI than in the general population, and, conversely, POI occurs more frequently in women affected by some autoimmune diseases than in other women. Approximately 15% of women with POI present with autoimmune thyroiditis (Hoek *et al*, 1997) and the frequency of POI is higher in women with T1DM than in the general population (Hoek *et al*, 1997). However, it must be noted that biochemical and/or ultrasound signs of thyroiditis can be detected in 10-15% women in the general population and that the concomitant association of POI and thyroiditis or POI and T1DM in the same woman does not justify *per se* a diagnosis of "autoimmune POI". Surely more relevant is the association between POI and AAD (Betterle *et al*, 2002; Hoek *et al*, 1997; Falorni *et al*, 2002b). Approximately 4-8% of women with POI are positive for circulating adrenal autoantibodies, a frequency significantly higher than that expected in the general population (<0.5%) (Betterle *et al*, 2002; Falorni *et al*, 2002b). On the other hand, 10-20% of women with AAD develop POI before the age of 40 years (Betterle *et al*, 2002).

The existence of ovarian autoantibodies was first shown in the 1960's in studies that used indirect immunofluorescence on cryostatic sections of adrenal, ovary, testis and placenta (Blizzard *et al*, 1967; Irvine & Barnes, 1974). Subsequent studies have repeatedly confirmed the existence of ovarian autoantibodies in women with POI (Sotsiou *et al*, 1980; Elder *et al*, 1981; Ahonen *et al*, 1987; Betterle *et al*, 1993). Ovarian autoantibodies detected by indirect immunofluorescence cross-react with autoantigens expressed in other tissues, mainly the adrenal cortex, the testis and the placenta, which indicates that the autoantigen(s) recognized by these autoantibodies are not restricted to the ovary, but expressed also in other organs. Hence, a more correct definition of these autoantibodies is that of Steroid-Cell Autoantibodies (StCA). Interestingly, although all the tissue components are present in the ovarian cryostatic sections used for the autoantibody assay, the immunofluorescence pattern of StCA is restricted to the theca cells of the growing follicle with no staining of primary follicles or granulosa cells in secondary and tertiary follicles. The same autoantibodies stain specifically Leydig cells of the testis.

Although indirect immunofluorescence is still the most widely used method to detect ovarian autoantibodies in clinical practice, the accuracy of this method has been questioned, mostly because of a low diagnostic specificity (Novosad et al, 2003). Some of the autoantigens recognised by StCA have been identified as the steroidogenic enzymes 17α-hydroxylase (17OH) and side-chain cleavage (P450scc) (Chen et al, 1996; Perniola et al, 2000; Falorni et al, 2002b). The development of immunoradiometric assays, using in vitro translated recombinant human 35S-radiolabelled autoantigens, have enabled the estimate of the diagnostic sensitivity and specificity of 17OHAb and P450sccAb for autoimmune POI (Chen et al, 1996; Perniola et al, 2000; Falorni et al, 2002b).

17OHAb and P450sccAb are each present in 50 to 80% of women positive for StCA (Chen et al, 1996; Perniola et al, 2000; Falorni et al, 2002b). Over 90% of StCA-positive women are positive for 17OHAb and/or P450sccAb, which is demonstrating that 17OH and P450scc are major targets of StCA, but other autoantigens may also be recognized by a subset of StCA.

StCA, 17OHAb and/or P450sccAb can be detected almost exclusively in women with POI who are also positive for adrenal autoantibodies, most specifically 21OHAb. The association of steroid-cell autoimmunity with adrenal autoimmunity is so strong that 21OHAb appear to be the marker at highest diagnostic sensitivity for autoimmune POI (Perniola et al, 2000; Falorni et al, 2002b, Bakalov et al, 2005). Since only less than 0.5% of women with POI can be found positive for StCA in the absence of 21OHAb, 17OHAb or P450sccAb, we can conclude that unequivocal biochemical signs of ovarian autoimmunity against steroidogenic enzymes are present almost exclusively in women with clinical or pre-clinical AAD.

Several studies have demonstrated that an autoimmune oophoritis can be found at ovarian biopsy only in women positive for ovarian and/or adrenal autoantibodies (Irvine, 1980; Gloor & Hurlimann, 1984; Sedmak et al, 1987; Bannatyne et al, 1990; Hoek et al, 1997; Bakalov et al, 2005), thus confirming that steroidogenic cell autoantibodies identify women with an ongoing ovarian autoimmune process. On the other hand, in the absence of ovarian and adrenal autoantibodies, no histological sign of autoimmune infiltration can typically be detected at ovarian biopsy, even in women who present with other autoimmune diseases, such as thyroiditis, T1DM, inflammatory bowel disease or systemic lupus erithematosus. Accordingly, a classification of autoimmune POI cannot be based only on the presence of other autoimmune manifestations, in the absence of specific autoantibodies in the serum.

Autoimmune oophoritis is characterized by a selective mononuclear cell infiltration into the theca layer of large, antral follicles, with earlier stage follicles consistently free of lymphocytic infiltration (Hoek et al, 1997; Bakalov et al, 2005). This finding is in line with the selective staining of theca cells at the indirect immunofluorescence assay and confirms that the steroidogenic cell ovarian autoimmune process is mainly directed against theca cells.

The absence of steroidogenic cell autoantibodies does not exclude the possibility that other autoantibodies may be present and other autoimmune mechanisms may be active. Many other potential autoantigens, such as LH receptor (Moncayo et al, 1989), FSH receptor (Ryan & Jones, 2004), zona pellucida (Kelkar et al, 2005), 82-86 kDa Ags and 52-63 kDa Ags (Wheatcroft et al, 1997) have been proposed as markers of ovarian autoimmunity, but the association of these autoantibodies with POI has not been confirmed (Anasti et al, 1995;

Tonacchera *et al*, 2004). Only detection of autoantibodies against steroidogenic enzymes can, accordingly, ensure, at present, an accurate identification of women with autoimmune oophoritis. Using these autoantibody markers, autoimmunity accounts for approximately 4-5% of all POI cases.

Along with the decline of serum concentrations of estradiol, POI is typically characterized with a reduction in synthesis and secretion of inhibins (Petraglia *et al*, 1998) and anti-müllerian hormone (AMH) (Méduri *et al*, 2007), as a result of the progressive decline in ovarian function. In an initial study of three women with autoimmune POI (Welt *et al*, 2005) this general paradigma was however questioned, as increased serum concentrations of inhibin B were detected. This initial finding was confirmed in a subsequent larger study (Tsigkou *et al*, 2008) that demonstrated increased levels of serum inhibin B and total inhibin in a group of 22 women with autoimmune POI, as compared to 71 women with idiopathic, non-autoimmune POI and 90 healthy fertile women. The results of these studies (Welt *et al*, 2005; Tsigkou *et al*, 2008) led to the formulation of a novel hypothesis of the pathophysiology of autoimmune POI. Differently from other forms of ovarian insufficiency, in which a general reduction of ovarian function can be observed, autoimmune POI is characterized by the selective autoimmune destruction of theca cells with preservation of granulosa cells that produce low amounts of estradiol because of lack of substrates. The subsequent increase in FSH levels stimulates viable granulosa cells that, in return, produce increased amounts of inhibins.

AMH levels have been found to be normal in women with hypogonadotrophic amenorrhea while they are very low or undetectable in women with physiological menopause or hypergonadotrophic amenorrhea (POI) (Méduri *et al*, 2007; La Marca *et al*, 2006; Knauff *et al*, 2009). AMH is exclusively produced by primary and pre-antral/small antral follicles, and the immunohistochemical findings of the absence of an inflammatory reaction around primary follicles (Hoek *et al*, 1997; Bakalov *et al*, 2005) provided a sound rationale to estimate AMH production in women with autoimmune POI. We recently documented normal serum AMH concentrations in two-thirds of women with recently diagnosed autoimmune POI (La Marca *et al*, 2009), which provides the first demonstration of the existence of a subgroup of women with POI with a preserved ovarian follicle pool for several years. Since AMH is the best biochemical marker of residual follicle pool, the results of our study (La Marca *et al*, 2009) are highly relevant for the future planning of clinical trials of immunotherapy aimed at preserving the residual functional tissue and/or delay the progression of the destructive ovarian autoimmune process in women with autoimmune POI.

6. Conclusions

Autoimmune Addison's disease is made evident by the apperance of circulating 21OHAb, the gold immune marker for the identification of subjects with an ongoing adrenal autoimmune process. The appearance of 21OHAb marks pre-clinical autoimmune Addison's disease, in asymptomatic subjects. In these individuals, the response to the ACTH-stimulation test enables the discrimination of an early, potentially reversible phase, from an irreversible phase of the disease.

POI affects around 1% of women below the age of 40 years and the detection of steroid cell autoantibodies enables the identification of autoimmune cases. At present, only the detection of 21OHAb and 17OHAb or P450sccAb may accurately identify autoimmune cases of POI.

Although autoantibodies are widely used in clinical practice, they have no pathogenic role for either AAD or POI and these diseases are thought to be the consequence of a T-cell mediated autoimmune destruction.

Substitutive therapy of either AAD or POI is not influenced by presence or absence of autoantibodies, but identification of autoimmune forms of these disease is nevertheless important. Approximately two thirds of AAD patients have at least another associated autoimmune disease, either clinical or pre-clinical. Accordingly, screening for other autoimmune disorders is mandatory in autoimmune AAD, but not strictly necessary in other forms of PAI. More importantly, autoimmune POI has a distinct pathophysiology which differs from that of other forms of ovarian insufficiency. Detection of steroid-cell autoantibodies enables the identification of subjects with an initially preserved follicle pool.

No animal models of spontaneous steroid-cell autoimmunity are currently available, and there is strong need for the generation of such models that may enable the improvement of our understanding of the molecular mechanisms of these diseases.

During the next few years large multicentric studies are expected to be performed to identify subjects at high-risk for developing AAD and clinical trials are being planned with the aim of immunomodulate the adrenal autoimmune response and delay progression towards clinical AAD. The availability of novel immunological technologies will prove instrumental in the molecular characterization of the steroid cell autoantigens and peptides recognised by human autoreactive T cells responsible for the adrenocortical cell destruction. In addition, epidemiological studies are needed to provide novel insights on the role of putative environmental factors.

7. References

Ahonen P, Miettinen A, Perheentupa J. Adrenal and steroidal cell antibodies in patients with autoimmune polyglandular disease type I and risk of adrenocortical and ovarian failure. *J Clin Endocrinol Metab* 64:494–500 (1987).

Altuntas CZ, Johnson JM, Tuohy VK. Autoimmune targeted disruption of the pituitary-ovarian axis causes premature ovarian failure. *J Immunol* 177:1988-1996 (2006).

Anasti JN, Flack MR, Froehlich J, Nelson LM. The use of human recombinant gonadotropin receptors to search for immunoglobulin G-mediated premature ovarian failure. *J Clin Endocrinol Metab* 80:824-828 (1995).

Anderson JR, Goudie RB, Gray KG, Timbury GC. Autoantibodies in Addison's disease. *Lancet* 1:1123–1124 (1957).

Andrada JA, Bigazzi PL, Andrada E, Milgrom F, Witebsky E. Serological investigation on Addison's disease. *Clin Sci* 206:1535–1541 (1968).

Arvat E, Di Vito L, Laffranco F *et al.* Stimulatory effect of adrenocorticotropin on cortisol, aldosterone, and dehydroepiandrosterone secretion in normal humans: dose-response study. *J Clin Endocrinol Metab* 88:3141–3146 (2000).

Bakalov VK, Anasti JN, Calis KA, *et al.* Autoimmune oophoritis as a mechanism of follicular dysfunction in women with 46,XX spontaneous premature ovarian failure. *Fertil Steril* 84:958-965 (2005).

Bannatyne P, Russell P, Shearman RP. Autoimmune oöphoritis: a clinicopathologic assessment of 12 cases. *Int J Gynaecol Pathol* 9:191–207 (1990)

Barker JM, Ide A, Hostetler C *et al.* Endocrine and immunogenetic testing in individuals with type 1 diabetes and 21-hydroxylase autoantibodies: Addison's disease in a high-risk population. *J Clin Endocrinol Metab* 90:128-134 (2005).

Baumann-Antczak A, Wedlock N, Bednarek J *et al.* Autoimmune Addison's disease and 21-hydroxylase. *Lancet* 340:429-430 (1992).

Bednarek J, Furmaniak J, Wedlock N, *et al.* Steroid 21-hydroxylase is a major autoantigen involved in adult onset autoimmune Addison's disease. *FEBS Lett* 309:51-55 (1992).

Bellastella G, Rotondi M, Pane E, *et al.* Simultaneous evaluation of the circulating levels of both Th1 and Th2 chemokines in patients with Autoimmune Addison's Disease. *J Endocrinol Invest* (2011), in press

Betterle C, Scalici C, Presotto F, *et al.* The natural history of adrenal function in autoimmune patients with adrenal autoantibodies. *J Endocrinol* 117:467-475 (1988).

Betterle C, Rossi A, Dalla Pria S, et al. Premature ovarian failure: autoimmunity and natural history. *Clin Endocrinol (Oxf)* 39:53-43 (1993).

Betterle C, Volpato M, Rees-Smith B *et al.* I. Adrenal cortex and steroid 21-hydroxylase autoantibodies in adult patients with organ-specific autoimmune diseases: markers of low progression to clinical Addison's disease. *J Clin Endocrinol Metab* 82:932-938 (1997).

Betterle C, Volpato M, Pedini B, Chen S, Rees-Smith B, Furmaniak J.Adrenal-cortex autoantibodies (ACA) and steroid-producing cells autoantibodies (StCA) in patients with Addison's disease: comparison between immunofluorescence and immunoprecipitation assays. *J Clin Endocrinol Metab* 84:618-622 (1999).

Betterle C, Dal Pra C, Mantero F, Zanchetta R. Autoimmune adrenal insufficiency and autoimmune polyendocrine syndromes: autoantibodies, autoantigens, and their applicability in diagnosis and disease prediction. *Endocr Rev* 23:327-364 (2002).

Betterle C, Dal Pra C, Pedini B, *et al.* Assessment of adrenocortical function and autoantibodies in a baby born to a mother with autoimmune polyglandular syndrome Type 2. *J Endocrinol Invest* 27:618-21 (2004).

Björses P, Halonen M, Palvimo JJ *et al.* Mutations in the AIRE gene:effects on subcellular location and transactivation function of the autoimmune polyendocrinopathy-candidiasis-ectodermal dystrophy protein. *Am J Hum Genet* 66:378-392 (2000)

Blizzard RM, Kyle M. Studies of the adrenal antigens and autoantibodies in Addison's disease. *J Clin Invest* 42:1653-1660 (1963).

Blizzard RM, Chee D, Davis W. The incidence of adrenal and other autoantibodies in the sera of patients with idiopathic adrenal insufficiency (Addison's disease). *Clin Exp Immunol* 2:19-30 (1967).

Boscaro M, Betterle C, Volpato M, *et al.* Hormonal responses during various phases of autoimmune adrenal failure: no evidence for 21-hydroxylase enzyme activity block in vivo. *J Clin Endocrinol Metab* 81:2801-2804 (1996).

Bottomley MJ, Collard MW, Huggenvik JI *et al.* The SAND domain structure defines a novel DNA-binding fold in transcriptional regulation. *Nat Struct Biol* 8:626-33 (2001).

Brozzetti A, Marzotti S, La Torre D, *et al.* Autoantibody responses in autoimmune ovarian insufficiency and in Addison disease are IgG1-dominated and suggest a predominant, but not exclusive, Th1 type of response. *Eur. J. Endocrinol* 163:309-317 (2010a).

Brozzetti A, Marzotti S, Tortoioli C, *et al*. Cytotoxic T Lymphocyte Antigen-4 Ala17 polymorphism is a genetic marker of autoimmune adrenal insufficiency: Italian association study and meta-analysis of European studies. *Eur. J.Endocrinology* 162:361-9 (2010b).

Calongos G, Hasegawa A, Komori S, Koyama K. Harmful effects of anti-zona pellucida antibodies in folliculogenesis, oogenesis, and fertilization. *J. Reprod. Immunol.* 79:148-155 (2009).

Cetani F, Barbesino G, Borsari S *et al*. A novel mutation of the autoimmune regulator gene in an Italian kindred with autoimmune polyendocrinopathy-candidiasis ectodermal dystrophy, acting in a dominant fashion and strongly cosegregating with hypothyroid autoimmune thyroiditis. *J. Clin. Endocrinol. Metab.* 86:4747–4752 (2001).

Chen S, Sawicka J, Betterle C, *et al*. Autoantibodies to steroidogenic enzymes in autoimmune polyglandular syndrome, Addison's disease and premature ovarian failure. *J Clin Endocrinol Metab* 81:1871-1876 (1996).

Chen S, Sawicka J, Prentice L, *et al*. Analysis of autoantibody epitopes on steroid 21-hydroxylase (21-OH) using a panel of monoclonal antibodies. *J Clin Endocrinol Metab* 83:2977–2986 (1998).

Coco G, Dal Pra C, Presotto F, *et al*. Estimated risk for developing autoimmune Addison's disease in patients with adrenal cortex autoantibodies. *J Clin Endocrinol Metab* 91:1637-1645 (2006).

Coles AJ, Thompson S, Cox AL, Curran S, Gurnell EM, Chatterjee VK. Dehydroepiandrosterone replacement in patients with Addison's disease has a bimodal effect on regulatory (CD4+CD25hi and CD4+FoxP3+) T cells. *Eur J Immunol.* 35:3694-3703 (2005).

Colls J, Betterle C, Volpato M, Prentice L, Smith BR, Furmaniak J. Immunoprecipitation assay for autoantibodies to steroid 21-hydroxylase in autoimmune adrenal diseases. *Clin Chem* 41:375–380 (1995).

De Bellis A, Bizzarro A, Rossi R, *et al*. Remission of subclinical adrenocortical failure in subjects with adrenal autoantibodies. *J Clin Endocrinol Metab* 76:1002–1007 (1993).

De Rosa G, Corsello SM, Cecchini L, Della Casa S, Testa A. A clinical study of Addison's disease. *Exp Clin Endocrinol* 90:232–242 (1987).

do Carmo Silva R, Kater CE, Dib SA, *et al*. Autoantibodies against recombinant human steroidogenic enzyme 21-hydroxylase, side-chain cleavage and 17α-hydroxylase in Addison's disease and autoimmune polyendocrine syndrome type III. *Eur J Endocrinol* 142:187–194 (2000).

Durand B, Sperisen P, Emery P, Barras E, Zufferey M, Mach B, Reith W. RFXAP, a novel subunit of the RFX DNA binding complex is mutated in MHC class II deficiency. *EMBO J* 16: 1045-1055 (1997).

Elder M, Maclaren N, Riley W. Gonadal autoantibodies in patients with hypogonadism and/or Addison disease. *J Clin Endocrinol Metab* 52:1137–1142 (1981).

Falorni A, Nikoshkov A, Laureti S, et al. High diagnostic accuracy for idiopathic Addison's disease with a sensitive radiobinding assay for autoantibodies against recombinat human 21-hydroxylase. J Clin Endocrinol Metab 80:2752–2755 (1995).

Falorni A, Laureti S, Nikoshkov A, et al. 21-hydroxylase autoantibodies in adult patients with endocrine autoimmune diseases are highly specific for Addison's disease. Clin. Exper. Immunol. 107:341-345 (1997).

Falorni A, Laureti S, Candeloro P, et al. Steroid-cell autoantibodies are preferentially expressed in women with premature ovarian failure who have adrenal autoimmunity. Fertility & Sterility 78:270-279 (2002a).

Falorni A, Laureti S, Santeusanio F. Autoantibodies in autoimmune polyendocrine syndrome type II. Endocrinol.Metab.Clin.N.Am. 31:369-389 (2002b).

Falorni A, Laureti S, De Bellis A, et al. Italian Addison Network Study: Update of diagnostic criteria for the etiological classification of primary adrenal insufficiency. J Clin Endocrinol Metab 89:1598-1604 (2004).

Falorni A, Brozzetti A, La Torre D, Tortoioli C, Gambelunghe G. The association of genetic polymorphisms and autoimmune Addison's disease. Expert Review of Clinical Immunology 4:441-456 (2008).

Falorni A, Chen S, Zanchetta R et al. Measuring adrenal autoantibody response: interlaboratory concordance in the first international serum exchange for the determination of 21-hydroxylase autoantibodies. Clin Immunol (2011), in press, doi: 10.1016/j.clim.2011.04.012

Freeman M, Weetman AP. T and B cell reactivity to adrenal antigens in autoimmune Addison's disease. Clin Exp Immunol 88:275-279 (1992).

Furmaniak J, Talbot D, Reinwein D, Benker G, Creagh FM, Smith B. Immunoprecipitation of human adrenal microsomal antigen. FEBS Lett 232:25–28 (1988).

Furmaniak J, Kominami S, Asawa T, Wedlock N, Colls J, Rees-Smith B. Autoimmune Addison's disease. Evidence for a role of steroid 21-hydroxylase autoantibodies in adrenal insufficiency. J Clin Endocrinol Metab 79:1517–1521 (1994).

Gambelunghe G, Falorni A, Ghaderi M et al. Microsatellite polymorphism of the MHC class I chain-related (MIC-A and MIC-B) genes marks the risk for autoimmune Addison's disease. J Clin Endocrinol Metab 84:3701–3707 (1999).

Gambelunghe G, Kockum I, Bini V et al. Retrovirus-like long terminal repeat DQ-LTR13 and genetic susceptibility to type 1 diabetes mellitus and autoimmune Addison's disease. Diabetes 54:900-905 (2005).

Ghaderi M, Gambelunghe G, Tortoioli C et al. MHC2TA single nucleotide polymorphism and genetic risk for autoimmune adrenal insufficiency. J Clin Endocrinol Metab 91:4107-4111 (2006).

Gloor E, Hurlimann J. Autoimmune oöphoritis. Am J Clin Pathol 81:105–109 (1984).

Goudie RB, Anderson JR, Gray KK, Whyte WG 1966 Autoantibodies in Addison's disease. Lancet 1:1173–1176 (1966).

Hayashi Y, Hiyoshi T, Takemura T, Kurashima C, Hirokawa K. Focal lymphocytic infiltration in the adrenal cortex of the elderly: immunohistological analysis of infiltrating lymphocytes. Clin Exp Immunol 77:101-105 (1989).

Hoek A, Schoemaker J, Drexhage HA. Premature ovarian failure and ovarian autoimmunity. *Endocr Rev* 18:107-134 (1997).

Husebye ES, Bratland E, Bredholt G, Fridkin M, Dayan M, Mozes E. The substrate-binding domain of 21-hydroxylase, the main autoantigen in autoimmune Addison's disease, is an immunodminant T cell epitope. *Endocrinology* 147:2411-2416 (2006).

Irvine WJ, Stewart AG, Scarth L. A clinical and immunological study of adrenocortical insufficiency (Addison's disease). *Clin Exp Immunol* 2:31-69 (1967).

Irvine WJ, Barnes EW. Addison's disease and associated conditions: with particular references to premature ovarian failure, diabetes mellitus and hypoparathyroidism. In: Gell PH, Coombs RRA, Lachman P, eds. Clinical aspects of immunology. Oxford, UK: Blackwell; 1301-1354 (1974).

Irvine WJ, Toft AD, Feek CM. Addison's disease. In: James VHT, ed. The adrenal gland. New York: Raven Press; 131-164 (1979).

Irvine WJ. Autoimmunity in endocrine disease. *Recent Prog Horm Res* 36:509-556 (1980)

Karin M. New twists in gene regulation by glucocorticoid receptor: is DNA binding dispensable? *Cell* 93:487-490 (1998).

Kasperlik-Zaluska AA, Migdalska B, Czarnocka B, Drac-Kaniewska J, Niegowska E, Czech W. Association of Addison's disease with autoimmune disorders—a long-term observation of 180 patients. Postgrad Med J 67:984-987 (1991).

Kelkar RL, Meherji PK, Kadam SS, Gupta SK, Nandedkar TD. Circulating autoantibodies against the zona pellucida and thyroid microsomal antigen in women with premature ovarian failure. *J Repr Immunol* 66:53-67 (2005).

Knauff EAH, Eijkemans MJC, Lambalk CB, *et al.* Anti-müllerian hormone, inhibin B, and antral follicle count in young women with ovarian failure. *J Clin Endocrinol Metab* 94:786-792 (2009).

Kong MF, Jeffcoate W. Eighty-six cases of Addison's disease. *Clin Endocrinol (Oxf)* 41:757-761 (1994).

Kosowicz J, Gryczynska M, Bottazzo GF. A radioimmunoassay for the detection of adrenal autoantibodies. *Clin Exp Immunol* 63:671-679 (1986).

Kriegel MA, Lohmann T, Gabler C, Blank N, Kalden JR, Lorenz HM. Defective suppressor function of human CD4+ CD25+ regulatory T cells in autoimmune polyglandular syndrome type II. *J Exp Med* 199:1285-1291 (2004).

Krohn K, Uibo R, Aavik E, Peterson P, Savilahti K. Identification by molecular cloning of an autoantigen associated with Addison's disease as steroid 17α-hydroxylase. *Lancet* 339:770-773 (1992).

La Marca A, Pati M, Orvieto R, Stabile G, Carducci Artenisio A, Volpe A. Serum Anti-Mullerian Hormone levels in women with secondary amenorrhea. *Fertil Steril* 85:1547-1549 (2006).

La Marca A, Marzotti S, Brozzetti A, *et al.* Primary ovarian insufficiency due to steroidogenic cell autoimmunity is associated with preserved pool of functioning follicles. *J Clin Endocrinol Metab* 94:3816-3823 (2009).

Laureti S, De Bellis A, Muccitelli VI, *et al.* Levels of adrenocortical autoantibodies correlate with the degree of adrenal dysfunction in subjects with preclinical Addison's disease. *J Clin Endocrinol Metab* 83:3507-3511 (1998).

Laureti S, Vecchi L, Santeusanio F, Falorni A. Is the prevalence of Addison's disease underestimated? *J Clin Endocrinol Metab* 84:1762 (1999)

Laureti S, Arvat E, Candeloro P, *et al.* Low dose (1 μg) ACTH test in the evaluation of adrenal dysfunction in pre-clinical Addison's disease. *Clin Endocrinol (Oxf)* 53:107–115 (2000).

Laureti S, Candeloro P, Aglietti MC, *et al.* Dehydroepiandrosterone, 17α-hydroxyprogesterone and aldosterone responses to the low-dose (1 μg) ACTH test in subjects with preclinical adrenal autoimmunity. *Clin Endocrinol (Oxf)* 57:677-683 (2002).

Løvås K, Husebye ES. High prevalence and increasing incidence of Addison's disease in western Norway. *Clin Endocrinol (Oxf)* 56:787–791 (2002)

Magitta NF, Bøe Wolff AS, Johansson S *et al.* A coding polymorphism in NALP1 confers risk for autoimmune Addison's disease and type 1 diabetes. *Genes Immun.* 10:120-124 (2009).

Masternak K, Barras E, Zufferey M *et al.* A gene encoding a novel RFX-associated transactivator is mutated in the majority of MHC class II deficiency patients. *Nature Gen* 20:273-277 (1998).

McHardy-Young S, Lessof MH, Maisey MN. Serum TSH and thyroid studies in Addison's disease. *Clin Endocrinol (Oxf)* 1:45–56 (1974).

Méduri G, Massin N, Guibourdenche J, *et al.* Serum anti-Müllerian hormone expression in women with premature ovarian failure. Hum Reprod 22:117-123 (2007).

Meskhi A, Seif MW. Premature ovarian failure. *Curr. Opin. Obstet. Gynecol.* 18:418-426 (2006).

Moncayo H, Moncayo R, Benz R, Wolf A, Lauritzen C. Ovarian failure and autoimmunity. Detection of autoantibodies directed against both the unoccupied luteinizing hormone/human chorionic gonadotropin receptor and the hormonereceptor complex of bovine corpus luteum. *J Clin Invest* 84:1857-1865 (1989).

Myhre AG, Undlien DE, Løvås K *et al.* Autoimmune adrenocortical failure in Norway autoantibodies and human leukocyte antigen class II associations related to clinical features. *J Clin Endocrinol Metab* 87:618-623 (2002).

Nekrep N, Jabrane-Ferrat N, Wolf HM, Eibl MM, Geyer M, Peterlin BM. Mutation in a winged-helix DNA-binding motif causes atypical bare lymphocyte syndrome. *Nature Immunol.* 3:1075-1081 (2002).

Nerup J, Andersen V, Bendixen G. Anti-adrenal, cellular hypersensitivity in Addison's disease. *Clin Exp Immunol* 4:355-363 (1969).

Nerup J, Andersen V, Bendixen G. Anti-adrenal, cellular hypersensitivity in Addison's disease. IV. In vivo and in vitro investigations on the mitochondrial fraction. *Clin Exp Immunol* 6:733-739 (1970).

Nerup J. Addison's disease-clinical studies. A report of 108 cases. *Acta Endocrinol (Copenh)* 76:127–141 (1974).

Neufeld M, MacLaren NK, Blizzard RM. Two types of autoimmune Addison's disease associated with different polyglandular autoimmune (PGA) syndromes. *Medicine (Baltimore)* 60: 355–362 (1981).

Nikoshkov A, Falorni A, Lajic S, *et al.* A conformation-dependent epitope in Addison's disease and other endocrinological autoimmune diseases maps to a carboxyl-terminal functional domain of human steroid 21-hydroxylase. *J Immunol* 162:2422–2426 (1999).

Nomura K, Depura H, Saruta T. Addison's disease in Japan: characteristics and changes revealed in a nationwide survey. *Intern Med* 33:602–606 (1994).

Novosad JA, Kalantaridou SN, Tong ZB, Nelson LM. Ovarian antibodies as detected by indirect immunofluorescence are unreliable in the diagnosis of autoimmune premature ovarian failure: a controlled evaluation. *BMC Womens Health* 3:2 (2003)

Oelkers W. Adrenal insufficiency. *N Engl J Med* 335:1206–1212 (1996)

Papadopoulos KI, Hallengren B. Polyglandular autoimmune syndrome type II in patients with idiopathic Addison's disease. *Acta Endocrinol (Copenh)* 122:472–478 (1990).

Park YS, Sanjeevi CB, Robles D et al. Additional association of intra-MHC genes, MICA and D6S273, with Addison's disease. *Tissue Antigens* 60:155-163 (2002).

Perniola R, Falorni A, Clemente MG, Forini F, Accogli E, Lobreglio G. Organ-specific and non-organ-specific autoantibodies in children and young adults with autoimmune polyendocrinopathy-candidiasis-ectodermal dystrophy (APECED). *Eur J Endocrinol* 143:497-503 (2000).

Petraglia F, Hartmann B, Luisi S, et al. Low levels of serum inhibin A and inhibin B in women with hypergonadotropic amenhorrea and evidence of high levels of activin A in women with hypothalamic amenhorrea. *Fertil Steril* 70:907-912 (1998).

Pitkänen J, Doucas V, Sternsdorf T et al. The autoimmune regulator protein has transcriptional transactivating properties and interacts with the common coactivator CREB-binding protein. *J Biol Chem* 275:16802–16809 (2000).

Pitkänen J, Vähämurto P, Krohn K et al. Subcellular localization of the autoimmune regulator protein. characterization of nuclear targeting and transcriptional activation domain. *J Biol Chem* 276:19597–19602 (2001).

Rabinowe SL, Jackson RA, Dluhy RG, Williams GH. Ia-positive T lymphocytes in recently diagnosed idiopathic Addison's disease. *Am J Med* 77:597–601 (1984).

Reith W, Mach B. The bare lymphocyte syndrome and the regulation of mhc expression. *Annu. Rev. Immunol.* 19:331-373 (2001).

Rotondi M, Falorni A, De Bellis A et al. Elevated serum interferon-γ-inducible chemokine-10/CXC chemokine ligand-10 in autoimmune primary adrenal insufficiency and *in vitro* expression in human adrenal cells primary cultures after stimulation with proinflammatory cytokines. *J Clin Endocrinol Metab* 90:2357–2363 (2005).

Rotondi M, Chiovato L, Romagnani S, Serio M, Romagnani P. Role of chemokines in endocrine autoimmune diseases. *Endocrine Rev* 28:492-520 (2007).

Ryan MM, Jones HR Jr. Myasthenia gravis and premature ovarian failure. *Muscle Nerve* 30:231-233 (2004).

Samy ET, Parker LA, Sharp CP, Tung KSK. Continuous control of autoimmune disease by antigen-dependent polyclonal CD4+CD25+ regulatory T cells in the regional lymph node. *J Exp Med* 202:771-781 (2005).

Samy ET, Setiady YY, Ohno K, Pramoonjago P, Sharp C, Tung KSK. The role of physiological self-antigen in the acquisition and maintenance of regulatory T-cell function. *Immunol Rev* 212:170-84 (2006).

Sedmak DD, Hart WR, Tubbs RR. Autoimmune oöphoritis: a histopathologic study involved ovaries with immunologic characterization of the mononuclear cell infiltrate. *Int J Gynecol Pathol* 6:73–81 (1987).

Skinningsrud B, Husebye ES, Gervin K *et al*. Mutation screening of PTPN22: association of the 1858T-allele with Addison's disease. *Eur J Hum Genet*. 16:977-982 (2008a).

Skinningsrud B, Husebye E, Pearce SH et al. Polymorphisms in CLEC16A and CIITA at 16p13 are associated with primary adrenal insufficiency. *J Clin Endocrinol Metab* 93:3310-3317 (2008b).

Sotsiou F, Bottazzo GF, Doniach D. Immunofluorescence studies on autoantibodies to steroid-producing cells, and to germline cells in endocrine disease and infertility. *Clin Exp Immunol* 39:97–111 (1980).

Stechmesser E, Scherbaum WA, Grossman T, Berg PA. An ELISA method for the detection of autoantibodies to adrenal cortex. *J Immunol Methods* 80:67–76 (1985).

Su MA, Giang K, Zumer K *et al*. Mechanisms of an autoimmune syndrome in mice caused by a dominant mutation in Aire. *J Clin Invest* 118:1712-1726 (2008).

Söderbergh A, Winqvist O, Norheim I, *et al*. Adrenal autoantibodies and organ-specific autoimmunity in Addison disease. *Clin Endocrinol (Oxf)* 45:453–460 (1996).

Tanaka H, Perez MS, Powell M *et al*. Steroid 21-hydroxylase autoantibodies: measurements with a new immunoprecipitation assay. *J Clin Endocrinol Metab* 82:1440–1446 (1997).

The Finnish-German APECED Consortium. An autoimmune disease, APECED, caused by mutations in a novel gene featuring two PHD-type zinc-finger domains. Autoimmune Polyendocrinopathy-Candidiasis-Ectodermal Dystrophy. *Nat Genet* 17:399–403 (1997).

Tonacchera M, Ferrarini E, Dimida A, *et al*. Gonadotrophin receptor blocking antibodies measured by the use of cell lines stably expressing human gonadotrophin receptors are not detectable in women with 46,XX premature ovarian failure. *Clin Endocrinol (Oxf)* 61:376-381 (2004).

Tsigkou A, Marzotti S, Borges L, et al. High serum inhibin concentration discriminates autoimmune oophoritis from other forms of primary ovarian insufficiency. *J.Clin.Endocrinol.Metab.* 93:1263-1269 (2008).

Welt CK, Falorni A, Taylor AE, Martin KA, Hall JE. Selective theca cell dysfunction in autoimmune oophoritis results in multifollicular development, decreased estradiol, and elevated inhibin B levels. *J Clin Endocrinol Metab* 90:3069-3076 (2005).

Wheatcroft NJ, Salt C, Milford-Ward A, Cooke ID, Weetman AP. Identification of ovarian antibodies by immunofluorescence, enzyme-linked immunosorbent assay or immunoblotting in premature ovarian failure. *Hum Reprod* 12:2617-2622 (1997)

Winqvist O, Karlsson FA, Kämpe O. 21-Hydroxylase, a major autoantigen in idiopathic Addison's disease. *Lancet* 339:1559–1562 (1992).

Winqvist O, Gustafsson J, Rorsman F, Karlsson FA, Kämpe O. Two different cytochrome P450 enzymes are the adrenal antigens in autoimmune polyendocrine syndrome type I and Addison's disease. *J Clin Invest* 92:2377–2385 (1993).

Wuepper KD, Weigienka LC, Hugh Fudenberg H. Immunologic aspect of adrenocortical insufficiency. *Am J Med* 46:206–216 (1969).

Yu L, Brewer KW, Gates S *et al.* DRB1*04 and DQ alleles: expression of 21-hydroxylase
     autoantibodies and risk of progression to Addison's disease. *J Clin Endocrinol Metab*
     84:328-335 (1999).
Zelissen PM, Bast EJ, Croughs RJ. Associated autoimmunity in Addison's disease. *J
     Autoimmunity* 8:121–130 (1995).

4

Excretion of Steroid Hormones in Rodents: An Overview on Species Differences for New Biomedical Animal Research Models

Juan Manuel Busso[1,3] and Rubén Daniel Ruiz[2,3]
[1]Instituto de Ciencia y Tecnología de Alimentos, Facultad de Ciencias Exactas, Físicas y
Naturales (FCEFyN) – Universidad Nacional de Córdoba (UNC)/ Consejo Nacional
de Investigaciones Científicas y Técnicas (CONICET)
[2]Instituto de Fisiología, Facultad de Ciencias Médicas, UNC
[3] Established investigators from the CONICET
Argentina

1. Introduction

Living organisms have regular patterns and routines that involve obtaining food and carrying out life-history stages such as breeding, migrating, molting and hibernating. The acquisition, utilization, and storage of energy reserves (and other resources) are critical to lifetime reproductive success, and this reproductive process could be affected by predictable and unpredictable environmental changes (McEwen and Wingfield, 2003; Schneider, 2004). Allostasis is achieving physiological stability through change (see details in McEwen and Wingfield, 2003); the allostatic state refers to altered and sustained activity levels of the primary mediators, i.e., glucocorticosteroids that integrate physiology and associated behaviors in response to changing environments and challenges. Focused on these primary mediators, particularly in steroid hormones, it has been well accepted for a long time that variations (increases) of adrenal glucocorticoids are associated with stress responses. Moreover, measuring changes in glucocorticoid concentration (and also in levels of adrenaline and noradrenaline) has been the most frequently used strategy to monitor physiological responses to stress and distress challenges (Terlouw et al, 1997; Wielebnowski, 2003; Mormède et al, 2007; Sheriff et al., 2011). In terms of changes in steroid secretory patterns in response to a stressor, glucocorticoids are known to change over the course of minutes and those levels will subsequently (within hours to days) affect steroid reproductive hormones (such as testosterone, estradiol and progesterone) (Sapolsky et al., 2000).

While experiencing severe stress, animals, as humans, can succumb to disease or fail to reproduce or develop properly (Moberg, 2000). Therefore, animals have evolved a suite of physiological and behavioral strategies to cope with environmental changes as well as to survive in a particular given time and space (Buchanan, 2000; Romero, 2004). Therefore, "environmental endocrinology" has developed in response to the need to understand how hormones modulate and control physiological processes in animals exposed to the exigencies of their particular natural environment. This has only been possible through spectacular developments in hormone assay techniques, which now make feasible hormone measurements on microlitre volumes of body fluids (Bradshaw, 2007). Four biological samples have been employed up to the present: blood, saliva, excreta (feces and urine), and integumentary structures (hair and feathers), each of them having advantages and disadvantages for use with different species and research purposes (Sheriff et al., 2011).

Blood collection continues being an attractive and reliable technique for steroid analysis; several reports for different species are available in the literature, such as for Japanese quail (Arora, 1979) or chinchilla (Tappa et al, 1989); these *species-specific reports provide recommendations on safety, ease of collection and repeated collections.* However, in a study of endocrine dynamics this approach may be impractical because blood extraction is a powerful stressor and it is known that within minutes, glucocorticoid secretion is stimulated and gonadal steroid secretion declines. For example, blood samples collected only from birds reflect unstressed (baseline) glucocorticoid concentrations with a high degree of confidence within less than 2 minutes (Sapolsky et al., 2000; Romero and Reed, 2005). In addition, when experiments involve small animals it is usually difficult to obtain the necessary blood volume, and repeated blood sampling can interfere with subsequent hormone measurements, and it may even be harmful as it has been reported for chinchilla. In large-sized bird and mammalian species, such as Greater Rhea (Léche et al., 2009) and Clouded Leopard (Wielebnowsky et al., 2002), blood collection may be dangerous for the operator and certainly stressful for animals. Blood sample collection is always a critical procedure in the laboratory, and an impractical approach in nature without the aid of auxiliary techniques (such as anesthesia); therefore, these "Gold" microliters of plasma/serum are always appreciated by researchers.

Hormones secreted by adrenal and gonad glands go through the bloodstream to their target tissues and cells, where they initiate a change in cellular activity by attaching to a receptor protein. Thereafter, steroids are excreted into the bile to undergo metabolic changes in the intestinal tract due to the enzymatic activity of the intestinal microflora. Also, enterohepatic recirculation of steroid metabolites, with possible further metabolic changes in the liver, is known to occur in many species. The reabsorbed metabolites may be excreted in the bile again or pass into urine (Taylor, 1971). Evaluating steroid metabolite content and/or profiles in either urine or feces represents an alternative technical approach without perturbing individuals, populations or animal species. This experimental strategy has been applied to a wide range of research goals in captive and free-ranging wildlife, as well as domestic and laboratory species. Several reviews focusing on steroid metabolism and the validation of particularly fecal steroid assays have been published in the last years (Schwarzenberger et al., 1996; Brown and Wildt, 1997; Monfort, 2003; Palme et al., 2005; Schwarzenberger, 2007).

The obvious advantage of assessing urinary or fecal hormone concentrations is that adrenal and gonadal functions can be determined without even touching the animal: the waste is simply recovered from the adequately arranged ground or enclosure floor and analyzed in the laboratory. Resulting hormonal profiles are generally less "noisy" than those observed after analyzing blood because the excretory patterns represent a pool of metabolites rather than reflecting the often hour-to-hour fluctuating dynamism quantified in blood (Pukazhenthi and Wild, 2004). According to recent reviews, it seems that this approach, noninvasive monitoring, will be utilized more than ever when well-focused endocrine issues are addressed and some steroids are involved (Palme and Möstl, 2002; Pukazhenthi and Wildt, 2004; Palme, 2005; Schwarzenberger, 2007). In fact, international programs have trained science students, especially researches from Latin American PhD programs (Swanson and Brown, 2004), as it can found in the reports of Busso et al. (2005a, 2007), Ponzio et al. (2004) in Argentina, of Brousset Hernández-Jauregui et al. (2005) in Mexico, and of Moreira et al. (2007) in Brazil. Similarly, new studies fully developed in traditionally called developing countries are clear evidence of the usefulness of this non-invasive approach (Leche et al., 2009, 2011). Furthermore, national funds or grants in these developing countries are becoming available to develop this type of noninvasive hormone research; e.g., in Argentina, new doctoral fellowships are being granted to support these studies.

A particular disadvantage of fecal steroid analysis is the presence of a vast number of different fecal steroid metabolites even in closely related species. For the development of techniques for fecal steroid analysis, experiments on the metabolism of radioactively labeled steroids have provided a valuable insight into the metabolism and excretion of hormone metabolites via feces and urine (Schwarzenberger, 2007; see discussion below). By contrast, steroids voided into urine are not extremely degraded; however, the use of urine steroids has the particular disadvantage that urine collection in some animals requires restraint in a metabolic cage, surgical interference or rigorous surveillance to collect samples during urination (Peter et al., 1996; Monfort, 2003). In non-invasive monitoring of steroid activity, several aspects must be considered before undertaking a new study, and/or focusing on a new species, or applying a new immunoassay (Millspaugh and Washburn, 2004; Buchanan and Goldsmith, 2004; Palme, 2005; Touma and Palme, 2005; Wielebnowski and Watters, 2007; Hayward et al., 2010).

When we intend to measure steroid metabolites in excreta, firstly we need to obtain them, usually by an extraction technique that should be simple, safe and efficient. Secondly, we usually need an immunoassay to detect (accurately, precisely, and specifically) variation of steroid levels in the matrix of interest. All these laboratory and validation steps as well as interpretation of results are strongly affected by information about steroid metabolism and catabolism; animal biological characteristics must be also taken into account (individual development, reproductive stage, nutritional strategy, copying strategy, etc.) during result analysis. Although we have not focused our revision on these aspects, the reader must be aware of them and their importance in the application of non-invasive monitoring.

As we have addressed steroid excretion, we need to know some aspects about steroid excretion before employing some immunoassays to reveal steroid activity: 1) **route of excretion** of each hormone to be evaluated, 2) **time-course** of steroid secretion in blood-stream and its clearance into urine and feces, 3) **proportion of excreted metabolites during biological cycles**, 4) **identification of steroid metabolites in the matrix selected**. These variables may be determined by injecting the hormone, usually a radiolabeled steroid or, less frequently, a large amount of unlabeled steroid and tracking their metabolite excretion over time. For example, Wielebnowski and Watters (2007) indicate that the types of fecal steroid metabolites excreted, the main route of excretion, and the time it takes for metabolization and excretion to occur should be identified before selecting an antibody and assay system. Normative data on steroid excretion is essential for improving the application of non-invasive monitoring; in addition, this information would be an extraordinary source of knowledge to compare several aspects of animal environmental endocrinology.

Therefore, based on updated endocrine data from wild, laboratory and farmed rodents, we propose to develop a comparative endocrine survey of the routes of gonadal and adrenocortical steroid excretion. In our laboratory, chinchilla were subjected to radiometabolism studies of progesterone, corticosterone, testosterone and estradiol (Ponzio et al, 2004; Busso et al, 2005a, 2007). Since domesticated chinchilla still share some genomic characteristics with their counterparts in the wild, the analysis would serve as an adequate example of widely diverse interests (scientific, ecological, economic, cultural and emblematic values). Basically, our endocrinological studies contribute with some specific data from this particular large rodent to the existing data for other rodents. The information provided can be helpful for:

In situ studies: 1- assessment of ecological phenomena, focused on environmental endocrinology, i.e. by quantifying field concentrations of stress hormones in individual organisms; 2- identification of healthy individuals from endangered wild populations to develop reproductive *ex situ* programs.

Ex situ studies: 1- diagnosis of reproductive functions and dysfunctions of valuable farmed individuals 2- application of assisted reproductive techniques; 3- improvement of welfare of animal model for studying biomedical research; 4- development of new experimental biotypes for the study of hormonal disruptive effects of environmental pollute.

In general, reviews about those topics have apparently neglected information about rodents. These animals are not regarded as threatened mammals, and public appreciation about their biological importance is scarce and tends to overlook the ecological role and conservation problems of an order representing about 41% of mammalian species (Gippoliti and Amori, 1998; Amori and Gippoliti, 2001, 2003). However, the order Rodentia is a tremendous biodiversity example of life strategies, with more than 2000 species, which encompass a staggering diversity of form, behavior and physiology. Additionally, scientists have frequently employed several rodent species to conduct research, and have used rodents even as animal models for biomedical studies.

2. Excretion of steroid hormones

Nowadays, it is widely accepted that basic knowledge of the metabolism and excretion of glucocorticoids is necessary for the development of a non-invasive technique to monitor adrenocortical activity (Möstl and Palme, 2002). Similarly, information of sex steroid metabolism is essential to monitor steroidogenic activity of gonads (Brown et al, 1994). The first step in assay development is identifying the excretory routes for each hormone of interest; conducting an infusion study would be extremely valuable in domestic and nondomestic animals, if captive-held counterparts are available and the tests are feasible (Wielebnowski and Watters, 2007), such as the studies performed in domestic chinchilla to evaluate wild chinchilla (Busso et al, 2005a, 2007; see further details below). We also accept that, in practical terms, it is unnecessary to determine the specific molecular structure of the hormones being monitored in each species. However, it is critical to demonstrate that fluctuations in the hormone metabolites being measured provide physiologically relevant information (Monfort, 2003). Accordingly, it is well accepted that endocrine glands must be challenged to monitor their activation, e.g., by injecting ACTH or dexamethasone and measuring whether glucocorticoid levels in the tested matrix reflects the predicted changes in the blood. The use of a biological test or the so called "biologically relevant tests" (that expose an animal to a biological stressor to measure the glucocorticoids in samples) is also recommended; this ensures that the noninvasive monitoring will appropriately measure glucocorticoids in the field when animals are exposed to genuine stressors (Sheriff et al., 2011). Several reports may be useful to set up an experimental design for applying a non-invasive approach (Brown and Wildt, 1997; Wasser et al., 2000; Palme and Möstl, 2002;

Buchanan and Goldsmith, 2004; Millspaugh and Washburn, 2004; Palme, 2005; Goymann, 2005; Klasing, 2005; Palme et al., 2005; Wielebnowski and Watters, 2007).

Pharmacological and biological relevance tests are truly useful for validating non-invasive endocrine monitoring. Nevertheless, such validations should not miss the radiolabelling studies, since these allow us to discover, investigate and/or discuss the functional relevance of steroids. In fact, steroid receptors and the co-evolution of steroidogenic enzymes and steroid-inactivating enzymes had an important role in the evolution of complex regulatory networks in vertebrates, contributing to vertebrate survival and diversification in the last 500 million years (Baker, 1996, 2003).

Cholesterol is the precursor of the five major classes of steroid hormones. According to their number of carbon-atoms, these classes are: progestagens, glucocorticoids (and mineralcorticoids, C21); androgens (C19); and estrogens (C18). Because of their common precursor cholesterol, they are apparently all structurally related across birds and mammalian species; however, they show strong functional differences. Steroid hormones bind to intracellular proteins, termed receptors, which function as transcription factors. The receptors are specific for a given class of steroid. These receptors are members of the large superfamily of nuclear hormone receptors that include different hormones such as glucocorticoids, mineralocorticoids, vitamin A, thyroid and retinoids, as well as sex steroids (Brown, 1999). It is also well known that steroid hormones are synthesized in a number of endocrine tissues, mainly gonads, adrenals, and placenta.

Steroid hormones are dissociated from their receptors and metabolized by the target cell or the liver, which possess enzymes capable of altering the specific steroids and rendering them biologically inactive and water soluble. Typically, inactivation involves reduction or removal of side chain or attached groups or both, as well as the combination with other molecules (conjugation), such as glucose, to form a glucuronide or conjugation with sulfate. The relative emphasis on sulfate or glucuronide varies depending on the steroid and/or species (Norris, 2007). During this inactivation process, steroids are metabolized in the liver and excreted via the bile into the gut. Enterohepatic recirculation of steroid metabolites, with possible further metabolic changes in the liver, may facilitate steroid metabolite reabsorption; the reabsorbed metabolites would be excreted in the bile again or pass into urine. More than 40 years ago, Taylor (1971) revised studies on the excretion of steroid hormone metabolites in bile and feces. Regarding steroid metabolites, those of the less polar molecules tend to be excreted in bile to a greater extent than metabolites of polar steroids; e.g., progesterone metabolites are mainly present in bile (and feces). In contrast, hydrocorticortisone (cortisol) is almost completely excreted as urinary metabolites. On the basis of evidence reviewed, a hypothesis was postulated suggesting that the membrane of the bile canaliculi would have receptor sites specific for certain steroids metabolites (Taylor, 1971). The binding of these substances at the receptor sites is an obligatory step prior to active transfer of the substances across the canalicular membrane. In "primitive" mammals, such as rats and mice, the receptor sites have poor specificity and are therefore able to bind metabolites of most steroid hormones. In other species, evolution has resulted in a decrease in the number, specificity and binding capacity of these sites. Therefore, some steroid metabolites are partially bound and so excreted into bile (e.g., progesterone), whereas others are less firmly, or not, bound and therefore return to the blood by a passive or active transport. This hypothesis seems to go some way to explaining the difference in biliary excretion of steroid metabolites among species, and the excretion of different steroids by the same species. Radioinfusions have offered data as new evidence for increased caution in the inferences due to differences between species.

As pointed out above, it is possible to evaluate gut passage time using radiometabolism studies, in which radio-labeled steroids are usually injected and then clearance of radioactivity into urine and faecal compartments is monitored (Brown et al., 1994; Palme et al., 1996); this procedure reflects time delay quite precisely and therefore provides a rough estimate of the expected delay. The delay time between circulation of steroids in plasma and their appearance in urine samples is usually rather short (less than 5 h), but fecal steroid metabolites have an appreciable lag time (Palme et al., 1996; Schwarzenberger et al., 1996). For example, lag time or time course of fecal excretion may range from less than 30 minutes to more than one day, depending on the species, sometimes even within species, depending on the activity rhythms of animals (Palme and Möstl, 2002; Monfort, 2003; Palme, 2005). Recently, Touma et al. (2003) indicated that metabolism and excretion of corticosterone in urine and feces of mice are not only significantly affected by sex, but also by the time of day when the radioactive peak was observed (after administration). Several radiometabolism studies demonstrated that oestrogens in the form of estradiol and/or estrone are present in fecal samples; by contrast, testosterone, progesterone and, especially, cortisol/corticosterone are heavily metabolized and the original hormone is barely present in the feces (Schwarzenberger, 2007). Therefore, the route of excretion varies considerably among species, and among steroids within the same species.

This chapter focuses on the updated comparative endocrine analysis of the routes of excretion of gonadal and adrenocortical steroids, taking into account the published information on non-invasive analyses being used by a variety of scientists (e.g., conservation biologists, animal scientists) to examine glucocorticoid (i.e., stress hormone) and gonadal steroids (i.e. reproductive hormones) secretion in domestic and wild rodents. Also, radiolabeled procedures have also provided useful results for testing the efficiency of different protocols for extracting hormones from samples (Schwarzenberger et al, 1996).

3. Measurements of steroids in rodent excreta: Use of radiolobelled infusions for evaluation of corticosterone/cortisol, progesterone, testosterone and estradiol catabolism

Over 40% of mammal species belong to the order Rodentia. While rodents are often thought of as just mice and rats, more than 2000 species in this order encompass a staggering diversity of form, behavior and physiology. In fact, excluding the human species, the order Rodentia is the group of most prosperous modern mammals, occupying very different ecological niches in almost all the planet, mostly specialized in rapid reproduction that can be adjusted to different circumstances (Conaway, 1971; Young, 1985; Bronson, 1999). At present, based on rodent morphology of their lower jaw, living rodents are divided into two suborders: the Sciurognathi (squirrel and mouse-like forms) and the Hystriocognathi (cavy-like forms). Although this classification might still be a matter of debate as well as those based on the long-standing division of the insertion patterns of masseter muscles or the plane of incisor insertions (Mess et al., 2001; Huchon et al., 2002; Kay et al. 2008), these aspects are beyond the scope of present review. We currently support or choose the present classification of rodents as squirrel and mouse or cavy-like forms. It has been proposed that Rodentia is a monophyletic group; however, several molecular studies have suggested that the guinea pig and its relatives (such as Hystriocognathi or cavy-like forms) are closer to other orders of mammals than to families of rats and mice. For example, taking into account that insulin is a conservative molecule in mammals, as we might think of steroids,

Hystricognathi species represent an exception having a very divergent molecule with unusual physiological properties among rodents (Opazo et al, 2005).
In our laboratory, we have been studying aspects of reproductive biology in chinchilla (*Chinchilla lanigera*) for over 15 years (Ponce et al., 1998a, b; Carrascosa et al., 2002; Ponzio et al., 2004, 2007a, b, 2008; Busso et al., 2005a, b, c, 2007). This is an interesting taxon, since domesticated chinchilla used for the fur industry still share some genomic characteristics with their endangered (almost extinct) counterparts. Actually, *Chinchilla* spp. are critically endangered in South American wild populations according to the IUCN (IUCN/SSC Rodent Specialist Group):

Wild rodents
Chinchilla lanigera, a chinchillid from the Cordillera de la Costa and rocky Andean slopes of Chile (400-2500 m asl), which is threatened by the fur trade and habitat loss due to overgrazing, firewood collection, and mining. **Chinchilla brevicaudata**, another chincillid from the central Andean region of Peru, Bolivia, Argentina, and Chile. This species inhabits at higher altitudes (over 3,000 m asl), and is also threatened by the fur trade. Although its actual status is poorly known, it is already extinct in Argentina and Peru and probably is facing extinction in other parts of its range. The Convention on International Trade in Endangered Species of Wild Fauna and Flora (CITES), lists in Appendix I all South American populations of Chinchilla, but no other rodents. According to Lidicker (IUCN/SSC Rodent Specialist Group, 1989), these listings by IUCN and CITES do not mean for sure that the populations of most rodent species are in good health, but only that we know very little about them.

Box 1. a status in nature must be verified in CITES and IUCN before start a new radiolabelled steroid infusion

Back to steroid hormones, most of the knowledge about endocrine modulation of reproductive physiology in *Chinchilla* spp. has been derived from studies in females (Tam, 1971, 1972; Brookhyser and Aulerich, 1980; Gromadzka-Ostrowska and Sylarska-Gozdz, 1984; Gromadzka-Ostrowska et al., 1985). With respect to the male endocrine reproductive physiology, Cepeda et al. (2006) obtained a plasma testosterone profile during the annual reproductive cycle, showing that endocrine activity increased immediately before the breeding season. Other studies performed using blood sampling have also been reported in chinchilla (Brookhyser et al., 1977; Tappa et al., 1989); however, serial samples taken over time induced injury in some animals. Alternatively, we validated a tool for non-invasively assessing endocrine testicular and ovary activity as well as adrenocortical activity by detecting hormone changes in excreta (Ponzio et al., 2004; Busso et al., 2005a, 2007).
We subjected some males and females to radiometabolism studies of testosterone, and progesterone and estradiol, respectively; we also studied corticosterone excretion in males. Firstly, after assessing ^{14}C-testosterone metabolite excretion in male chinchilla (Busso et al., 2005a), several urinary and fecal androgen metabolites were separated by HPLC for their identification, but only fecal metabolites were associated with native testosterone. More than one metabolite derived from ^{14}C-testosterone showed   immunoreactivity and further

biochemical and biological tests demonstrated that the employment of excreta would be useful to assess endocrine testicular function in this species. In female chinchillas, we also performed radiolabeled infusion of ³H-estradiol and ¹⁴C-progesterone, but in contrast to testosterone assessment, natural steroids were evaluated (were separated by HPLC-UV) in urinary and fecal extracts from pregnant individuals. This is a particular protocol to avoid the use of radioactive material in technical procedures, as normally expected at present. Chromatographic analyses demonstrated that most peaks were associated with the polar mobile phase in urine, whereas in feces, there were both polar and non-polar peaks. All HPLC fractions were individually analyzed by UV detector and by estradiol or progesterone immunoassays. These experiments suggest that chinchillas excrete native forms of progesterone and estradiol in low concentrations in urine and feces, whereas only progesterone-derived metabolites appear to be present in both excreta (Busso et al., 2007). Figure 1 depicts reproductive endocrine normative data with respect to route of steroid excretion in chinchilla (Hystricognathi rodent).

Radioinfusion studies in chinchilla

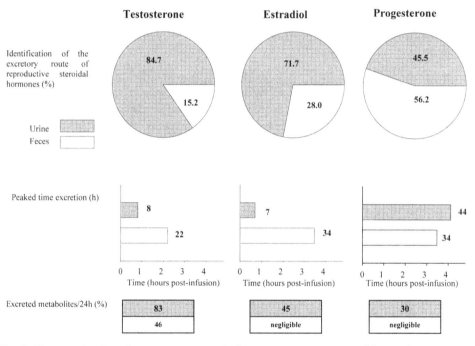

Fig. 1. Characterization of testosterone metabolite excretion in urine and feces after isotope administration (i.m.) in chinchilla males (n = 4; details in Busso et al. 2005a). Similarly, estradiol and progesterone metabolite excretion in excreta after isotope administration (i.p.) in chinchilla females (n = 4; details in Busso et al. 2007).

Furthermore, in the same experimental model, we also established that the urinary route of corticosterone excretion was predominant in male (Ponzio et al., 2004) and HPLC analysis revealed that most corticosteroids are excreted as readily hydrolysable steroid conjugates of cortisol. Results shown together with data on corticosterone excretion in Figure 1 clearly demonstrate that urine is the main route, except for progesterone, where radioactive metabolites were almost equally found in urinary (45.5 ± 13.5%) and fecal extracts (56.2 ± 4.9%). As expected, radioactive peaks generally appeared earlier in urine than in feces. However, estradiol and progesterone radioactive metabolite time-courses showed great individual differences between 24-48 h post infusions, the highest percentages of excreted radioactive metabolites being detected during 48h post-infusion.

Interestingly, based on these results from our radiometabolism studies and those reported for other rodents subjected to radiolabeled infusion up to this moment, we considered that the route of steroid metabolite excretion varies depending on the rodentia suborder. Therefore, it was proposed that the urinary route is preferential in Hystrichomorpha (chinchilla and guinea pigs; currently considered cavy-like forms) while in the Sciurognathi (squirrel and mouse-like forms, formerly considered Sciumorpha or Myormorpha suborders), the primary excretory route is the feces (Busso et al., 2006, Ponzio et al., 2006).

To our best knowledge, Taylor (1971) provided the best compilation of radiometabolism studies in mammalian species reported in the literature up to the present. Two of Taylor's major conclusions are relevant for our purposes: a) different steroids are excreted to different extents in urine and feces; this is evident, for example, in our comparative endocrinological studies in chinchilla (see Figure 1); and b) the same steroid is excreted to different extents in urine and feces of different species; reports revised by Taylor in the 1970s and most of the reports published thereafter are included in Figure 2. In this illustration our compilation is arranged according to our hypothesis of preferential route of steroid metabolite excretion in Rodentia suborders (see details in legend). It can be useful to take into account certain physical-chemical natural characteristics of steroids; considering the physico-chemical characteristics of steroid polarity, steroids are firstly shown in Figure 2 according to their water solubility (considering that steroids are heavily metabolized and the original hormone is barely present, particularly in the feces). Anyway, according to recent revisions, taxonomic relatedness does still little to predict the precise nature of metabolites or their relative routes of excretion (urine versus feces; Palme et al. 2005; Schwanzenberger, 2007).

3.1 Hystricognathi (cavy-like forms)
Both Guinea pigs and chinchilla are commonly employed as animal models in biomedical investigations. These species belong to the hystricomorph group of rodents that are well represented in South America, and have remarkably long reproductive cycles compared to other rodents.

Few studies on the comparative aspects of steroid metabolism and excretion in cavy-like forms (chinchilla and guinea pig) are available; published data of most reproductive steroids indicate that they are excreted mainly by urine (except for progesterone in chinchilla, see above). Fewer studies are available for sex steroids in this group of rodents; Bogdan and Monfort (2001) evaluated fecal estrogen and progesterone profiles in breeding and non-breeding females of the North American porcupine (*Erethizon dorsatum*; *Erethizontoidae family*). For glucocorticoids, cortisol is the main adrenal steroid hormone present in guinea pig plasma (Malinowska and Nathanielsz, 1974). No studies applying radiolabeled glucocorticoids in guinea pig have been conducted according to our last search, but apparently cortisol metabolites are found in large quantities in urine (Fajer and Vogt, 1963).

Results of the application of a non-invasive technique in chinchilla indicate that glucocorticoids would present mainly in urine (Ponzio et al., 2004), and that cortisol would also be the main adrenal steroid. Cortisol was also detected in an experiment employing a cortisol RIA in blood samples of *Octodon degus* (*Octodontoidae family*); in addition, an ACTH positive effect on blood cortisol profile and cortisol fecal metabolite excretion was detected (Soto Gamboa et al., 2009). However, in the latter study it is difficult for us to establish a close correlation between results from different matrices because of sampling regimens.

3.2 Sciurognathi (squirrel and mouse-like forms)

Rats and mice are also widely used as animal models of human diseases in biomedical research. Other rodents such as those in the sciurid group, e.g., ground squirrel, have been extensively used as mammalian models of ecology, population regulation, and behavior. Nevertheless, Lepschy et al. (2007), as other authors, argued that the small body size of rodents and difficulties involved in blood sampling make it difficult to apply an invasive procedure. We should keep in mind that stress is a significant source of experimental errors and a major cause of stress in laboratory animals, and reducing stressful conditions in normal husbandry and in application of methods is essential to achieve an adequate level of reliability in the experimental results (Dahlin et al., 2009). Therefore, a non-invasive technique to monitor stress hormones in these animals is highly desirable (Siswanto et al., 2008; Touma et al., 2004; Thanos et al, 2009; Kalliokoski et al., 2010).

Likewise, Harper and Austad (2000) developed a noninvasive method for measuring adrenal activity in house mice, deer mice, and red-back voles (*members of Muridae and Cricetidae families*), as other authors did in old field mice (*Cricetidae family;* Good et al., 2003), in spiny mice (*Acomys cahirinus; Muridade family*) (Nováková et al., 2008; Frynta et al., 2009), in agouti and non-agouti deer mice (*Peromyscus maniculatus; Cricetidae family*) (Hayssen et al., 2002), and in Columbian ground squirrel (*Sciuridae family*) (Bosson et al, 2009). Similarly, although most of those authors did not perform a previous radioinfusion study, a noninvasive assessment proved to be useful also in different reproductive studies conducted in others small rodents (DeCantanzaro et al., 2003; Kuznetzov et al., 2004; Cavigelli et al., 2005; Chelini et al., 2005).

In mice, corticosterone and testosterone are excreted mainly by feces. Although several reports showed aspects of steroid metabolism in some rodents such as mice during the 1960s and 1970s, new studies have contributed to increase that limited information. Touma et al. (2003) injected mice i.p. with ^{3}H-corticosterone; although males excreted significantly more radioactive metabolites via the feces than females (72 vs 56%), this study demonstrated once again that most corticosterone metabolite excretion was via the feces in both sexes. Conversely, Kalliokoski et al. (2010) reported that corticosterone metabolite content is about 50% higher in urine than in feces; therefore, they recommended that future studies should analyze primarily the output in urine, although this matrix is volatile and difficult to collect. Billiti et al. (1998) employed 3 mice and 3 deer mice (3–24 months of age) to perform radiolabeled   testosterone infusion (intraperitoneally), and found that the proportion of the injected testosterone excreted in feces was 62% for *Mus* spp. and 58% for *Peromyscus* spp. Noteworthy, it has been reported that in mice, the rate of excretion vs. time profile showed between two and three elimination phases in urine and feces (and more than 90% excreted testosterone metabolites were found during first 24 h). This information revealed that the first phase corresponded to radioactive testosterone that went directly to highly perfused tissues such as liver and kidney, and the second phase corresponded to a slower component in which hormone is sequestered in slowly perfused tissues such as adipose tissues; also, the route of administration, such as the intraperitoneal one, may favor the excretion of testosterone in one phase over another. All these are important considerations not only for future experiments but also for application in field studies.

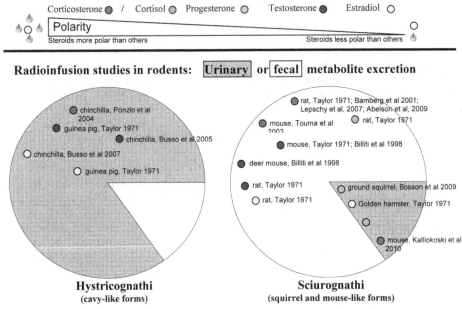

Hystricognathi
(cavy-like forms)

Sciurognathi
(squirrel and mouse-like forms)

Fig. 2. Compilation of radiometabolism studies in rodent species reported in the literature. Firstly, adrenal and sex steroids are ordered according to solubility in aqueous phase in an "ideal" physical chemistry system in the laboratory. Pie charts are illustrated according to that hypothesis that postulates that in Hystricognathi rodents the urinary route (gray) is preferential, whereas in Sciurognathi, feces (white) is the primary excretory route (details in the text); the size of gray and white portions in both pie charts is only illustrative. Colors of circles are associated with steroids; in addition, circles as well as references were located according to the main route of excretion of each hormone of interest in the studied species, i.e. in Sicurognathi: feces: corticosterone in rat: similar results are revealed by different reports, e.g., Taylor, 1971; Bamberg et al., 2001; Lepschy et al., 2007 and Abelson et al., 2009.

Recently, cortisol radioinfusions were informed for squirrel species (Bosson et al., 2009; Dantzer et al., 2010) as well the application of noninvasive monitoring in Cape ground squirrel (Pettitt et al., 2007). In Columbian ground squirrel, this glucocorticoid is highly metabolized, with virtually none being excreted. The percentages of radioactive cortisol recovered were 31% and 6.5% in urine and feces, respectively; it can be argued that these values are low. The authors accepted this problem but, because of the characteristics of excreta collection, results were certain only for feces. Similar results were obtained by Dantzer et al. (2010), who injected radiolabeled cortisol in North American red squirrel; the hormone was entirely metabolized and excreted in both urine (70.3 ± 0.02%) and feces (29.7 ± 0.02%), with a lag time to peak excretion of 10.9 ± 2.3 h in feces. With respect to cortisol excretion in mouse-like forms, we found only one reference (for rat, Taylor, 1971); the main route was feces, as well as for corticosterone in other Sciurognathi rodents. Since squirrels belong to the Sciuridade family, which is closer to Lagomorpha than the Muridae family (rat and mouse, etc.), this genetic proximity would explain these results. Accordingly, low fecal excretion of glucocorticoid metabolites (about 8%) has also been found in European hares (*Lepus europaeus*; Teskey- Gerstl et al., 2000). In fact, Taylor (1971) informed (another species of Lagomorpha order) that only between 3-5% of testosterone or 4% of estradiol are excreted in rabbit feces.

Similarly to the studies analyzed above, different techniques have been applied in rats to monitor the route, time-course and proportions of excreted steroid metabolites. Bamberg et al. (2001) employed male Sprague-Dawley 8 week-old rats which were injected i.p. with ^{3}H-corticosterone (16 μCi) at 09:00. Meanwhile, Lepschy et al. (2007) started an experiment at the same time as the former study; however, each rat (both sexes were employed in this study; 12 week-old individuals) was intravenously injected with different doses of ^{3}H-corticosterone (62.1 μCi). Both studies showed that the main route of corticosterone excretion in the male was feces. It is quite difficult to compare both studies since a different sample collection technique was applied. Firstly, when employing only males, during the first day, urine or feces samples were collected at different time schedule. Lepschy et al. (2007) collected all voided excreta from both sexes during the first day (probably the most recommended). Both radioactive urinary peaks were detected earlier than feces peaks, but there was a great variability in urine: 1-6h and 4-10h, respectively. Technical differences in the study of the same steroid in the same species were further reported by Abelson et al. (2009), who studied male Sprague-Dawley rats after intravenous administration of a low dose (1μCi) of radioactive corticosterone. The amount of radioactivity detected in feces was highest and displayed a more pronounced peak 12h after injection when the substance was administered through a jugular vein catheter than through tail vein injection.

As expected, it is evident that there were great differences in the profiles of radioactive excretion among individuals in rodents, particularly in well studied species such rats and mice, as in others mammals (Brown et al, 1994; Palme et al, 1996), i.e., time course may change with the route and time of administration, even between sexes in some species (see detailed studies on rats: Touma et al., 2003; Eriksson et al., 2004; Abelson et al., 2009). Similarly, in chinchilla, Busso et al. (2005a, 2007) also indicated that radioactive urinary estradiol peaked between 24-48h, the radioactive peak being at 34h post-infusion. Several technical aspects, rather than biological ones, must be taken into account before deciding to undertake a new investigation; from molecular structure of interested hormone (free marked or conjugated steroid), through animal state and development, up to sample collection regimen, etc. Further studies are necessary to standardize how to obtain endocrinological information from animal "waste" as soon as possible.

A key advantage of measuring hormones in excreta is that this procedure integrates hormone levels over time, instead of measuring a single time point (as in snapshot) represented by hormone levels in blood. We consider that time peak excretion after radioinfusion or steroid hormone increase after gland has been stimulated is not a robust measure because there are too many sources of variation. Several variables, such as dietary preferences, gastrointestinal anatomy, digestive physiology, biochemical capabilities, and commensal microflora, called "nutritional strategy" by Klasing (2005) in birds, may affect retention time and consequently time course of excreted steroids among species and/or individuals of the same population. Besides, a different sample collection schedule also seriously affects interpretation of time course or hormonal profiles; collecting naturally all voided urine or feces is advisable, as it has been observed in many reports. Therefore, in attempting to collect all samples, some problems may arise, i.e., in the study of testosterone excretion in chinchilla, an "animal effect" associated with each hormonal profiles was found. This effect evoked a delayed excretion of testosterone metabolites in some males with respect to others; a constipation process was a probable source of variation that has previously been detected in other farmed animals (Palme et al., 1996; Busso et al., 2005a). It is advisable to use each animal as its own control, thereby minimizing the problems of individual differences in basal and peak levels (Touma and Palme, 2005).

Urinary and fecal excretion frequency may be affected by other factors, such as some stressors effects on different individuals. Nowadays, increasing evidence indicates considerable variation between individuals in the magnitude and pattern of their corticosterone responses (called "personalities"). Furthermore, regularity of food intake and resulting defecation frequency has not been investigated sufficiently and needs to be considered as a potential variable for steroid metabolite analyses. In addition, changes in defecation frequency and patterns due to seasonal variation, reproduction, or even stress may alter elimination rate and therefore systematically affect the amount of metabolites excreted per sample (Wielebnowski and Watters, 2007). Further experiments are necessary to enhance our understanding of kinetic parameters; these variables are still significant research topics or unresolved issues that will allow us to elucidate the relationship between physiological events and detection of changes in excreta.

Elimination of steroids via the urine is usually very rapid as maximal concentration is found within a few hours after administration of radioactive tracer and/or peak natural concentrations in the plasma; the first urinary samples collected usually exhibit most of the excreted metabolites. In feces, peak concentrations of radioactivity were observed after a certain lag time (usually after 24 h or up to 48h) (Monfort, 2003; Palme, 2005; Schwanzenberger, 2007). However, this is not a particularly useful or informative measure as it is highly dependent on the sampling regimen, and fails to account for differences in the general shape of the hormone excretion-time profile (Kalliokoski et al. 2010). Thus, we consider that proportion of total metabolites excreted per activity phase (such as dark/light cycle; endocrine cycles, etc.) would be more informative than the exact time of peak excretion; however, most importantly, hormone monitoring must be performed in repeated long-term studies.

The reviewed information is significantly useful because when monitoring stress and/or reproductive endocrine responses in a long-term study, competitive immunoassays will be used in different matrices (urine, feces, etc) to reveal adrenal and/or gonadal endocrine activities. Thus, depending on the species, the hormone, and the research question, it is relevant to "pick" the appropriate antibody and assay design that allows for detection of most, or at least a considerable amount, of the immunoreactive metabolites involved (Wielebnowski and Watters, 2007). Otherwise, some problems may arise when working with a matrix that exhibits lowest concentration of excreted metabolites. For example, an assay for testosterone fecal metabolites in guinea pig failed to clearly discriminate among intact males, castrated males, and females (Bauer et al., 2008). In addition, it was not possible to detect fecal progestagen changes throughout pregnancy, pre-partum and post-partum stages in chinchilla compared with results obtained from urine samples (Busso et al., 2007).

This does not mean that we do not recommend working with samples with low steroid concentrations. In fact, there are good examples like the report of Muir et al. (2001), involving urinary samples of female and male mice, since this mouse species excretes reproductive steroids mainly by feces. However, greatest efforts are needed when samples are collected from the less quantitative route of steroid excretion in a given species.

4. Remarkable issues for a precise assessment of steroid hormone excretion in rodents

Steroid hormones have demonstrated a major regulatory role in vertebrate physiology (affecting, for example, fetal and postnatal growth and development, and maintaining allostasis, particularly, progesterone or glucocorticoids, as other examples, which are important in female reproduction or are involved in the "fight or flight" response). The physiological changes mediated by adrenal and sex steroids receptors provided early vertebrates with an advantage in competing with the diverse organisms that evolved during the Cambrian explosion (Baker, 1997). Therefore, it is of great importance and interest to study how these hormonal modulators respond to different environmental conditions, such as the studies of chemical disruptors on endocrine activity with implications in normal neuroendocrine responses (Crews et al., 2000; Dickerson and Gore, 2007)

Let´s remember that rodents are eutherian mammals (Short, 1985) and that one obvious way of increasing or decreasing an animal's reproductive potential is by altering its gestation length. Three groups stand out with respect to gestation length/maternal weight ratio: hystricomorph rodents as well as primates have relatively long gestations, and whales with relatively short gestations. Hystricomorph rodents, here called cavy-like form, have evidently developed a different reproductive strategy than other rodents. By contrast, Sciurognathi species generally exhibit small body size, short lifespan, short gestation (21 days in mice and rats),numerous litters, and rapid rates of development, as well as short birth intervals (all these species called "r" strategist in ecology). All rodent species together amount to 2000 different taxa; however, information mostly comes from few species of two families (Muridae: Old World mice, rats, gerbils and relatives or Cricetidae: New World rat, mice, voles, hamsters and relatives). These families are genetically closely related and have been well studied: they display differences of degree but not of kind.

Contrarily, Hystricomorph rodents (about 170 species) appear to be more diversified in their patterns of reproduction than any other group of related mammals. The hystricomorph rodents, which are particularly well represented in South America, have colonized harsh environments at either high altitude or high latitudes. Under such conditions, it would be advantageous for a species like the chinchilla to prolong gestation (more than 100 days) so as to allow birth during clement weather. However, this environmental explanation cannot account for the long gestations of those hystricomorphs that live in subtropical forests, or those that live in underground burrows as the plains viscacha (Weir and Rowlands, 1973; Short, 1985; Bronson, 1999). Therefore, this group of mammals (rodents), excluding the human species, is the group of most prosperous modern mammals, occupying very different ecological niches almost worldwide, mostly specialized in different rhythms of reproduction that can be adjusted to different circumstances. This biodiversity offers several phenotypes or biotypes of animals to study general and comparative endocrinological aspects. Finally, how these animals have synchronized to cope with habitats and face environmental challenges up to present is one of our major research concerns.

Regarding our research work that focused on chinchilla, we considered only steroid excretion in rodents in this chapter. It was not our goal to thoroughly review the details of each species. We found out that few species of rodents were subjected to radiolabeled studies of steroid excretion. According to the latest publications, taxonomic relatedness does little to predict the precise nature of metabolites or their relative routes of excretion (urine versus feces; Palme et al. 2005; Schwanzenberger, 2007). The best way to clarify these questions is to perform radiometabolism experiments and a physiological and biological validation of the immunoassay, such as the work conducted in Columbian ground squirrel (Bosson et al., 2009). However, at present, radioinfusion as an experimental approach to the noninvasive study of adrenal and/or gonadal activity seems "old-fashioned". Accordingly, we did our best to include in the present revision as many reports of application of non-invasive hormone monitoring in rodents species as possible. We also know that it may not be possible to elucidate why different steroids are excreted in urine and feces to different extents; however, a better framework for rodents is now available with respect to differences among species in terms of the same steroid being excreted in urine and feces to different extents. In the assessment of adrenal and gonadal endocrine activities using non-invasive techniques, several extensive considerations should be taken into account (Buchanan and Goldsmith, 2004; Millspaugh and Washburn, 2004; Palme, 2005; Touma and Palme, 2005; Schwarzenberger, 2007; Wilebnowski and Watters, 2007); however, these aspects are beyond the scope of the present revision, but all of them may be affected by the ranking of the excretory routes.

Accordingly, multidisciplinary scientific efforts might be useful to increase our knowledge on comparative endocrinology in rodents, using different species as biotypes or new animal models for the studies. Some concerns about it have already been stated. Smale et al. (2005) pointed out that the study of neuroendocrinology in nontraditional mammals is an essential approach that complements methodologies (such as knock-out mouse) by taking advantage of allelic variation produced by natural selection. Obviously, the technical advantages of non-invasive hormonal monitoring with repeated measures in long-term studies have strongly encouraged biologists (and specialists such as ecologists, ethologists, etc.) as well as other professionals in human and veterinary medicine, zoological exhibition and/or animal production managers.

In summary, the application of noninvasive hormonal monitoring has proven very useful for the generation of normative data (for the species, reproductive cycles, stress responses, etc.) and particularly for the assessment of individual endocrine state. All the aspects shown in Box 2 must be addressed for a precise assessment of steroid hormone excretion.

Finally, one of the main advantages of measuring steroids in blood is the study of the dynamics of hormone secretion; however, great efforts must be made to meet the technical requirements for obtaining a blood sample for an accurate and reliable measurement (route of blood extraction, minimal obtained blood volume, extraction time to avoid stress interference in steroid profiles, etc.). Therefore, hormonal quantification in different biological matrices such urine and feces is an alternative approach. But also, this approach does not exclude technical disadvantages involved in sample collection, such as frequency of elimination of excreta, volume of excreta (which can affect the distribution of hormone metabolites, etc.). Therefore, both types of samples, blood and excreta, are seriously affected by the sampling protocol. Laboratories should continue reviewing (and possibly standardizing) this aspect. In addition, there are extra sources of variation affecting sampling protocol such as nutritional strategy, which also seriously alter the precise hormonal determination. Moreover the fact that an individual may be studied without being disturbed, another interesting aspect in the use of non-invasive hormone monitoring is that metabolite concentrations frequently are 2 to 4 times higher than plasma levels (Peter et al., 1996). However, this quantitative advantage is lost when the route of steroid excretion is unknown.

"Keys for a precise assessment of steroid hormone excretion"

- **Who?** ID of steroids of interest; particularly it is necessary to know species differences and to identify the main glucocorticoid by the adrenal gland in rodents (cortisol or corticosterone).
- **How much?** Percentage of hormone metabolite excretion into urine or feces; route of excretion may be determined by radiolabeled or unlabeled infusion of each hormone of interest.
- **When it happened?** Time course of steroid secretion in blood-stream and its clearance into urine and feces. The best approach is to collect all voided urine and excreted feces, because there is still no standardization with respect to sampling protocols. In the future, it seems that proportion of excreted metabolites during activity cycles (day/night; elimination phases) may be a better approach to understanding steroid excretion with respect to individual endocrine state.
- **Which matrix?** After choosing the biological matrix (urine or feces), identification of steroid metabolite in the matrix of interest is essential to obtain the best results in immunoassay performance. Each matrix has advantages and disadvantages.
- **How are results expressed?** To follow the endocrine gland activity in the best way possible, it would be useful to express hormone excretion rated by fixed period of time (i.e. hour of sample collection) and to inform total volume or weight/period of time of voided urine and excreted feces, respectively.
- **What else?** Sex, life stages (juvenile, adult, aging change), environmental characteristics (photoperiod, temperature, feeding strategy, coping strategy) must be taken into account to improve our knowledge.

ID: identification.

Box 2. Recycling information from excretes about animal stress and reproductive endocrine states in rodents.

5. Acknowledgements

J. M. Busso jmbusso@conicet.gov.ar and R. D. Ruiz are Established Investigators from CONICET, Argentina and their contributions were supported by CONICET, Agencia Córdoba Ciencia, SECyT-UNC and FONCyT, Argentina.

6. References

Abelson, KSP, Fard SS, Nyman J, Goldkuhl R, Hau J. (2009). Distribution of (^{3}H)-corticosterone in urine, feces and blood of male Sprague-Dawley rats after tail vein and jugular vein injection. In Vivo: 23: 381-386.

Amori G and Gippoliti S, (2003) A higher–taxon approach to rodent conservation priorities for the 21st century. Animal Biodiversity and Conservation, 26: 2: 1-18

Amori, G Gippoliti, S. (2001). Identifying priority ecoregions for rodent conservation at the genus level. Oryx 35, 158-165

Baker, ME. (1997). Steroid receptor phylogeny and vertebrate origins. Mol Cell Endocrinol, 135: 101-107.

Baker, ME. (2003). Evolution of adrenal and sex steroid action in vertebrates: a ligand-based mechanism for complexity. BioEssays, 25: 396-400.

Biddlecombe R.A. and Law B., (1996). Validation of an immunoassay. In Brian Law (ed): Immunoassay a practical guide. Taylor and Francis Ltd, London, pp 171-203.

Blanga-Kanfi S, Miranda H, Penn O, Pupko T, DeBry RW, Huchon D. (2009). Rodent phylogeny revised: analysis of six nuclear genes from all major rodents clades. BMC Evolutionary Biology 9:71, 2148-9-71.

Bosson CO, Palme R, Boonstra R. (2009). Assessment of the stress response in Columbian Ground Squirrels: laboratory and Field validation of an enzyme immunoassay for fecal cortisol metabolites. Physiol Biochem Zool 82: 291-301.

Bogdan D, Monfort SL. (2001). Faecal oestrogen and progesterone profiles in breeding and non-breeding female north American porcupine (*Erethizon dorsatum*). Mammalia 65, 73-82.

Bradshaw D. (2007). Enviromental endocrinology. Gen Comp Endocrinol, 152: 125–141.

Bronson FH. (1999). Rodentia. In Knobil E, Neill JD (eds): Encyclopedia of reproduction. Academic Press, New York, pp 282-289.

Brookhyser KM, Aulerich RJ, Vomachka AJ. (1977). Adaptation of the orbital sinus bleeding technique to the chinchilla (*Chinchilla laniger*). Lab. Anim. Sci. 27: 251-254.

Brousset Hernández-Jauregui DM, Galind Maldonado F, Valdez Pérez RA, Romano Pardo M, Schuneman de Aluja A. (2005). Cortisol in saliva, urine, and feces: non-invasive assessment of wild mammals. Vet Mex 36: 325-337.

Brown JL, Wildt DE. (1997). Assessing reproductive status in wild felids by noninvasive faecal steroid monitoring. Int. Zoo Yb. 35, 173-191.

Brown JL, Wasser SK, Wildt DE, Graham LH. (1994). Comparative aspects of steroid hormone metabolism and ovarian activity in felids, measured noninvasively in feces. Biol. Reprod. 51, 776-786.

Brown JL. Steroids hormones-Overview (1999): In Knobil E, Neill JD (eds): Encyclopedia of reproduction. Academic Press, New York, pp 282-289.

Buchanan KL (2000). Stress and the evolution of condition-dependent signals. TREE, 15: 156-160.

Buchanan K, Goldsmith A. (2004). Noninvasive endocrine data for behavioural studies: the importance of validation. Anim. Behav. 67: 183–185.

Busso JM, Ponzio MF, Dabbene V, Fiol de Cuneo M, Ruiz RD. (2005a) Assessment of urine and fecal testosterone metabolite excretion in *Chinchilla lanigera* males. Anim. Reprod. Sci. 86, 339-351.

Busso JM, Ponzio MF, Chiaraviglio M, Fiol de Cuneo M, Ruiz RD. (2005b). Elecroejaculation in the Chinchilla (*Chinchilla lanigera*): effects of anesthesia on seminal characteristics. Res. Vet. Sci. 78, 93-97.

Busso JM, Ponzio MF, Fiol de Cuneo M, Ruiz RD. (2005c). Year-round testicular volume and semen quality evaluations in captive *Chinchilla lanigera*. Anim. Reprod. Sci. 90, 127-134.

Busso JM. Estudio de la función reproductora y optimización de biotecnología para mejorar la eficacia reproductiva del género chinchillla. Fac Cs Ex, Fis y Nat-UNC, Córdoba-Argentina; Ph D Thesis 2006.

Busso JM, Ponzio MF, Fiol de Cuneo M, Ruiz RD,. (2007) Noninvasive monitoring of ovarian endocrine activity in the chinchilla (Chinchilla lanigera). Gen Comp Endocr; 150: 288-297.

Carrascosa RE, Martini AC, Ponzio MF, Busso JM, Ponce AA, Lacuara JL. (2001). Storage of *Chinchilla laniger* semen at 4°C for 24 or 72 h with two different cryoprotectants. Cryobiology 42, 301-306.

Cavigelli SA, Monfort SL, Whitney TK, Mechref YS, Novotny M, McClintock MK. (2005). Frequent serial fecal corticoid measures from rats reflect circadian and ovarian corticosterone rhytms. J. Endocrinol. 184, 153-163.

Chelini MOM, Souza NL, Rocha AM, Felippe ECG, Oliveira CA. (2005). Quantification of fecal estradiol and progesterone metabolites in Syrian hamsters (Mesocricetus auratus). Brazilian J of Medical and Biological Research, 38: 1711-1717.

Cepeda R, Adaro L, Peñailillo G. (2006) Morphometric Variations of Chinchilla laniger Prostate and Plasmatic Testosterone Concentration During its Annual Reproductive Cycle. Int J Morphol; 24: 89-97.

Conaway C.H. (1971). Ecological adaptation and mammalian reproduction. Biol. Reprod. 4, 239-247.

Crews D, Willingham E, Skipper JK. (2000). Endocrine disruptors: present issues, future directions. Q Rev Biol 75: 243-260.

Dahlin J, Lam J, Hau J, Astuti P, Siswanto H, Abelson KSP.(2009). Body weight and faecal corticosterone metabolite excretion in male Sprague-Dawley rats following short transportation and transfer from Group-housing to single-housing. Scand. J. Lab. Anim. Sci. 36: 205-213.

Dantzer B, McAdam AG, Palme R, Fletcher QE, Boutin S, Humphries MM, Boonstra R. (2010). Fecal cortisol metabolite levels in free-ranging North American red squirrels: Assay validation and the effects of reproductive condition. Gen Comp Endocrinol 167: 279–286

DeCantanzaro D, Muir C, Beaton EA, Jetha M. (2004). Non-invasive repeated measurement of urinary progesterone, 17 -estradiol, and testosterone in developing, cycling, pregnant, and postpartum female mice. Steroids 69, 687-696.

Dickerson SM, Gore AC. (2007). Estrogenic envrionmental endocrine-disrupting chemical effects on reproductive neuroendocrine function and dysfunction across the life cycle. Rev Endocr Metab Disord 8: 143-159.

Eriksson E, Royo F, Lyberg K, Carlsson H-E, Hau J. (2004). Effect of metabolic cage housing on immunoglobulin A and corticosterone excretion in faeces and urine of young male rats. Exp Physiol 89, pp 427-433

Fajer AB, Vogt M. (1963). Adrenocortical secretion in the Guinea-pig. J Physiol, 169: 373-385.

Frynta D, Nováková M, Kutalová H, Palme R, Sedlácek. (2009). Apparatus for collection of fecal samples from undisturbed Spiny mice (Acomys cahirinus)living in a complex social group. J Am Assoc Lab Anim Sci. 48: 196–201.

Gippoliti S, Amori G. (1998). Rodent conservation, zoos, and the importance of the "common species". Zoo Biol. 17, 263-265.

Good T, Khan MZ, Lynch WL. (2003). Biochemical and physiology validation of a corticosteroid radioimmunoassay for plasma and fecal samples in oldfield mice (Peromyscus polionotus). Physiol and Behav 80: 405- 411.

Goymann, W. (2005). Noninvasive monitoring of hormones in bird droppings. Physiological validation, sampling, extraction, sex differences, and the influence of diet on hormone metabolite levels. Ann NY Acad Sci 1046; 35-53.

Gromadzka-Osrttowska J, Zalewka B, Szylarska-Gozdz E. (1985). Peripheral plasma progesterone concentration and hematological indices during normal pregnancy of Chinchillas (Chinchilla laniger). Comp. Biochem. Physiol. 82 A, 661-665.

Gromadzka-Ostrowska, Zalewska B. (1984). Progesterone concentration and their seasonal changes during the estrus cycle of chinchilla. Acta. Theriogenology. 20: 251-258.

Harper JM, Austad SN. (2000). Fecal glucocorticoids: a noninvasive method of measuring adrenal activity in wild and captive rodents. Physiol. Biochem. Zool. 73, 12-22.

Hayssen V, Harper JM, DeFina R. (2002). Fecal corticosteroids in agouti and non-agouti deer mice (Peromyscus maniculatus). Comp. Biochem. Physiol., A, 132: 439- 446.

Hayward LS, Booth R, Wasser S. (2010). Eliminating the artificial effect of sample mass on avian fecal hormone metabolite concentration. Gen Comp Endocrinol, 169: 117-122

Homyack JA. (2010). Evaluating habitat quality of vertebrates using conservation physiology tools. Wildlife Res, 37: 332-342.

Huchon D, Madsen O, Sibbald MJJB, Ament K, Stanhope MJ, Catzeflis F, de Jong WW, Douzery EJP (2002). Rodent phylogeny and timescale for the evolution of glires: evidence from an extensive taxon sampling using three nuclear genes. Mol. Biol. Evol. 19: 1053–1065.

Kalliokoski O, Hua J, Jacobsen KR, Schumacher-Petersen C, Abelson KSP. (2010). Distribution and time course of corticosterone excretion in faces and urine of female mice with varying systemic concentrations. Gen Comp Endocrinol, 168: 450-454.

Kay EH, Hoekstra HE. (2008). Rodents. Current Biol, 18 R406-R410.

Klasing, KC (2005). Potential impact of nutritional strategy on noninvasive measurements of hormones in birds. Ann. N Y Acad. Sci. 1046: 5–16.

Kuznetsov VA, Tchabovsky AVT, Kolosova IE, Moshkin MP. (2004). Effect of habitat type and population density on the stress levels of Midday Gerbils (Meriones meridianus Pall) in free-living populations. Biol Bull Russ Acad Sci, 31: 628-632.

Arora KL. (1979). Blood sampling and intravenous injections in Japanese quail (Coturnix coturnix japonica). Lab Anim Sci. 29:114-118.

Lèche A, Busso JM, Navarro JL, Hansen C, Marín RH, Martella MB. (2011). Non-invasive monitoring of adrenocortical activity in Greater Rhea (Rhea americana) by measuring fecal glucocorticoid metabolites. Journal of Ornithology, in press.

Lèche A, Busso JM, Hansen C, Navarro JL, Marín RH, Martella MB (2009) Physiological stress in captive Greater rheas (Rhea americana): Highly sensitive plasma corticosterone response to an ACTH challenge. Gen Comp Endocrinol 162: 188-192

Malinowska KW, Nathanielsz PW. (1974). Plasma aldosterone, cortisol and corticosterone in the new-born guinea-pig. J. Physiol. 236: 83-93.

McEwen BS, Wingfield JC (2003). The concept of allostasis in biology and biomedicine. Horm and Behavior, 43: 2-15.

Mess A, Mohr B, Martin T. (2001). Evolutionary transformations of hystricognath rodentia and the climantic change in the Eocene to late Oligocene time interval. Zoossystmatics and Evol, 77: 193-206

Millspaugh J.J., Washburn B.E. (2004). Use of fecal glucocorticoid metabolite measures in conservation biology research: considerations for application and interpration. Gen. Comp. Endocrinol. 138, 189-199.

Moberg GP. (2000). Biological response to stress: implications for animal welfare. Chapter 1, in: Moberg GP, Mench JA (eds). The biology of animal stress. Basic principles and implications for animal welfare. CAB International, pp 1-22.

Monfort SL. (2003). Non-invasive endocrine measures of reproduction and stress in wild population. In Holt WV, Pickard AR, Rodger JC, Wild DE. (eds). Reproductive Science and integrated Conservation, Cambridge, London, pp 146-165.

Moreira N, Brown JL, Moraes W, Swanson WF, Monteiro-Filho EL. (2007). Effect of housing and environmental enrichment on adrenocortical activity, behavior and reproductive cyclicity in the female tigrina (Leopardus tigrinus) and margay (Leopardus wiedii). Zoo Biol, 26:441-60

Mormède P, Andanson S, Aupérin B, Beerda B, Guémené D, Malmkvist J, Manteca X, Manteuffel G, Prunet P, Van Reenen CG, Richard S, Veissier I. (2007). Exploration of the hypothalamic–pituitary–adrenal function as a tool to evaluate animal welfare. Physiol and Behav, 92: 317–339.

Möstl E., Palme R. (2002). Hormones as indicators of stress. Domest Anim Endocrinol 23: 67–74

Muir C, Spironello-Vella E, Pisani N, deCatanzaro D. (2001). Enzyme immunoassay of 17ß-Estradiol, estrone conjugates, and T in urinary and fecal samples from males and female mice. Horm. Metab. Res. 33,653-658.

Norris DO. (2007). Synthesis, Metabolism, and Actions of Bioregulators. In Vertebrate endocrinology, Fourth Edition. Elsevier Academic Press, pp 46-105.

Nováková M, Palme R, Kutalová H, Jansky L, Frynta D. (2008). The effects of sex, age and commensal way of life on levels of fecal glucocorticoid metabolites in spiny mice (Acomys cahirinus). Physiology and Behavior, 95: 187–193.

Opazo JC, Palma RE, Melo F, Lessa EP. (2005). Adaptative evolution of the insulin gene in Caviomorph Rodents. Mol. Biol. Evol. 22:1290-1298.

Pettitt BA, Wheaton CJ, Waterman JM. (2007). Effects of storage treatment on fecal steroid hormone concentrations of a rodent, the Cape ground squirrel (Xerus inauris). Gen Comp Endocrinol 150: 1-11.

Palme R, Fischer P, Schildorfer H, Ismail MN. (1996). Excretion of infused 14C-steroid hormones via faeces and urine in domestic livestock. Anim Reprod Sci, 43: 43-63.

Palme R., S. Rettenbacher, C. Touma, S.M. El-Bahr, and Möstl E. 2005. Stress hormones in mammals and birds: comparative aspects regarding metabolism, excretion, and noninvasive measurement in fecal samples. Ann N Y Acad Sci 1040:162–171.

Palme, R. (2005). Measuring fecal steroids: guidelines for practical application. Ann. N.Y. Acad. Sci. 1046: 75–80.

Peter, A. T., N. Kapustin, and J. K. Critser. (1996). Analysis of sex steroid metabolites excreted in the feces and urine of nondomesticated animals. Compend Contin Educ Pract Vet 18:781–789.

Ponce AA, Carrascosa RE, Aires VA, Fiol de Cuneo M, Ruiz RD, Ponzio MF Lacuara JL. (1998a) Activity of Chinchilla laniger spermatozoa collected by electroejaculation and cryopreserved. Theriogenology 50, 1239-1249.

Ponce AA, Aires VA, Carrascosa RE, Fiol de Cuneo M, Ruiz RD, Lacuara JL. (1998b). Functional activity of epididymal Chinchilla laniger spermatozoa cryopreserved in different extenders. Res. Vet. Sci. 64, 239-243.

Ponzio MF, Monfort SL, Busso JM, Dabbene VG, Ruiz RD, Fiol de Cuneo M. (2004). A non-invasive method for assessing adrenal activity in the chinchilla (Chinchilla lanigera). J. Exp. Zool. 3, 218-227.

Ponzio MF. "Detección de situaciones potencialmente estresantes y su repercusión sobre la fisiología reproductiva en un modelo animal (Chinchilla laniger)". Fac Cs Ex, Fis y Nat-UNC, Córdoba-Argentina; Ph D Thesis 2006.

Ponzio MF; Busso JM, Ruiz RD, Fiol de Cuneo, M. (2007) Time-related changes in functional activity and capacitation of chinchilla (Chinchilla lanigera) spermatozoa during in vitro incubation. Anim Reprod Sci; 102: 343-349.

Ponzio MF; Busso JM, Ruiz RD, Fiol de Cuneo, MF, Ponce, AA (2008). Functional activity of frozen thawed Chinchilla lanigera spermatozoa cryopreserved with glycerol or ethyleneglycol. Reprod Dom Anim; 43: 228-233.

Pukazhenthi BS, Wild DE. (2004). Which reproductive technologies are most relevant to studying, managing and conserving wildlife? Reprod Fert and Develp 16: 33-46.

Romero LM. (2004). Physiological stress in ecology: lessons from biomedial research. Trends in Ecol Evol, 19: 249-255.

Romero LM, Reed JM. (2005). Collecting baseline corticosterone samples in the field: is under 3 min good enough? Comp Biochem Physiol, Part A 140: 73– 79.

Sapolsky RM, Romero LM, Munck AU. (2000). How do glucocorticoids influence stress responses? Integrating permissive, suppressive, stimulatory, and preparative actions. Endocr. Rev. 21:55-89.

Schneider JE. (2004). Energy balance and reproduction. Physiol and Behav, 81: 289-317.

Schwarzenberger F, Möstl E, Palme R, Bamberg E. (1996). Faecal steroid analysis for on-invasive monitoring of reproductive status in farm, wild and zoo animals. I, Anim Reprod Sci 42: 515-526.

Schwarzenberger F. (2007) The many uses of non-invasive faecal steroid monitoring in zoo and wildlife species. Inter Zoo Yearbook; 41: 52 – 74

Sheriff MJ, Dantzer B, Delehanty B, Palme R, Boonstra R. (2011). Measuring stress in wildlife: techniques for quantifying glucocorticoids. Oecologia Feb 23. [Epub ahead of print]

Short, RV. Species differences in reproductive mechanisms. (1985). In Austin CR, and Short RV (eds): chapter 2, Reproduction in mammals. Cambridge University Press, pp 62-101.

Siswanto H, Hau J, Carlsson H-E, Goldkuhl R, Abelson KSP. (2008). Corticosterone concentration in blood and excretion in faces after ACTH administration in male Sprague-Dawley rats. In Vivo (International Journal of Experimental and Clinical Pathophysiology and Drug Research), 22:435-440.

Soto Gamboa M, Gonzalez S. (2009). Validation of a radioimmunoassay for measuring fecal cortisol metabolites in the hystricomorph rodent, Octodon degus. J Exp Zool, 311A:496–503.

Smale L, Heideman PD, French JA. (2005). Behavioral neuroendocrinology in nontraditional species of mammals: things the 'knockout' mouse CAN'T tell us. Horm Behav, 48: 474-483.

Swanson WF, Brown JL. (2004). Internation training programs in reproductive sciences for conservation of Latin American felids. Anim Reprod Sci, 82-83: 21-34.

Tam W.H. (1971). The production of hormonal steroids by ovarian tissues of the chinchilla (*Chinchilla lanigera*). J. Endocr. 50, 267-279.

Tam WH (1972). Steroid metabolic pathways in the ovary of the chinchilla (Chinchilla laniger). J Endocr; 52: 37-50.

Tappa B, Amao H, Takahashi KW (1989). A simple method for intravenous injection and blood collection in the chinchilla (Chinchilla laniger). Lab Anim 23: 73-75.

Taylor W., (1971). The excretion of steroid hormone metabolites in bile and feces. Vitam. Horm. N.Y. 29, 201-285.

Thanos PK, Cavigelli SA, Michaelides M, Olvet DM, Patel U, Diep MN, Volkow. (2009). A non-invasive method for detecting the metabolite stress response in rodents: characterization and disruption of the circadian corticosterone rhythm. Physiol Res 58: 219-228.

Terlouw EMC. Schouten WGP, Ladewig J. Physiology (1997). In: Appleby MC, Hughes Bo (eds), chapter 10 Animal Welfare. CABI International, pp 143-158.

Teskey-Gerstl A, Bamberg E, Steineck T, Palme R. (2000). Excretion of corticosteroids in urine and faeces of hares (*Lepus europaeus*). J. Comp. Physiol. B. 170, 163-168.

Touma C., Sachser N., Mostl E., and Palme R., (2003). Effects of sex and time of day on metabolism and excretion of corticosterone in urine and feces of mice. Gen. Comp. Endocrinol. 130, 267-278.

Touma C, Palme R. (2005). Measuring fecal glucocorticoid metabolites in mammals and birds: the importance of validation. Ann N Y Acad Sci 1046:54-74.

Touma C, Palme R, Sachser N. (2005). Analyzing corticosterone metabolites in fecal samples of mice: a noninvasive technique to monitor stress hormone. Horm and Behav, 45: 10- 22.

Wasser SK, Kathleen EH, Brown JL, Cooper K, Crockett CM, Bechert U, Millspaugh JJ, Larson S, Monfort SL. (2000). A generalized fecal glucocorticoid assay for use in a diverse array of nondomestic mammalian and avian species. Gen. Comp. Endocr. 120, 260-275.

Weir BJ, Rowland IW. (1973). Reproductive strategies of mammals. Annu Rev Ecol Syst 4: 139-163.

Wielebnowski N. (2003). Stress and distress: evaluating their impact for the well-being of zoo animals. J. Am. Vet. Med. Assoc. 223, 973-977.

Wielebnowski NC, Fletchall N, Carlstead K, Busso JM, Brown JL. (2002). Noninvasive assessment of adrenal activity associated with husbandry and behavioral factors in the North American clouded leopard population. Zoo Biol. 21, 77-98.

Wielebnowski N, Watters J. (2007). Applying fecal endocrine monitoring to conservation and behavior studies of wild mammals: important considerations and preliminary tests. Israel J Ecology and Evolution, 53: 439-460.

Young JZ. (1985). Roedores y lagomorfos. En: La vida de los vertebrados. Ediciones Omega, Barcelona, pp 533-542.

Part 2

Metabolic Bone Disease

5

New Trends in Calcium and Phosphorus Metabolism Disorders – Hypoparathyroidism

Gonzalo Díaz-Soto[1] and Manuel Puig-Domingo[2]
[1]Servicio de Endocrinología y Nutrición, Hospital Clínico de Valladolid.
Centro de Investigación de Endocrinología y Nutrición Clínica (IEN). Facultad
de Medicina de Valladolid
[2]Servei de Endocrinologia i Nutrició. Hospital Germans Trias i Pujol. Badalona
Universitat Autònoma de Barcelona.
Spain

1. Introduction

Numerous physiological functions are regulated by calcium. In fact, ionized intracellular calcium (Ca2+) is the most common signal transduction element, a universal cofactor for various enzymes and a crucial participant in different physiologically relevant pathways at the cell membrane level. Thus, ensuring a stable level of extracellular Ca2+ is a priority for preserving many cell functions as automatism of nerve and muscle activity, contraction of cardiac, skeletal and smooth muscle, release of neurotransmitters and secretion of endocrine and exocrine hormones, among others.

The levels of extracellular Ca2+ and phosphorus (P) are tightly regulated by complex mechanisms that have evolved from a phylogenetic perspective, in order to maintain their extracellular concentrations within relatively narrow limits. Among key participants in the regulation of Ca2+, parathyroid hormone (PTH), calcitonin and 1-25 dihydroxyvitamin D are major hormones involved in mineral ion homeostasis, through their effects on parathyroid glands, bone, kidney and intestine.

Although, injury or removal of the parathyroid glands during neck surgery is by far the most common cause of acute and chronic hypoparathyroidism, there are other no so common causes as parathyroid hormones or vitamin D related disorders that may contribute to an impaired parathyroid function.

Conventional treatment of chronic hypocalcemia, particularly hypoparathyroidism, is based on calcium salts, vitamin D (mainly calcitriol), and drugs that increase renal tubular reabsorption of calcium as thiazides. Recently, new treatments have been developed, increasing the therapeutic armamentarium for hypocalcemic disorders, as synthetic recombinant human parathyroid hormone (rhPTH) 1–34 administered once or twice daily in patients with hypoparathyroidism. This treatment modality has proved to reduce urinary calcium excretion compared with calcitriol therapy and to maintain serum calcium in the normal range, thus avoiding chronic hypercalciuria that may lead to renal function impairment, nephrocalcinosis and renal insufficiency in the long term. What is more, new rhPTH release formulations are currently under investigation, opening a new field to explore for the treatment of hypoparathyroidism.

In this chapter, we will discuss the regulation of the metabolism of calcium and phosphorus and their integrated pathways to maintain their levels within physiological limits with special focus on hypocalcemic disorders and new treatment approaches.

2. Physiological regulation of calcium and phosphorus metabolism

Extracellular Ca2+ participates in the regulation of numerous physiological functions, as automatism of nerve and muscle activity, contraction of cardiac, skeletal and smooth muscle, release of neurotransmitters and secretion of endocrine and exocrine hormones among others; thus, physiological concentrations of extracellular ionized Ca2+ remain virtually constant at 1.2 mM (5 mg/dL) (Brown, 1991). For these reason, different physiological mechanisms are involved for maintaining extracellular Ca2+ level whiting these narrow limits that includes parathyroid hormone (PTH), calcitonin and 1-25 dihydroxyvitamin D as major hormones participating in mineral ion homeostasis, through their effects on parathyroid glands, bone, kidney and intestine.

2.1 General Homeostasis of calcium and phosphorus metabolism

The bone acts as a true storehouse of Ca2+ and P, containing nearly the total Ca2+ and P of the body in its mineral structure. Only 1% of Ca2+ from the bone is in constant exchange with extracellular Ca2+ and under tight regulation as this quantitatively minor amounts play a crucial physiological role (Kronenberg et al, 2007).

Extracellular Ca2+ not bound to proteins (albumin and globulins mainly), called as ionized Ca2+, acts as the biological active fraction. Its physiological concentration remains virtually constant at 1.2 mM tightly controlled by hormonal mechanisms.

In contrast, resting cytosollic calcium concentration is about 100 nM but fluctuations allow increases up to 1 microM (100 folders) through cellular activation by releasing Ca2+ from intracellular stores (endoplasmic reticulum, mitochondria) and through activated channels thanks to a very large chemical gradient (10,000:1). Intracellular Ca2+ acts as a key intracellular messenger and cofactor for various enzymes and biological functions (Valero et al, 2008).

On the other hand, organic P is a main constituent and coenzyme for numerous physiological processes as replication, differentiation, development, energy expenditure and storage. Any alteration on P homeostasis cause severe disorders that affect global organ functions (Figure 1).

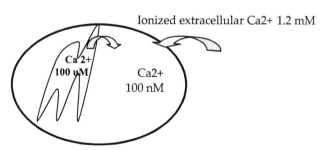

Fig. 1. Calcium concentration in the cell, plasma and intracellular stores and main fluxes (endoplasmic reticulum).

The levels of extracellular Ca2+ and P are tightly regulated by complex mechanisms in a coordinated way that has evolved from a phylogenetic perspective in order to maintain their extracellular concentrations within relatively narrow limits.

2.2 Parathyroid hormone

The parathyroid cell is a prototypical extracellular Ca2+ sensing cell (Brown, 1998). This characteristic allows the constant monitoring of extracellular ionized Ca2+ levels, thus, increasing extracellular Ca2+ is sensed by plasma membrane receptor of parathyroid glands cells (the calcium sensing receptor –CaSR-) that mediates the reduction of PTH hormone secretion (Figure 2) (Riccardi & Gamba, 1999).

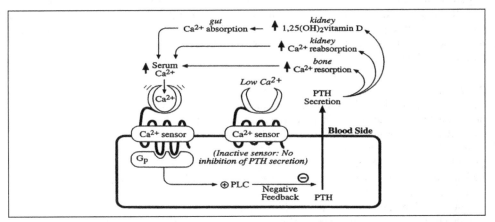

Fig. 2. PTH regulation on parathyroid gland by extracellular Ca2+ levels through CaSR http://chemistry.gravitywaves.com/CHE452/20_Calcium%20Homeostasis16.htm March 15 2011. Dr Noel Sturm

In last years, inherited diseases caused by mutations of the CaSR have been studied (Health et al, 1996). Loss-of-function mutations induce a loose of sensitivity to extracellular Ca2+ levels and a disruption of the downregulation mechanism of PTH secretion as in familiar hypocalciuric hypercalcemia and neonatal severe hyperparathyroidism. These inherited diseases are characterized by mild or severe hypercalcemia. Gain of function mutations have been described in recent years, and in these conditions the hypersensitivity to Ca2+ levels cause hypocalcemia due to a premature inhibition of PTH secretion by the parathyroid gland as in autosomal dominant hypoparathyroidism (Polak et al, 1994).

Parathyroid hormone (PTH) is secreted by parathyroid glands regulated by ionized extracellular Ca2+ through CaSR. PTH is a 84 amino acids peptide hormone synthesized as a large pre-prohormone that exerts its biological effects on its intact configuration or by different amino terminal fragments. A continuous PTH high level as seen in hyperparathyroidism induces stimulation of bone resorption and the release of Ca2+ and P to plasma, and consequently leads to a decrease of bone mineral density. On the other hand, intermittent administration of PTH has the opposite effect and it is the basis of its use in the treatment of severe osteoporosis. In the kidney, PTH acts stimulating Ca2+ reabsorption and P urinary excretion. Indirectly, PTH provides active vitamin D by hydroxylation of 25(OH)D3 in position 1 (1,25(OH)2D3) which increases calcium absorption at the gut level.

In summary, PTH acts as a Ca2+ rising hormone and a major regulatory of Ca2+ metabolism; conversely, increasing levels of Ca2+ exert a downregulation feed back effect on PTH secretion (Shoback, 2008).

2.3 Calcitonin

Calcitonin is a 32 amino acid peptide hormone secreted by parafollicular cells (C cells) of the thyroid gland. Despite of its important role in few vertebrae animals, in humans its role on Ca2+ and P metabolism is less important. However, it is used in the treatment of hypercalcemia due to its decreasing Ca2+ renal reabsorption effect and its inhibition Ca2+ bone resorption; thus, calcitonin has a net hypocalcemic effect on plasma Ca2+ levels in hypercalcemic disorders. Its regulation is mediated by Ca2+ ionized extracellular levels in part through the CaSR as in parathyroid glands, although other hormone and vitamin factors could also play an important role. Finally, calcitonin is also secreted by different neuroendocrine tumours, as medullary thyroid carcinoma, and it used as tumour marker (Kudo et al, 2011).

2.4 Vitamin D

Vitamin D acts as a real hormone. Its synthesis and tissue concentration is more dependent of seasonal and sun exposure factors rather than oral intake. Endogenous inactive vitamin D (colecalciferol-Vitamin D3) is synthesized by ultraviolet radiation, although nutritional alternative sources (supplemented dairy products, fat fish and liver) could eventually provide sufficient quantities for covering daily needs. Vitamin D3 activation requires hydroxylation of the 25th and 1st positions to get full biological activity (1,25(OH)2D3); this process takes place in the liver and kidney where hydroxylation is successively performed and at the kidney level activation of 1-hydroxilase is partially dependent of PTH. Vitamin D can also be hydroxilated at position 24 which renders inactive the molecule.

The main effect of vitamin D on Ca2+ and P metabolism is to stimulate calcium absorption in the bowel by means of the binding of its active form 1,25(OH)2D3 to the vitamin D nuclear receptor (VDR) (Shiohara et al, 2005). A less pronounced but also an important effect of vitamin D is to promote Ca2+ and P apposition in the bone and to stimulate calcium excretion in the kidney. The VDR is a ubiquitous receptor which is expressed in most tissues and cell lines and in fact vitamin D has been implicated in numerous biological actions as activation of the immune system, autoimmune diseases, cardiovascular risk, proliferation and differentiation of cancer cell lines among others (Fernandez et al, 2009; Mathieu & Adorini, 2002; Nagpal et al, 2005).

Calcium and vitamin D intake is currently though to be under normal requirements, especially in old populations due to loss of efficiency of vitamin D synthesis and age-related down regulation of 1alpha kidney hydroxylation in relation with kidney function, as well as insufficient sun exposure in aged people. At the moment, a worldwide high prevalence of vitamin D deficiency has been described (Rosen, 2011).

2.5 Integrated homeostasis of calcium metabolism

The levels of extracellular Ca2+ and P are tightly regulated by complex interrelation of PTH, calcitonin and 1-25 dihydroxyvitamin D through their balanced effects on parathyroid glands, bone, kidney and intestine target organs (Figure 3).

PTH secretion is regulated by extracellular Ca2+ levels and activation of 25(OH)D3 to 1,25(OH)2D3 is regulated by PTH action on kidney. 1,25(OH)2D3 enhances calcium absorption on gut. On the same way, calcitonin regulation is mediated by Ca2+ ionized extracellular level. These complex mechanisms work in concert to keep Ca2+ and P+ in a constant concentration for maintaining under optimal conditions some critical physiological functions as automatism of nerve and muscle activity, contraction of cardiac, skeletal and smooth muscle, release of neurotransmitters and secretion of endocrine and exocrine hormones among others.

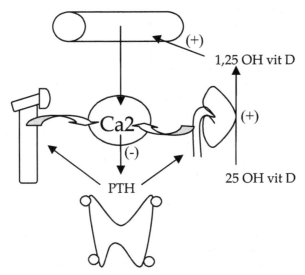

Fig. 3. Integrated physiological homeostasis of calcium metabolism.

Calcium and vitamin D insufficiency leads to an increase in calcium intestinal absorption, renal uptake and calcium bone reabsorption. The first step to reach the new equilibrium is initiated by the low extracellular calcium concentration which is sensed by CaSR and triggers PTH secretion by the parathyroid glands. The increment of PTH level increases the synthesis of the activated form of vitamin D and stimulates absorption of tubular calcium on kidney. On the other hand, 1,25 OH vitamin D acts on the nuclear pathways of the entherocytes to increase absorption of dietary calcium, which is quantitatively the most important response to calcium and vitamin D insufficiency. To summarize, chronic calcium and vitamin D insufficiency provoques a continuous compensatory hyperparathyroidism aimed to maintain Ca2+ and P+ into the physiological levels; this chronic hyperactivation of the parathyroid glands may have deleterious consequences at the long term.

3. Hypocalcemic disorders

Any alteration of this close balance between the hormones involved in calcium metabolism could originate disorders characterized by the presence hypocalcemia.

Although, injury or removal of the parathyroid glands during neck surgery is the most common cause of acute and chronic hypoparathyroidism, other not so common causes should be evaluated and ruled out, mainly caused by alteration in intestinal absorption (vitamin D related) or by decrease reabsorption at the bone and kidney levels (parathyroid hormones related).

3.1 Parathyroid hormones related disorders

Parathyroid hormones related hypocalcaemia could be differentiated from other causes by a low or inappropriately normal PTH level in the presence of low calcium levels, mild hyperphosphatemia and low 1,25(OH)2D3.

PTH related causes of hypocalcemia include:

3.1.1 Parathyroid glands destruction

Injury or removal of the parathyroid glands during neck surgery is the most common cause of acute and chronic hypoparathyroidism. Its incidence rate is usually related to surgeon's experience, the type of pathology and the surgical technique performed (Sthepen, 2000). Although postsurgical hypoparathyroidism is usually a transitory problem, occasionally, it persists in 0.4%-33% of cases depending on the series (Page & Strunsky 2007; Torregrosa et al, 2005). It may be caused by vascular interruption or involuntary removal during surgery and it uses to be permanent if there is no remission after 6-9 months after surgery.

After hyperparathyroidism adenoma removal, a transient suppressive hypoparathyroidism can occur in the first 48 hours after surgery of functional nature. In these cases, hungry bone syndrome should be ruled out and could be identified as hypophosphatemia is virtually always an associated feature after surgery of a severe and of long duration hyperpathyroidism.

However, any infiltrative or autoimmune disease that affects all parathyroid glands could cause hypoparathyroidism. Wilson disease, hemochromatosis, metastic disease can infiltrate parathyroid glands causing their dysfunction (Angelopoulos et al, 2006). Autosomal recessive autoimmunity hypoparathyroidism can be part of autoimmunity polyglandular syndrome type 1, in which Addison disease and mucocutaneous candidiasis are found together with hypocalcemia (Husebye et al, 2009). This syndrome has been related to the autoimmunity regulatory gene AIRE. Autoimmunity antibodies against parathyroid glands and CaSR can support this diagnosis (Dittmar & Kahaly, 2003).

3.1.2 Congenital/inherited parathyroid disorders

Transient neonatal hypocalcaemia is a quite frequent disorder that is usually resolved during the first days after birth. Hyperparathyroidism and diabetes of the mother are the most common causes. However, hypocalcemia disorders that are not resolved during first 4 weeks or life require a more extended diagnosis work-up. Inactivating mutations of some transcription factors as glial cell missing factor (GCM) and SOX3 have been related to neonatal hypoparathyroidism.

In some cases, hypoparathyroidism is part of more complex malformative syndromes arising during the embryonic development, as Di George's syndrome. Di George's syndrome or velo-cardio-facial syndrome is the most frequent severe malformation (1/3000) and it is caused by embryonic disorder of third, fourth and fifth branchial pouches, resulting in the absence of parathyroid glands associated with cardiac malformations, abnormal facies, thymus hypoplasia, and cleft palate. It is caused by deletions in 22q11, and less frequently in 10p (Kobrynski & Sullivan, 2007). Other not so common causes of neonatal/inherited hypoparathyroidism are Kenny-Caffey syndrome and Barakat syndrome among others.

Gain of function mutations of CaSR amino-terminal domain have been published in recent years; in these cases, hypersensitive sensing to Ca2+ levels cause hypocalcemia by premature inhibition of PTH secretion by the parathyroid glands expressed as an autosomal dominant hypoparathyroidism (Pollak et al, 1994). In these patients hypocalcemia is found together with hypercalciuria and normal PTH. In such a situation, treatment with vitamin D results in the development of hypercalcemia which may lead to nephrocalcinosis and renal failure; thus, treatment is aimed to avoid symptoms of hypocalcemia and not to achieve normocalcemia (Pearce et al, 1996).

3.1.3 Pseudohypoparathyroidism
Pseudohypoparathyroidism is characterized by peripheral PTH resistance despite of elevated PTH levels, and hypocalcaemia plus hiperphophatemia plasma levels similar to what is found in hypoparathyroidism after having ruled out magnesium deficiency and renal failure. It may be associated to a characteristic morphotype called Albright´s hereditary osteodysthophy. Its genetic bases and clinical features will be described in detail in another chapter.

3.2 Vitamin D related hypocalcemia
Hypocalcemia syndrome due to vitamin D related disorders is mainly caused by alterations in intestinal absorption of dietary calcium. Hypocalcemic disorders in the context of vitamin D deficiency are characterized by elevated PTH plasma levels and hypophosphatemia with an increased renal phosphate clearance (Figure 4). Increased PTH is of compensatory nature aimed to maintain Ca2+ and P+ within the physiological levels by calcium mobilization from skeleton, increased renal reabsorption of calcium and increased renal 1alpha hydroxylation.

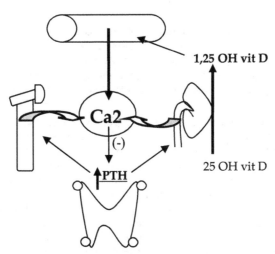

Fig. 4. Adaptation to vitamin D and calcium insufficiency (adaptation pathways on bold type).

Vitamin D related hypocalcaemia could be caused by:

3.2.1 Vitamin D absorption/synthesis deficiency
Vitamin D deficiency is mostly seen in old people, although younger populations may also suffer from this condition. As vitamin D could be sourced by skin synthesis under

ultraviolet irradiation and/or dietary intake, any deficiency on dietary intake or reduction on intestinal fat-soluble vitamin D absorption (gastrectomy, intestinal illness, chronic hepatic insufficiency) and any decrease in skin synthesis due to insufficient solar irradiation or used of high solar protective factor sun blocks, could cause a vitamin D deficiency. It also causes a compensatory hyperparathyroidism and has been correlated with seasonal psychiatric and immune disorders in northern countries (Rosen, 2011).

Modern food industry has supplemented dairy products with vitamin D although it has not been correlated with improvements in general population vitamin D levels.

3.2.2 Impaired 1 or 25 alpha hydroxilation of Vitamin D

Any alteration on hepatic or kidney functions could lead on deficient hydroxylation of vitamin D, as in renal or liver failure. This would cause an intestinal calcium absorption and a compensatory increase in circulating PTH.

It is a common clinical entity especially in chronic renal failure under dialysis. The failure of 1alpha hydroxilation at the kidney level causes a decrease in plasma calcium by malabsorption of dietary calcium intake and a compensatory elevation of PTH (secondary hyperparathyroidism) without an increased phosphate clearance because of kidney failure. Treatment of compensatory hyperparathyroidism is based on the administration of the active form of vitamin D (1-25(OH)2 Vit D) to cover 1alpha hydroxilase deficit, an increase in calcium intake and phosphate binders (Messa et al, 2010). Regulation of PTH secretion with non hypercalcemic Vitamin D analogs and calcimimetics (parathyroid CaSR sensitizers) has been a revolution in the treatment of secondary hyperparathyroidism associated to renal failure (Borstand et al, 2010).

3.2.3 Impaired entero-hepatic circulation of vitamin D

Vitamin D is a fat-soluble vitamin, so it is under entero-hepatic circulation and adiposity and hepatic deposit. Any alteration on entero-hepatic circulation or accelerated hepatic metabolism and its nature is mainly drug-induced: anticonvulsants, tuberculostatic treatment, and bile acid sequestrants; any of these could cause an accelerated loss of vitamin D.

3.2.4 Calcitriol resistance-Hereditary vitamin D resistant rickets

Some inherited disorders have been described to be associated with vitamin D resistance; their frequency is very low. They are characterized by a biochemical profile concordant with vitamin D deficiency and compensatory hyperparathyroidism with normal or even elevated levels of vitamin D that indicates a resistance vitamin D status. Most mutations described in vitamin D resistant rickets involve intranuclear vitamin D receptor (VDR) at the DNA binding domain and it affects the regulation of gene expression (Mallory et al, 2004).

Clinical features are variable but it uses to appear during childhood with hypocalcaemia and hypophosphatemia, associated with alopecia, bone deformations and short stature. Treatment with high doses of calcitriol do not use to be successful, although it depends on the specific mutations on VDR. Vitamin D analogues have opened new therapeutic possibilities on this rare illness. Treatment with sequestrant compounds could cause an accelerated loss of vitamin D.

3.3 Other causes

Other hypocalcaemia causes include: bone apposition in osteoblastic metastasis; sequestration by intravascular drugs or by acute hyperphosphatemic states (rhabdomyolysis, chemotherapy); treatment or ion alterations and vitamin D insufficiency in HIV infected patients; critical illness as acute pancreatitis.

4. Acute hypocalcaemia treatment

Acute hypocalcaemia is a medical emergency that requires a quick diagnosis and treatment. However, chronic hypocalcaemia is frequently asymptomatic and treatment must be aiming to normalization of calcium levels without increasing complications (Cooper & Gottoes, 2008).

Acute hypocalcaemia can be diagnosed by measuring total calcium levels using protein correction to calculate free extracellular calcium (a decrease in calcium of 0.8 mg/dl for every 1 g/dL decrease in albumin) or by direct monitoring of ionized $Ca2+$ (Kronenberg et al, 2007).

Symptoms are correlated with acute instauration and magnitude of the deficiency, especially in relation to neuromuscular excitability as carpopedal spasm. In acute and severe cases of hypocalcemia general tetany, broncospasm and serious cardiac arrhythmias have been described, thus serum calcium levels must be measured frequently in this period, and electrocardiographic monitoring must be done during initial replacement therapy.

Acute hypocalcemia treatment requires prompt normalisation of calcium plasma levels using intravenous calcium infusion; other ions alterations are particularly important, i.e. the correction of hypomagnesaemia that causes impaired secretion of PTH from parathyroid glands and precludes the correction of hypocalcemia.

5. Chronic hypocalcemia treatment

The conventional treatment of chronic hypocalcemia and hypoparathyroidism is based on calcium salts, vitamin D (mainly calcitriol), and drugs that increase renal tubular reabsorption of calcium as thiazides. However, over the past few years, the administration of synthetic recombinant human parathyroid hormone (rhPTH) 1–34 once or twice daily, even with more physiological releasing devices in patients with hypoparathyroidism has proved to reduce urinary calcium excretion compared with calcitriol therapy, and to maintain serum calcium in the normal range, thus avoiding chronic hypercalciuria that may lead to renal function impairment, nephrocalcinosis and renal insufficiency in the long term. On the other hand, new vitamin D analogues have been investigated to maintain calcium levels on normal range without hypercalciuria complications.

In this section we will describe conventional and new treatment approaches of chronic hypocalcemia mainly focused on post surgical hypoparathyroidism, due to the important innovations appeared in last years.

5.1 Conventional treatments

The conventional treatment of chronic hypocalcaemia and hypoparathyroidism is based on calcium salts, vitamin D (mainly calcitriol), and drugs that increase renal tubular reabsorption of calcium as thiazides.

Treatment objectives are to maintain free ionized calcium levels within the normal interval or plasma calcium in the lower half or slightly below the normal range (8.0-8.5 mg/dL), and to avoid hypercalciuria (< 250 mg urine calcium/24 hours) and other treatment complications. It should be directed at the underlying disorder (Shoback, 2008).

5.2 Calcium salts

Long-term treatment of patients with chronic hypocalcemia is warranty with 1 to 3 g of elementary calcium per day in the various forms of salts available (table 1) because of the increased excretion of calcium. Interrupting the supplement can rapidly lower an elevated calcium value. It should be must be scheduled in 3-4 doses with meals to facilitates its absorption. Calcium carbonate is by far the most used calcium salts due to its low cost, despite of gastrointestinal adverse effects and that it requires gastric acidification to assure its absorption; thus achlorhydric patients or under proton-pump inhibitors treatment should be avoid unlike citrate calcium and should be taken with food or citrus drinks to promote maximal absorption. Besides, calcium citrate is preferable because it increases urinary citrate thus helping calcium to stay in solution (Harvey et al, 1988). Of the calcium preparations available, only the carbonate and citrate salts contain sufficient elemental calcium (per tablet) for the efficient treatment of most patients with hypoparathyroidism. Other preparations may be used in patients who cannot tolerate citrate and carbonate salts. The percentage of elemental calcium is lower in these other preparations, and do not adds any benefit (Maeda et al, 2006; Shoback, 2008).

Calcium Salts	Ca element content	Milligrams of salt needed 1 g preparation elementary calcium
Calcium Carbonate	40%	2500
Calcium Phospathe	38%	2631
Calcium Chloride	27%	3700
Calcium Citrate	21%	4762
Calcium Lactate	13%	7700
Calcium Gluconate	9%	11100

Table 1. Calcium salts available. Calcium carbonate: constipation is a common side effect; calcium carbonate is best absorbed with meals and with acid present in the stomach. Calcium citrated: Recommended in patients who have achlorhydria or who are taking a proton-pump inhibitor, in order to achieve sufficient absorption of calcium (Maeda et al, 2006).

5.3 Vitamin D

All patients with hypoparathyroidism must be treated with vitamin D or analogues in addition to calcium. Vitamin D chosen must be selected depending on the underlying disorder, thus impaired renal 1alpha hydroxylation should be treated with 1alpha hydroxilated analogues, but vitamin D insufficiency could be treated with non hydroxilated vitamin D metabolites (Cooper & Gittoes, 2008).

Compared to PTH, replacement with calciferol steroids leads to a higher urinary excretion of Ca with an increased risk of nephrocalcinosis. Vitamin D toxicity is an important concern and may occur at any time. Manifestations may include altered mental status, fatigue, thirst, dehydration, reduced renal function, nephrolithiasis, and constipation. Treatment involves discontinuation of the vitamin D preparation and the calcium salt intake. Depending on the severity, and especially if the toxic effects are related to treatment with vitamin D metabolites with long half-lives, intravenous saline infusion and possibly oral glucocorticoids may quickly antagonize vitamin D action and restore normocalcemia in a short period of time. Levels of 25-hydroxyvitamin D must be monitored, even in patients receiving calcitrol and alfacalcidiol to assess vitamin D dosage adequacy. The target 25-hydroxyvitamin D level is 30 ng/ml.

The current most used drugs are dihydrotachysterol (average half-time 7 days), alphacalcidol (average half life-2 days) and calcitriol (average half life-1 day) depending on underlying pathology (table 2). Not all drugs are available in all countries and short half-life compound are more recommendable due to its higher security. Theorically, for patients with labile calcemia, dihydrotachysterol may be preferable because it provides better stability but a higher risk of intoxication. When an additional rapid effect is needed or security is the priority short-acting drugs can be added. (Maeda et al, 2006).

On hypoparathyroidism, calcitriol is preferred over vitamin D2/D3 because of its potency, rapid onset and offset of action. The vast majority of patients require calcitriol in dosages of 0.25 µg, taken twice daily, and extremely rare cases up to 0.5 µg four times daily. However, vitamin D and calcium dosage show a remarkable variability so straight monitoring and titration is warranted at the beginning of the treatment.

Vitamin D metabolites	25/1a hydroxilation required	Dosage per day	Onset of action	Offset of action
Vitamin D2 (ergocalciferol)/ Vitamin D3 (cholecalciferol)	+/+	25,000-100,000 UI once daily	10-14 days	14-25 days
1, 25 OH Vitamin D (Calcitriol)	-/-	0.25-1 ug twice daily	1-2 days	2-3 days
1a hydroxivitamin D (alfacalcidiol)	+/-	0.5-3.0 ug daily	1-2 days	5-7 days
Dihydrotachysterol	-/-	0.2-1.0 mg once daily	4-7 days	7-21 days
25 (OH) vitamin D (Calcidiol)	-/+	0.625-5 mg	4-8 weeks	6-12 weeks

Table 2: Vitamin D metabolites and actions (Maeda et al, 2006; Shoback, 2008).

5.4 Enhanced calcium renal tubular reabsorption: Thiazides

Hypoparathyroidism causes increased excretion of urinary calcium in relation to serum calcium and chronic vitamin D treatment predisposes to hypercalciuria, nephrolithiasis, and nephrocalcinosis. The use of drugs that increase renal tubular reabsorption of calcium as thiazides could be useful in hypocalcemia as complementary treatment and may help to control hypercalciuria (Porter et al, 1978). In fact, patients should be evaluated annually to rule out complications of vitamin D chronic treatment as nephrocalcinosis by imaging techniques and cataracts with an ophthalmic revision (Levine , 2001), besides high water intake is recommended, at least 1.5–2.5 L/day.

5.5 New treatment approaches

Treatment of hypoparathyroidism/hypocalcemia with vitamin D metabolites and calcium salts are usually well tolerated. However, quality of life studies suggest that despite optimization or normalization of biochemical values, patients with treated hypoparathyroidism show scores of depression, anxiety and somatisation higher than matched controls (Arlt et al, 2002). What is more, vitamin D and calcium salts are not an absolutely safe treatment. In fact, treatment is aimed to target low-normal calcium levels in order to prevent hypercalciuria and deterioration of renal function at long term.

In last years, the administration of synthetic human PTH 1-34 once or twice-daily in patients having hypoparathyroidism has proved to reduce the level of urinary calcium excretion compared with calcitriol therapy as well as maintaining serum calcium in the normal range, avoiding chronic hypercalciuria that may lead to impairment of renal function, nephrocalcinosis and renal insufficiency. Cost and inconvenience of injection treatment in the case of rPTH are the reasons why currently classic treatment with vitamin D plus calcium is preferred, despite the risk of hypercalciuria and long term impairment of renal function. However, in recent years, successful rhPTH treatment has been reported in cases of hypocalcemia and hypoparathyroidism not controlled by conventional therapy, thus indicating its usefulness is such a resistant cases (Angelopolulos et al, 2007; Mahajan et al, 2009; Puig-Domingo et al, 2008, Sanda et al, 2008, Shiohara et al, 2006; Winer et al, 2008).

On the other hand, research on calcium sensing receptor and vitamin D analogues have opened new and promising investigation in future treatments. In fact, in last years clinical availability of cinacalcet, the agonist of Calcium Sensing Receptor has proved to be effective for the treatment of hyperparathyroidism (Marcocci et al, 2009). Research on antagonists of calcium sensing receptor (calcilytic agents) may be used to promote inactivation of the receptor in the parathyroid glands and increase PTH secretion, specially in those hypocalcemic patients with activated CaSR mutations (Nemeth et al, 2001; Leth et al, 2010).

5.6 Recombinant human PTH

Hypoparathyroidism is one of the few endocrine diseases for which hormone-replacement therapy is not the treatment approach. Over the last 10 years, some clinical assays using synthetic recombinant human parathyroid hormone 1–34 (rhPTH) administered once or twice daily in adults and children with hypoparathyroidism, have proved to maintain serum calcium in the normal range as well as reducing urinary calcium excretion compared with conventional treatment with vitamin D (Winer et al, 1993, 1996, 1998, 2003, 2008, 2010). This treatment modality may prevent renal function impairment, nephrocalcinosis and renal insufficiency in the long term as it avoids the chronic hypercalciuric state associated to vitamin D administration. On the other hand, many studies have shown that rhPTH treatment in adult subjects with osteoporosis produces a rapid rise in bone mineralization, which may contribute to a faster recovery of lost bone mineral content of these patients (Farocki et al, 2007).

Despite these advantages, rhPTH has not become the treatment of choice for hypoparathyroidism, because conventional treatment with vitamin D and calcium salts is usually well tolerated, and rhPTH injection is more expensive. However, in recent years, successful rhPTH treatment has been reported in cases of hypocalcaemia and hypoparathyroidism not controlled by conventional therapy as an off-label treatment.

Only a few small, randomized trials have assessed the use of injectable PTH (1-34) and supplemental calcium in patients with this condition in a relative short period of follow-up of 3 years. In those trials, rhPTH has proved to maintain calcium levels between normal or slightly below normal range but with a significantly reduction of urinary calcium excretion. Twice-daily rhPTH versus once allowed a marked reduction in the total daily PTH 1–34 dose, with less fluctuations in serum calcium, normalization of urine calcium and significantly improved metabolic control both in adults and children. Also, rhPTH efficacy has been extensively published in case reports dealing with hypocalcemic disorders not controlled under conventional treatment, some of them trying to mimic more physiological delivery as using multipulse subcutaneous pump PTH delivery (Puig-Domingo et al, 2008). Major concerns of rhPTH use are related to safety; those data have been obtained mainly from osteoporosis treatment studies. Animal toxicity studies have raised concerns regarding dose-dependent PTH effects on the bone (Sato et al, 2002). Long-term, supraphysiological doses of recombinant human PTH 1-34 (rhPTH), given under continuous delivery rather than in a pulsatile way to rats with normal functioning parathyroid glands, was associated to an increased risc of osteosarcoma development. However, this higher risk has been associated to a particular effect on rat bones and does not seem relevant to PTH-deficient patients receiving physiological replacement doses. In fact, post commercialisation follow-up has not detected an increase in human osteosarcoma diagnosis until now (Harper et al, 2007). Anyway, more physiological release of PTH as using subcutaneous pumps delivery or patch could be even a safer alternative (Horwitz & Stewart, 2008).

5.7 Calcium sensing receptor antagonists

PTH secretion is regulated by a cell surface receptor that detects small changes in the level of plasma calcium, the calcium sensing receptor (figure 2). This receptor provides a particularly interesting and new molecular target for drugs useful for treating calcium and bone disorders. At the moment, a calcimimetic (compounds that mimic or potentiate the effects of extracellular calcium at the CaSR) is commercialized as cinacalcet (Mimpara ®) and it is approved and used in non surgical or tertiary hyperparathyroidism (Marcocci et al, 2009).

In the same way, molecules that blocked CaSR activity will stimulate PTH secretion. Although, there is no calcilytic compound available yet for therapeutic human use, some of them are under research with promising preliminary results, especially for the treatment of patients with CaSR activating mutations whose treatment with vitamin D and calcium does not correct the underlying pathophysiological defect, and they often worsen hypercalciuria and accelerate kidney stone formation or nephrocalcinosis resulting in impaired renal function under conventional treatment (Letz et al, 2010).

6. Conclusion

Numerous physiological functions are regulated by calcium metabolism, thus, ensuring a stable level of extracellular Ca2+ is a priority for preserving normal homeostasis. In this respect, levels of extracellular Ca2+ and phosphorus are tightly regulated by complex mechanisms in which key participants are parathyroid hormone, calcitonin and 1-25 dihydroxyvitamin D through their effects over parathyroid glands, bone, kidney and intestine. Any alteration of this close balance between the hormones involved in calcium metabolism could originate hypocalcemia.

Although post surgical hypoparathyroidism is the most common cause, diagnosis and treatment of hypocalcemic disorders require a detailed study and infrequent causes should also be evaluated and ruled out. Hypoparathyroidism could be classified into two main groups: vitamin D related causes and parathyroid hormone related causes. Although, conventional treatment of chronic hypocalcaemia and hypoparathyroidism is based on calcium salts, vitamin D (mainly calcitriol) and drugs that enhance renal tubular reabsorption of calcium, the administration of synthetic recombinant human parathyroid hormone (rhPTH) 1–34 and research in calcium sensing receptor have opened new promising fields in the last few years.

7. References

Angelopoulos NG, Goula A, Rombopoulos G, Kaltzidou V, Katounda E, Kaltsas D, Tolis G. (2006) Hypoparathyroidism in transfusion-dependent patients with beta-thalassemia. J Bone Miner Metab.24(2):138-45.

Angelopoulos NG, Goula A, Tolis G. 2007 Sporadic hypoparathyroidism treated with teriparatide: a case report and literature review. Exp Clin Endocrinol Diabetes. Jan;115(1):50-4..

Arlt W, Fremerey C, Callies FReincke M, Schneider P, Timmermann W, Allolio B. (2002) Well-being, mood and calcium homeostasis in patients with hypoparathyroidism receiving standard treatment with calcium and vitamin D. Eur J Endocrinol 146:215-22.

Borstnar S, Erzen B, Gmeiner Stopar T, Kocjan T, Arnol M, Kandus A, Kovac D. (2010) Treatment of hyperparathyroidism with cinacalcet in kidney transplant recipients. Transplant Proc. Dec;42(10):4078-82.

Brown, EM. (1991) Extracellular Ca2+ sensing, regulation of parathyroid cell function, and role of Ca2+ and other ions as extracellular (first) messengers. Physiological Review. 71: 371-411

Brown EM, Pollak M, Hebert SC (1998) The extracellular calcium-sensing receptor: its role in health and disease. Annu Rev Med.;49:15-29..

Cooper MS, Gittoes NJ.(2008) Diagnosis and management of hypocalcaemia. BMJ Jun 7;336(7656):1298-302.

Dittmar M, Kahaly GJ. (2003) Polyglandular autoimmune syndromes: immunogenetics and long-term follow-up. J Clin Endocrinol Metab. Jul;88(7):2983-92.

Harvey JA, Zobitz MM, Pak CY (1998) Dose dependency of calcium absorption: a comparison of calcium carbonate and calcium citrate. J Bone Miner Res. Jun;3(3):253-8.

Heath H 3rd, Odelberg S, Jackson CE, Teh BT, Hayward N, Larsson C, Buist NR, Krapcho KJ, Hung BC, Capuano IV, Garrett JE, Leppert MF. (1996) Clustered inactivating mutations and benign polymorphisms of the calcium receptor gene in familial benign hypocalciuric hypercalcemia suggest receptor functional domains.J Clin Endocrinol Metab. Apr;81(4):1312-7.

Horwitz MJ, Stewart AF. (2008) Hypoparathyroidism: is it time for replacement therapy? J Clin Endocrinol Metab. Sep;93(9):3307-9.

Husebye ES, Perheentupa J, Rautemaa R, Kämpe O. (2009) Clinical manifestations and management of patients with autoimmune polyendocrine syndrome type I. J Intern Med. May;265(5):514-29.

Kobrynski LJ, Sullivan KE.(2007) Velocardiofacial syndrome, DiGeorge syndrome: the chromosome 22q11.2 deletion syndromes. Lancet.Oct 20;370(9596):1443-52.

Kronenberg HM, Melme S, Polonsky KS. Larsen, PR. Williams Textbook Of Endocrinology. Elsevier Saunders pp 1202-1204

Kudo T, Miyauchi A, Ito Y, Yabuta T, Inoue H, Higashiyama T, Tomoda C, Hirokawa M, Amino N. (2011) Serum calcitonin levels with calcium loading tests before and after total thyroidectomy in patients with thyroid diseases other than medullary thyroid carcinoma. Endocr J. 2011 Feb 24

Farooki A, Fornier M & Girotra M. 2007 Anabolic therapies for osteoporosis. New England Journal of Medicine 357 2410–2411.

Fernández CA, Puig-Domingo M, Lomeña F, Estorch M, Camacho Martí V, Bittini AL, Marazuela M, Santamaría J, Castro J, Martínez de Icaya P, Moraga I, Martín T, Megía A, Porta M, Mauricio D, Halperin I. Effectiveness of retinoic acid treatment for redifferentiation of thyroid cancer in relation to recovery of radioiodine uptake. J Endocrinol Invest. 32(3):228-33.

Harper KD, Krege JH, Marcus R, Mitlak BH. 2007 Osteosarcoma and teriparatide? J Bone Miner Res. Feb;22(2):334.

Letz S, Rus R, Haag C, Dörr HG, Schnabel D, Möhlig M, Schulze E, Frank-Raue K, Raue F, Mayr B, Schöfl C. (2010) Novel activating mutations of the calcium-sensing receptor: the calcilytic NPS-2143 mitigates excessive signal transduction of mutant receptors. J Clin Endocrinol Metab. Oct;95(10):E229-33.

Levine M. 2001 Hypoparathyroidism and pseudohypoparathyroidism. In: DeGroot LJ, Jameson JL. Endocrinology, 4th ed. Philadelphia: WB Saunders. pp. 1133-53.

Maeda SS, Fortes EM, Oliveira UM, Borba VC, Lazaretti-Castro M. (2006) Hypoparathyroidism and pseudohypoparathyroidism. Arq Bras Endocrinol Metabol. 2006 Aug;50(4):664-73.

Mahajan A, Narayanan M, Jaffers G, Concepcion L. 2009 Hypoparathyroidism associated with severe mineral bone disease postrenal transplantation, treated successfully with recombinant PTH. Hemodial Int. Oct;13(4):547-50.

Malloy PJ, Xu R, Peng L, Peleg S, Al-Ashwal A, Feldman D. 2004. Hereditary 1,25-dihydroxyvitamin D resistant rickets due to a mutation causing multiple defects in vitamin D receptor function. Endocrinology. 45(11):5106-14.

Marcocci C, Chanson P, Shoback D, Bilezikian J, Fernandez-Cruz L, Orgiazzi J, Henzen C, Cheng S, Sterling LR, Lu J, Peacock M. (2009) Cinacalcet reduces serum calcium concentrations in patients with intractable primary hyperparathyroidism. J Clin Endocrinol Metab. 2009 Aug;94(8):2766-72.

Mathieu C, Adorini L. 2002. The coming of age of 1,25-dihydroxyvitamin D(3) analogs as immunomodulatory agents. Trends Mol Med.8(4):174-9.

Messa P, Cafforio C, Alfieri C. (2010) Calcium and phosphate changes after renal transplantation. J Nephrol. Nov-Dec;23 Suppl 16:S175-81.

Nagpal S, Na S, Rathnachalam R. 2005 Noncalcemic actions of vitamin D receptor ligands. Endocr Rev.26(5):662-87.

Nemeth EF, Delmar EG, Heaton WL, Miller MA, Lambert LD, Conklin RL, Gowen M, Gleason JG, Bhatnagar PK, Fox J. (2001) Calcilytic compounds: potent and selective Ca2+ receptor antagonists that stimulate secretion of parathyroid hormone. J Pharmacol Exp Ther. Oct;299(1):323-31.

Page C, Strunski V. 2007 Parathyroid risk in total thyroidectomy for bilateral, benign, multinodular goitre: report of 351 surgical cases. J Laryngol Otol.;121(3):237-41.

Pearce SH, Williamson C, Kifor O, Bai M, Coulthard MG, Davies M, Lewis-Barned N, McCredie D, Powell H, Kendall-Taylor P, Brown EM, Thakker RV. (1996) A familial syndrome of hypocalcemia with hypercalciuria due to mutations in the calcium-sensing receptor. N Engl J Med. Oct 10;335(15):1115-22.

Pollak MR, Brown EM, Estep HL, McLaine PN, Kifor O, Park J, Hebert SC, Seidman CE, Seidman JG. (1994) Autosomal dominant hypocalcaemia caused by a Ca(2+)-sensing receptor gene mutation. Nat Genet. Nov;8(3):303-7.

Porter RH, Cox BG, Heaney D, Hostetter TH, Stinebaugh BJ, Suki WN. (1978) Treatment of hypoparathyroid patients with chlorthalidone. N Engl J Med. Mar 16;298(11):577-81.

Puig-Domingo M, Díaz G, Nicolau J, Fernández C, Rueda S, Halperin I. (2008) Successful treatment of vitamin D unresponsive hypoparathyroidism with multipulse subcutaneous infusion of teriparatide. Eur J Endocrinol. Nov;159(5):653-7.

Riccardi D, Gamba G. (1999) The many roles of the calcium-sensing receptor in health and disease. Arch Med Res. Nov-Dec;30(6):436-48.

Rosen CJ. 2011 Clinical practice. Vitamin D insufficiency. N Engl J Med. 20;364(3):248-

Sanda S, Schlingmann KP, Newfield RS. 2008 Autosomal dominant hypoparathyroidism with severe hypomagnesemia and hypocalcemia, successfully treated with recombinant PTH and continuous subcutaneous magnesium infusion. J Pediatr Endocrinol Metab. Apr;21(4):385-91.

Sato M, Ma YL, Hock JM, Westmore MS, Vahle J, Villanueva A , Turner CH. 2002 Skeletal efficacy with parathyroid hormone in rats was not entirely beneficial with long-term treatment. Journal of Pharmacological and Experimental Therapeutics 302 304–313.

Shiohara M, Shiozawa R, Kurata K, Matsuura H, Arai F, Yasuda T, Koike K. Effect of parathyroid hormone administration in a patient with severe hypoparathyroidism caused by gain-of-function mutation of calcium-sensing receptor. Endocr J.53(6):797-802.

Shoback D. (2008) Clinical practice. Hypoparathyroidism.N Engl J Med. Jul 24;359(4):391-403.

Sthephen J. 2000 Hyperparathyroid and hypoparathyroid disorders. N Engl J Med. 343(25):1863-75.

Torregrosa NM, Rodríguez JM, Llorente S, Balsalobre MD, Rios A, Jimeno L, Parrilla P. 2005 Definitive treatment for persistent hypoparathyroidism in a kidney transplant patient: parathyroid allotransplantation. Thyroid. 15(11):1299-302.

Valero RA, Senovilla L, Núñez L, Villalobos C. The role of mitochondrial potential in control of calcium signals involved in cell proliferation. Cell Calcium. Vol. 44, n° 3 (September 2008) pp 259-69.

Winer KK, Yanovski JA, Cutler GB Jr. (1996) Synthetic human parathyroid hormone 1-34 vs calcitriol and calcium in the treatment of hypoparathyroidism. JAMA. Aug 276(8):631-6.

Winer KK, Yanovski JA, Sarani B, Cutler GB Jr.(1998) A randomized, cross-over trial of once-daily versus twice-daily parathyroid hormone 1-34 in treatment of hypoparathyroidism. J Clin Endocrinol Metab. 1998 Oct;83(10):3480-6.

Winer KK, Ko CW, Reynolds JC, Dowdy K, Keil M, Peterson D, Gerber LH, McGarvey C, Cutler GB Jr. (2003) Long-term treatment of hypoparathyroidism: a randomized controlled study comparing parathyroid hormone-(1-34) versus calcitriol and calcium. J Clin Endocrinol Metab. 2003 Sep;88(9):4214-20

Winer KK, Sinaii N, Peterson D, Sainz B Jr, Cutler GB Jr. 2008 Effects of once versus twice-daily parathyroid hormone 1-34 therapy in children with hypoparathyroidism. J Clin Endocrinol Metab. Sep;93(9):3389-95.

Winer KK, Sinaii N, Reynolds J, Peterson D, Dowdy K, Cutler GB Jr.(2010) Long-term treatment of 12 children with chronic hypoparathyroidism: a randomized trial comparing synthetic human parathyroid hormone 1-34 versus calcitriol and calcium. J Clin Endocrinol Metab. 2010 Jun;95(6):2680-8.

6

Pseudohypoparathyroidism in Children

Benjamin U. Nwosu
University of Massachusetts Medical School
Worcester, Massachusetts,
USA

1. Introduction

Albright hereditary osteodystrophy (AHO) is a genetic syndrome characterized by a distinctive set of developmental and skeletal defects that may easily be misdiagnosed as exogenous obesity in children. There are very few publications detailing the comprehensive management of children and adolescents with this disorder. This chapter provides a comprehensive discussion of the various aspects of this disorder. At the end, the reader should be able to: (1) List the clinical features of Albright hereditary osteodystrophy, (2) Identify the genetic and molecular abnormalities of AHO, (3) List the clinical features of pseudohypoparathyroidism type 1a (PHP 1a), (4) Describe the management of children and adolescents with PHP 1a.

2. Genetics of Albright hereditary osteodystrophy

The molecular basis for AHO is a heterozygous mutation of the gene that encodes the G-stimulatory subunit ($G_s\alpha$) of guanine nucleotide-binding protein—the *GNAS* gene—that is located at chromosome 20q13.2. This type of mutation leads to a loss of expression or function of the $G_s\alpha$ which impairs the transmission of stimulatory signals to adenylate cyclase, limiting cyclic AMP generation necessary for hormone action(Lietman, 2008).

The *GNAS* gene is subject to imprinting. Patients with AHO who have *GNAS* mutations on maternally inherited alleles manifest resistance to multiple hormones, such as parathyroid hormone (PTH), thyroid stimulating hormone (TSH), gonadotropins, growth-hormone-releasing hormone (GHRH), and glucagon(Brickman, 1986; Weinstein, 2004). These defects lead to PHP 1a. On the other hand, patients with AHO who have *GNAS* mutations on paternally inherited alleles have only the phenotypic features of AHO without hormonal resistance, a condition termed pseudopseudohypoparathyroidism (PPHP) (Lietman, 2008). PHP 1b is an autosomal dominant disorder that is associated with the presence of hormone resistance that is limited to PTH target organs, normal $G_s\alpha$ activity, and the absence of features of AHO(Levine, 1983). PHP 1c is associated with features of AHO, resistance to multiple hormones, and normal GNAS activity while PHP type 2 is associated with renal resistance to PTH action and the absence of AHO phenotype(Levine, 2000).

More than 50 different loss-of-function mutations of *GNAS* have been reported in more than 70 affected individuals. Pohlenz *et al.*(Pohlenz, 2003) have reported a missense mutation, which results in the amino-acid substitution (Lys338Asn) in codon 338 of exon 12 of the *GNAS* gene associated with congenital hypothyroidism in AHO, though they did not state the precise mechanism by which this mutation leads to hypothyroidism. A Q35X mutation in exon 1 has been associated with growth-hormone deficiency(Germain-Lee, 2003), whereas a *de novo*, missense mutation, W281R in exon 11, has been linked to progressive osseous heteroplasia, a rare, autosomal-dominant condition that presents in childhood as dermal ossification that progresses to involve deep skeletal muscles(Chan, 2004). Germain-Lee *et al*.(Germain-Lee, 2003) identified a patient with a Q29X mutation, and Nwosu *et al*. (Nwosu, 2009) reported the association of Q29X mutation with a phenotype that includes Albright hereditary osteodystrophy, morbid obesity, acanthosis nigricans, insulin resistance, growth-hormone deficiency, hypothyroidism, and subcutaneous calcification.

3. Clinical features

3.1 General appearance
The developmental and skeletal defects that characterize AHO include short stocky physique (Figure 1a), round face, mental deficiency, heterotopic ossification, and brachymetaphalangism(Weinstein, 1993) (Figure 1 b, c). AHO is present in types 1a and 1c and PPHP. Hormonal resistance is seen in PHP 1a, PHP 1c and PHP type 2.

3.2 Stature
The prevalence of short adult height in PHP 1a is reported to be as high as 80%(Nagant de Deuschaisnes, 2007). Although height during childhood may be normal, adult height is often subnormal. The reason for the short stature in PHP 1a is multifactorial and includes GHRH resistance and chondrocytic dysfunction as explained below in section 3.8.

3.3 Mental deficiency
Learning disabilities and psychomotor retardation have been described in PHP 1a(Chen, 2005). The mechanism of this mental deficiency is unknown and early institution of thyroid hormone replacement does not seem to prevent the development of mental deficiency(Weisman, 1985). There appears to be a correlation with reduced $G_s\alpha$ since patients with PHP 1b do not present with mental deficiency in spite of equivalent serum calcium and phosphate abnormalities(Wilson, 1994). This mental deficiency is generally mild, but ranges from moderately severe delay to normal educational ability.

3.4 Ectopic calcification
In patients with PHP 1a, soft-tissue calcification has been reported in various body parts, especially in the subcutaneous tissues, and rarely in the brain and cardiac septum(Schuster, 1992). Persistent hyperparathyroidism is believed to have some causative role in this abnormal calcification. This situation is distinct from progressive osseous heteroplasia (Chan, 2004), a rare condition that causes dermal ossification.

3.5 Brachymetaphalangism
The hand abnormalities in the PHP and PPHP forms of AHO are indistinguishable (Poznanski, 1977). The malformations involve both the phalanges and metacarpals and are often symmetrical(Wilson, 1994) (Figure 1b). Shortening of the distal phalanx of the thumb is estimated to occur in 75% of AHO patients(Poznanski, 1977). Similar shortening occur in the metacarpals. Metacarpal shortening often involves the fourth and the fifth

metacarpals(Poznanski, 1977; Steinbach, 1965). Shortening of the metatarsals (Figure 1c), especially the third and fourth, is seen in about 70% of persons with AHO(Steinbach, 1966).

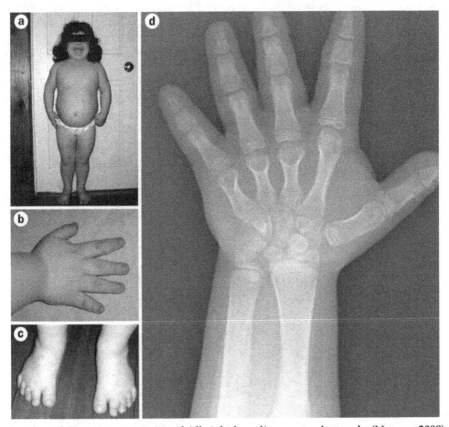

Fig. 1. a, b, c, d. Features suggestive of Albright hereditary osteodystrophy(Nwosu, 2009)
Figure 1 | Features suggestive of Albright hereditary osteodystrophy in the patient. a | Photo of a patient at 5 years of age showing an obese phenotype, round face, broad chest, short neck and digits consistent with pseudohypoparathyroidism type 1a. b | Photo of the patient's hand at 5 years of age showing brachyphalangism of the fingers, especially the third through fifth digits. c | Photo of the patient's feet at 5 years of age showing brachyphalangism of the toes. d | Bone age radiograph of the patient at 7 years of age showing premature fusion of the epiphyses of the distal phalanges of the thumb, midphalanges of both the second and fifth fingers, and shortening of the third through fifth metacarpals. Her bone age was read as 13 years at a chronological age of 7 years and 8 months.

3.6 Obesity and insulin resistance
Insulin resistance has not been described in patients with PHP 1a, and acanthosis nigricans is not a typical finding in AHO. Germain-Lee et al(Germain-Lee, 2003) reported a patient with acanthosis nigricans in a cohort of 13 patients with PHP 1a who had normal

hemoglobin A1c and fasting insulin levels. Nwosu et al(Nwosu, 2009) described a child with PHP 1a with acanthosis nigricans and insulin resistance (Figure 2).

A patient with Albright hereditary osteodystrophy-like syndrome with a normal *GNAS* gene that was complicated by type 2 diabetes mellitus with severe insulin resistance, growth-hormone deficiency and diabetes insipidus has been described(Sakaguchi, 1998). Long *et al.*(Long, 2007) reported that obesity is a more prominent feature of PHP 1a than of PPHP, and that severe obesity is characteristic of PHP 1a. They postulated that paternal imprinting of $G_s\alpha$ occurs in the hypothalamus such that maternal, but not paternal, $G_s\alpha$ mutations lead to loss of the melanocortin signaling cascade, which is important for signaling satiety. This loss of satiety signaling then leads to greater alteration in energy balance and notably greater insulin resistance in individuals with PHP 1a (as shown in Figure 2) than in those with PPHP.

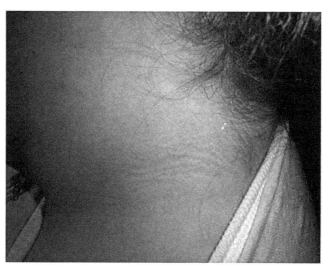

Fig. 2. Acanthosis nigricans of the neck folds in a patient with Albright Hereditary Osteodystrophy(Nwosu, 2009)

The insulin receptor belongs to a large class of tyrosine kinase receptors, and is structurally distinct from the heptahelical G_s receptors. The development of insulin resistance in the patient shown in Figure 2 most probably resulted from the combined effects of obesity, growth-hormone treatment, a family history of type 2 diabetes mellitus, and abnormal melanocortin signaling, as noted above. Obesity is the most common cause of insulin resistance in children(Caprio, 2002). It is postulated to represent a subclinical inflammatory state that promotes the production of proinflammatory factors, such as interleukin 6 and tumor necrosis factor, which are involved in the pathogenesis of insulin resistance(Bastard, 2006). Growth hormone antagonizes insulin's effects on glucose metabolism by inhibiting insulin-induced glucose uptake through the inhibition of insulin receptor substrate-2-associated phosphatidylinositol-3-kinase activity, without affecting glucose transporter 4 translocation(Sasaka-Suzuki N, 2009). A family history of type 2 diabetes mellitus conveys not only heritable genetic information, but also reveals familial behaviors and social norms that may exacerbate the individual's risk for insulin resistance and frank diabetes(Meigs, 2008).

3.7 Biochemical profile

The biochemical profile in patients with PHP 1a shows evidence of PTH resistance, with elevated serum concentrations of PTH and phosphate, and low or normal serum levels of ionized calcium. Serum TSH concentrations are elevated from infancy indicating TSH resistance at the receptor-complex level. Subnormal peak growth-hormone levels of <7.5 µg/l are commonly found when growth-hormone stimulation tests are carried out(Scott, 1995). Serum gonadotropins are either normal or slightly elevated in women with AHO despite their hypoestrogenic status(Namnoum, 1998). This is believed to be due to partial resistance to gonadotropins in the granulosa and theca cells of the ovary(Namnoum, 1998).

3.8 Bone age and other skeletal and radiologic features

The bone ages of children with PHP 1a are more advanced than would be expected for their stage of sexual maturation. Premature epiphyseal fusion occurs selectively in the hands and feet of affected patients(de Wijn, 1982; Steinbach, 1966). Furthermore, the phalanges of patients either lack epiphyses or have epiphyses that are partially fused when they first develop, which makes accurate assessments of bone age very difficult(Steinbach, 1966). This abnormal epiphyseal fusion is postulated to result from the loss of $G_s\alpha$, which induces resistance to parathyroid-hormone-related protein which, in turn, promotes premature differentiation of proliferating chondrocytes into hypertrophic chondrocytes(Kobayashi, 2002; Tavella, 2004; van der Eerden, 2000). This series of events leads to early closure of the growth plate and limb-reduction defects. Despite early fusion of the epiphyses in the phalanges, the epiphyses of long bones may remain open, thus an increase in height with growth-hormone therapy is still possible.

Other radiological features of PHP 1a in children include rickets which results from low levels of 1,25-dihydroxyvitamin D as a result of PTH resistance(Wilson, 1994). Generalized osteoporosis and osteitis fibrosa cystica(Burnstein, 1985; Steinbach, 1966) can be seen, and these pathologies are suggestive of some preservation of the skeletal remodeling response to the raised levels of circulating PTH(Kerr, 1987). Some of the skeletal abnormalities associated with AHO include shortened ulna, radial and tibial bowing, coxa vara, coxa valga and caudal narrowing of interpedicular distance(Wilson, 1994).

3.9 Hormonal defects and manifestations

In addition to the AHO phenotype, biochemical and hormonal derangements in PHP 1a lead to characteristic patterns of presentation. PHP 1a is associated with resistance to multiple hormones, such as PTH, TSH, gonadotropins, growth-hormone-releasing hormone, and glucagon(Brickman, 1986; Weinstein, 2004).

PHP 1a accompanied by growth-hormone deficiency was first described in 1995(Scott, 1995). The short stature of patients with PHP 1a results from a combination of several factors, such as epiphyseal defects and resistance to GHRH(Scott, 1995). This hormone resistance results in the inability of GHRH to stimulate pituitary somatotropes to produce growth hormone. Many patients with PHP 1a present with subclinical hypothyroidism in infancy (Pohlenz, 2003; Scott, 1995), as a result of resistance to TSH action. Resistance to PTH action could lead to hypocalcemia which could be complicated by hypocalcemic seizures, and/or muscle spasms. Resistance to the actions of the gonadotropins results in hypogonadism or menstrual irregularities in women with PHP 1a. The mechanism of this reproductive dysfunction is believed to be due to a partial resistance of the theca and granulosa cells of the ovary to gonadotropins due to deficient $G_s\alpha$ activity (Namnoum, 1998).

Whereas resistance to PTH, TSH, growth-hormone-releasing hormone, follicle-stimulating hormone, and luteinizing hormone may lead to clinical manifestations, the blunted cyclic AMP response to glucagon documented by Brickman *et al.*(Brickman, 1986) in patients with PHP 1a is apparently subclinical, as the glucose response is intact.

4. Differential diagnosis

The differential diagnoses of a child with this AHO phenotype include exogenous obesity, Cushing syndrome, severe hypoparathyroidism, Prader–Willi syndrome, and Laurence–Moon–Biedl–Bardet syndrome.

The generalized metacarpal and phalangeal shortening characteristics of acrodysostosis has been observed in cases of AHO(Ablow, 1977). Acrodysostosis presents with similar features as AHO including short stature, brachymetaphalangism, advanced bone age, mental deficiency and other radiologic features. However, cutaneous ossification does not occur in acrodysostosis, and pronounced nasal hypoplasia is a distinguishing feature of acrodysostosis, but has been described in PHP 1a(Ablow, 1977).

Turner syndrome and multiple familial exostoses are associated with short stature and metacarpal shortening but are easily distinguished from AHO(Wilson, 1994).

A diagnosis is usually reached by reviewing patient's family history, establishing the components of the AHO phenotype, such as short fourth metacarpals, and connecting these findings to the existing hormonal defects such as a history of subclinical hypothyroidism or parathyroid hormone resistance.

5. Treatment and management

The defect in PHP 1a leads to resistance to multiple hormones that mediate their actions through cyclic AMP(Spiegel, 1982). These include PTH, TSH, growth-hormone-releasing hormone, gonadotropins, glucagon, and possibly TSH-releasing hormone(Balavoine, 2008). Patients with $G_s\alpha$ deficiency could, therefore, develop hypothyroidism, hypogonadism, growth-hormone deficiency, and pseudohypoparathyroidism, depending on the degree of $G_s\alpha$ activity in specific tissues(Scott, 1995).

5.1 Hypoparathyroidism

The initial medical management of all patients with severe, symptomatic hypocalcemia should be with intravenous calcium. The recommended initial dose for newborn babies , infants and children is 0.5–1.0 ml/kg of 10% calcium gluconate administered over 5 min. Administration of oral calcium and 1α-hydroxylated vitamin D metabolites, such as calcitriol, is recommended for patients with symptomatic hypocalcemia. The goals of therapy are to maintain serum total and ionized calcium levels within the reference range and to reduce PTH levels to near normal. This normalization is important because elevated PTH levels in patients with PHP 1a could cause increased bone remodeling and lead to secondary hyperparathyroid bone disease(Abraham, 2007).

5.2 Growth-hormone deficiency

Some children with PHP 1a have hypothalamic growth-hormone deficiency and may benefit from therapy with recombinant human growth hormone to achieve optimal adult height. In those patients in whom defective growth-hormone secretion is suspected, the epiphyseal defects, commonly mischaracterized as bone-age advancement, should not disqualify these children from being considered for growth-hormone therapy. In addition to its effect on statural growth, growth-hormone therapy also seems to improve body composition in patients with PHP 1a(Nwosu, 2009).

5.3 Hypothyroidism

Most patients with PHP 1a present with subclinical hypothyroidism before the onset of hypocalcemia. Hypothyroidism is treated with thyroid hormone replacement using levothyroxine at age-appropriate and weight-appropriate doses. The aim of management is to normalize serum concentrations of TSH and free T_4.

5.4 Hypogonadism

Common reproductive dysfunctions in persons with PHP 1a include delayed puberty, oligomenorrhea and infertility(Abraham, 2007). Each condition requires age-appropriate therapy; for example, low-dose estrogenic formulations are used to induce puberty in adolescent girls with delayed puberty.

5.5 Obesity and insulin resistance

Patients with PHP 1a who also have a family history of type 2 diabetes mellitus may have familial risk factors for development of insulin resistance, prediabetes and type 2 diabetes mellitus. Growth-hormone therapy improves body composition, but may worsen insulin resistance. Lifestyle modifications should be incorporated in the management of patients with PHP 1a phenotype who may be at risk of metabolic syndrome. Early introduction of oral insulin-sensitizing agents, such as metformin, may be necessary when lifestyle modification is ineffective, especially in patients with prediabetes.

6. Conclusion

Accurate understanding of the features of AHO will prevent its misdiagnosis as exogenous obesity. Children diagnosed with PHP 1a should be further evaluated for associated endocrinopathies, such as resistance to growth-hormone-releasing hormone, which may lead to growth-hormone deficiency. Preliminary data suggest that the short stature in patients with PHP 1a may be ameliorated with growth-hormone therapy in some cases(Scott, 1995). The advanced bone age seen in PHP 1a is due to a chondrocytic signaling defect, and not due to excess production of sex hormones; therefore, bone-age advancement should not preclude affected children from being considered for growth-hormone therapy. However, a combination of growth-hormone therapy, family history of type 2 diabetes mellitus, and obesity in these children might lead to metabolic complications, such as insulin resistance, prediabetes and type 2 diabetes mellitus.

7. Future directions

A comprehensive management of a child with PHP 1a must address the controversies surrounding authorization of growth hormone therapy for these patients. This is because most health insurance carriers decline authorization for GH therapy in these patients because of the apparent bone age advancement that affects the digital bones but not the long bones.

It is equally important to address increasing weight gain in these patients as they are at risk for obesity and its co-morbidities. Even though insulin resistance is not part of the syndrome, there are increasing reports of worsening insulin resistance in these patients which predisposes them to frank diabetes mellitus. This is due to the synergistic effects of prevalent obesity and the pre-existing AHO phenotype.

The presence of delayed puberty may indicate LH and FSH resistance in these patients. There is no clear protocol for initiating sex hormone therapy in these patients. Most pediatric endocrinologists address this problem by adopting similar therapeutic modalities for the induction of the development of secondary sexual characteristics as in patients with Turner syndrome.

Most patients with PHP 1a have variable levels of mental deficiency. It is important to address this problem very early in life by recommending additional classroom supervision, and in severe cases, instituting an individualized educational plan.

In summary, a comprehensive management of a patient with PHP 1a includes a thorough assessment for associated hormonal defects, the obese phenotype and its comorbidities, and the degree of intellectual deficiency.

8. Acknowledgement

We thank Ms. Jessica Kowaleski for her clerical assistance. This work was supported in part by a grant to Dr Nwosu by the Faculty Scholars Diversity Program, University of Massachusetts Medical School.

9. References

Ablow, R. C., Hsia, Y. E., & Brandt, I. K. (1977). Acrodysostosis coinciding with pseudohypoparathyroidism and pseudo-pseudohypoparathyroidism. *AJR Am J Roentgenol, 128*(1), 95-99.

Abraham, M. R., & Khadori, R. K. (2007). Pseudohypoparathyroidism. *eMedicine,* http://www.emedicine.com/med/TOPIC1940.HTM.

Balavoine, A. S., Ladsous, M., Velayoudom, F. L., Vlaeminck, V., Cardot-Bauters, C., d'Herbomez, M., & Wemeau, J. L. (2008). Hypothyroidism in patients with pseudohypoparathyroidism type ia: Clinical evidence of resistance to tsh and trh. *Eur J Endocrinol, 159*(4), 431-437.

Bastard, J. P., Maachi, M., Lagathu, C., Kim, M. J., Caron, M., Vidal, H., Capeau, J., & Feve, B. (2006). Recent advances in the relationship between obesity, inflammation, and insulin resistance. *Eur Cytokine Netw, 17*(1), 4-12.

Brickman, A. S., Carlson, H. E., & Levin, S. R. (1986). Responses to glucagon infusion in pseudohypoparathyroidism. *J Clin Endocrinol Metab, 63*(6), 1354-1360.

Burnstein, M. I., Kottamasu, S. R., Pettifor, J. M., Sochett, E., Ellis, B. I., & Frame, B. (1985). Metabolic bone disease in pseudohypoparathyroidism: Radiologic features. *Radiology, 155*(2), 351-356.

Caprio, S. (2002). Insulin resistance in childhood obesity. *J Pediatr Endocrinol Metab, 15 Suppl 1*, 487-492.

Chan, I., Hamada, T., Hardman, C., McGrath, J. A., & Child, F. J. (2004). Progressive osseous heteroplasia resulting from a new mutation in the gnas1 gene. *Clin Exp Dermatol, 29*(1), 77-80.

Chen, Y. J., Shu, S. G., & Chi, C. S. (2005). Pseudohypoparathyroidism: Report of seven cases. *Acta Paediatr Taiwan, 46*(6), 374-380.

de Wijn, E. M., & Steendijk, R. (1982). Growth and maturation in pseudo-hypoparathyroidism: A longitudinal study in 5 patients. *Acta Endocrinol (Copenh), 101*(2), 223-226.

Germain-Lee, E. L., Groman, J., Crane, J. L., Jan de Beur, S. M., & Levine, M. A. (2003). Growth hormone deficiency in pseudohypoparathyroidism type 1a: Another manifestation of multihormone resistance. *J Clin Endocrinol Metab, 88*(9), 4059-4069.

Kerr, D., & Hosking, D. J. (1987). Pseudohypoparathyroidism: Clinical expression of pth resistance. *Q J Med, 65*(247), 889-894.

Kobayashi, T., Chung, U. I., Schipani, E., Starbuck, M., Karsenty, G., Katagiri, T., Goad, D. L., Lanske, B., & Kronenberg, H. M. (2002). Pthrp and indian hedgehog control differentiation of growth plate chondrocytes at multiple steps. *Development, 129*(12), 2977-2986.

Levine, M. A. (2000). Clinical spectrum and pathogenesis of pseudohypoparathyroidism. *Rev Endocr Metab Disord, 1*(4), 265-274.

Levine, M. A., Downs, R. W., Jr., Moses, A. M., Breslau, N. A., Marx, S. J., Lasker, R. D., Rizzoli, R. E., Aurbach, G. D., & Spiegel, A. M. (1983). Resistance to multiple hormones in patients with pseudohypoparathyroidism. Association with deficient activity of guanine nucleotide regulatory protein. *Am J Med, 74*(4), 545-556.

Lietman, S. A., Goldfarb, J., Desai, N., & Levine, M. A. (2008). Preimplantation genetic diagnosis for severe albright hereditary osteodystrophy. *J Clin Endocrinol Metab, 93*(3), 901-904.

Long, D. N., McGuire, S., Levine, M. A., Weinstein, L. S., & Germain-Lee, E. L. (2007). Body mass index differences in pseudohypoparathyroidism type 1a versus pseudopseudohypoparathyroidism may implicate paternal imprinting of galpha(s) in the development of human obesity. *J Clin Endocrinol Metab, 92*(3), 1073-1079.

Meigs, J. B., Shrader, P., Sullivan, L. M., McAteer, J. B., Fox, C. S., Dupuis, J., Manning, A. K., Florez, J. C., Wilson, P. W., D'Agostino, R. B., Sr., & Cupples, L. A. (2008). Genotype score in addition to common risk factors for prediction of type 2 diabetes. *N Engl J Med, 359*(21), 2208-2219.

Nagant de Deuschaisnes, C., Krane, SM. (2007). *Hypoparathyroidism* (3rd ed.). San Diego: Academic Press.

Namnoum, A. B., Merriam, G. R., Moses, A. M., & Levine, M. A. (1998). Reproductive dysfunction in women with albright's hereditary osteodystrophy. *J Clin Endocrinol Metab, 83*(3), 824-829.

Nwosu, B. U., & Lee, M. M. (2009). Pseudohypoparathyroidism type 1a and insulin resistance in a child. *Nat Rev Endocrinol, 5*(6), 345-350.

Pohlenz, J., Ahrens, W., & Hiort, O. (2003). A new heterozygous mutation (l338n) in the human gsalpha (gnas1) gene as a cause for congenital hypothyroidism in albright's hereditary osteodystrophy. *Eur J Endocrinol, 148*(4), 463-468.

Poznanski, A. K., Werder, E. A., Giedion, A., Martin, A., & Shaw, H. (1977). The pattern of shortening of the bones of the hand in php and pphp--a comparison with brachydactyly e, turner syndrome, and acrodysostosis. *Radiology, 123*(3), 707-718.

Sakaguchi, H., Sanke, T., Ohagi, S., Iiri, T., & Nanjo, K. (1998). A case of albright's hereditary osteodystrophy-like syndrome complicated by several endocrinopathies: Normal gs alpha gene and chromosome 2q37. *J Clin Endocrinol Metab, 83*(5), 1563-1565.

Sasaka-Suzuki N, A. K., Ogata T, Kasahara K. (2009). Gh inhibition of glucose uptake in adipocytes occurs without affecting glut-4 translocation thorugh an irs-2pi 3-kinase-dependent pathway. *J. Biol. Chem.*

Schuster, V., & Sandhage, K. (1992). Intracardiac calcifications in a case of pseudohypoparathyroidism type ia (php-ia). *Pediatr Cardiol, 13*(4), 237-239.

Scott, D. C., & Hung, W. (1995). Pseudohypoparathyroidism type ia and growth hormone deficiency in two siblings. *J Pediatr Endocrinol Metab, 8*(3), 205-207.

Spiegel, A. M., Levine, M. A., Aurbach, G. D., Downs, R. W., Jr., Marx, S. J., Lasker, R. D., Moses, A. M., & Breslau, N. A. (1982). Deficiency of hormone receptor-adenylate cyclase coupling protein: Basis for hormone resistance in pseudohypoparathyroidism. *Am J Physiol, 243*(1), E37-42.

Steinbach, H. L., Rudhe, U., Jonsson, M., & Young, D. A. (1965). Evolution of skeletal lesions in pseudohypoparathyroidism. *Radiology, 85*(4), 670-676.

Steinbach, H. L., & Young, D. A. (1966). The roentgen appearance of pseudohypoparathyroidism (ph) and pseudo-pseudohypoparathyroidism (pph). Differentiation from other syndromes associated with short metacarpals, metatarsals, and phalanges. *Am J Roentgenol Radium Ther Nucl Med, 97*(1), 49-66.

Tavella, S., Biticchi, R., Schito, A., Minina, E., Di Martino, D., Pagano, A., Vortkamp, A., Horton, W. A., Cancedda, R., & Garofalo, S. (2004). Targeted expression of shh affects chondrocyte differentiation, growth plate organization, and sox9 expression. *J Bone Miner Res, 19*(10), 1678-1688.

van der Eerden, B. C., Karperien, M., Gevers, E. F., Lowik, C. W., & Wit, J. M. (2000). Expression of indian hedgehog, parathyroid hormone-related protein, and their receptors in the postnatal growth plate of the rat: Evidence for a locally acting growth restraining feedback loop after birth. *J Bone Miner Res, 15*(6), 1045-1055.

Weinstein, L. S., Liu, J., Sakamoto, A., Xie, T., & Chen, M. (2004). Minireview: Gnas: Normal and abnormal functions. *Endocrinology, 145*(12), 5459-5464.

Weinstein, L. S., & Shenker, A. (1993). G protein mutations in human disease. *Clin Biochem, 26*(5), 333-338.

Weisman, Y., Golander, A., Spirer, Z., & Farfel, Z. (1985). Pseudohypoparathyroidism type 1a presenting as congenital hypothyroidism. *J Pediatr, 107*(3), 413-415.

Wilson, L. C., & Trembath, R. C. (1994). Albright's hereditary osteodystrophy. *J Med Genet, 31*(10), 779-784.

7

Retinoids and Bone

H. Herschel Conaway[1] and Ulf H. Lerner[2,3]

[1]*Department of Physiology and Biophysics, University of Arkansas for Medical Sciences,*
[2]*Department of Molecular Periodontology, Umeå University*
[3]*Center for Bone and Arthritis Research at Institute of Medicine, Sahlgrenska Academy at University of Gothenburg,*
[1]*USA*
[2,3]*Sweden*

1. Introduction

Vitamin A (retinol) can be produced in the body by hydrolysis of retinyl esters or reduction of retinal. Liver and eggs, which are good animal sources of vitamin A, contain retinyl esters. Plant sources such as carrots and spinach contain pro-vitamin A carotenoids, which can be cleaved to retinal. Retinal, also called retinaldehyde, is interconvertible with retinol (Fig. 1). Retinal also serves as an intermediate in the irreversible production of all-trans-retinoic acid (ATRA), which is considered the major biologically active derivative of vitamin A [Moise *et al.* 2007, Chambon 1996]. Another important derivative of vitamin A is the visual chromophore 11-cis-retinal [Wald 1968]. Binding of 11-cis-retinal to proteins called opsins is the chemical basis of vision. Vitamin A formed from retinyl esters or carotenoids in the normal diet, or ingested in fortified foods or dietary supplements, is stored in the liver and transported to tissues as a complex bound to retinol binding protein [Moise *et al.* 2007].

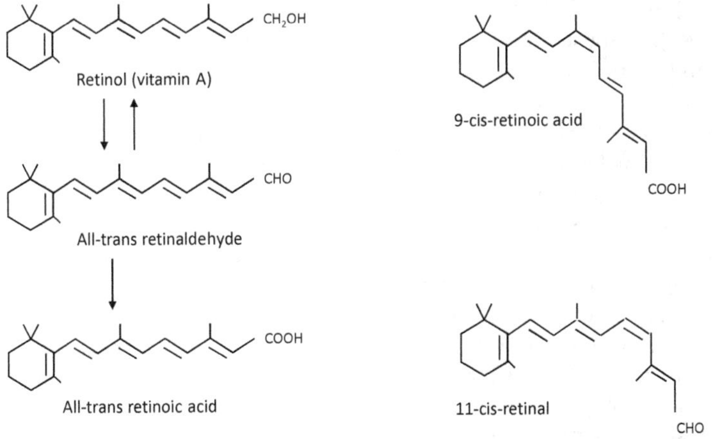

Fig. 1. Formation of all-trans retinoic acid from vitamin A and structures of 9-cis retinoic acid and 11-cis-retinal.

Effects of retinoids are mediated primarily by two families of nuclear hormone receptors, retinoic acid receptors (RARs) and the retinoid X receptors (RXRs) [Bastein *et al.* 2004]. Each receptor family is made up of three isoforms (α, β and γ), produced by separate genes. RARs can be activated by ATRA and the isomer 9-*cis* retinoic acid (9-cis RA), while RXRs are activated by 9-*cis* RA. RARs form heterodimers with RXRs and these heterodimers and RXR homodimers function as transcription factors, activating RAREs in the promoter regions of target genes. Most retinol signaling in cells is thought to be mediated by ATRA binding RAR in RAR/RXR heterodimers [Mic *et al.* 2003]. It is still not clear if 9-*cis* RA is formed physiologically in cells and what role this isomer may play as a specific ligand for RXR [Mic *et al.* 2003]. Activated retinoid receptors function as transcription factors, activating specific RA response elements (RAREs) for transcriptional regulation of target genes [Bastein *et al.* 2004, Mic *et al.* 2003].

Peroxisome proliferator-activated receptors (PPARs), α, β/δ, and γ, represent another group of nuclear hormone receptors that forms heterodimers with RXR. PPAR/RXR heterodimers also function as transcription factors, activating specific response elements of target genes [Mangelsdorf and Evans 1995, Bocher *et al.* 2002, Wilson *et al.* 2000]. Recent studies have indicated that ATRA not only can bind RARs, but can serve as a ligand for PPAR β/δ as well [Berry *et al.* 2007]. Channelling of ATRA to RARs or PPAR β/δ is suggested to depend on the intracellular binding proteins, RA binding protein II or keratinocyte fatty acid binding protein 5, which deliver ATRA to either RAR or PPAR β/δ, respectively [Schug *et al.* 2007].

Vitamin A plays an essential role in numerous biological processes, including vision, cellular proliferation, differentiation, and apoptosis, organ development and function, and immunity [Moise *et al.* 2007, Mark *et al.* 2006, Mark *et al.* 2009]. Numerous malformations and impaired vision, growth, organ function, and reproduction have been noted with vitamin A deficiency. Vitamin A is used in developing countries to help correct vitamin A deficiency [Moise *et al.* 2007]. Supplementation with vitamin A has had an enormous worldwide impact, saving countless lives, at minimal costs per patient. There is also widespread use of vitamin A derivatives (retinoids) for treatment of various skin conditions, such as acne [Peck *et al.* 1979], and for different cancers, including acute promyelocytic leukemia (APL), Kaposi's sarcoma, head and neck squamous cell carcinoma, ovarian carcinoma, and neuroblastoma [Siddikuzzaman *et al.* 2010]. Use of retinoids has proved particularly useful for treatment of APL [Siddikuzzaman *et al.* 2010]. Pharmacological concentrations (10^{-7} - 10^{-6}M) of ATRA block repression by a PML- RARα fusion protein that interferes with normal RARα transcriptional regulation in APL.

Besides serving as an intermediate in retinoic acid formation, recent studies have shown that retinal (retinaldehyde) is present at biologically active concentrations in fat tissue, where it antagonizes PPAR-γ activity, inhibits adipogenesis, and improves insulin sensitivity [Ziouzenkova *et al.* 2007]. These observations suggest that retinal may be an additional vitamin A derivative that plays an important role as a mediator of biological processes.

Hypervitaminosis A in experimental animals has been linked to increased bone resorption, decreased bone mass, and increased fractures [Frankel *et al.* 1986, Hough *et al.* 1988, Johansson *et al.* 2002]. There are also case studies in humans showing that significantly increased intake of vitamin A increases bone resorption, causes hypercalcemia, and induces skeletal pain [Frame *et al.* 1974]. Supplementation of the diet with vitamins is a common occurrence in developed countries and there is presently debate over whether more modest increases in vitamin A might promote skeletal abnormalities. Some studies have shown that increased vitamin A intake or elevated serum retinol levels [Michaelsson et al. 2003] are associated with an increased incidence of hip fracture or decreased bone mass [Melhaus et al. 1998, Feskanich et al. 2002, Promislow et al. 2002]; however, other studies have shown no deleterious effect on bone mass or fracture risk, and, in some instances, protection from bone loss because of increased vitamin A has been reported [Ribaya-Mercado and Blumberg 2007, Caire-Juvera et al. 2009]. In studies where vitamin A analogues have been evaluated, decreases in bone mass have been reported following isotretinoin and acitretin usage in some instances, but a recent, large scale, case-control study has found no increased risk of fracture with these agents [Vestergaard et al. 2010].

2. Bone tissue

Skeletal tissue is comprised primarily of either cortical (compact) or trabecular (cancellous) bone. In the adult, approximately 80% of skeletal mass is cortical bone and 20% trabecular bone. Cortical bone is found in the shafts of long bones and the outer surfaces of all other bones in the body. It is organized around blood vessels into cylinders of consolidated bone called osteons, or Haversian systems. Unlike trabecular bone, cortical bone does not contain bone marrow. Trabecular bone is characterized as a network of thin spicules of bone ("spongy bone"), which is found in the interior of vertebrae, flat bones in the skull, the pelvis and sacrum, and the distal and proximal parts of long bones. Both cortical and trabecular bone are important for bone strength. In the adult skeleton, both types of bone are remodelled and modelled [Martin and Seeman 2008]. Modelling of bone is a process that changes the size and shape of bone either by bone resorption without subsequent bone formation, or bone formation without prior bone resorption. Remodelling of bone is the process by which old bone is replaced by new bone. It is initiated by bone resorption to remove damaged bone, followed by new bone formation in the area resorbed. Remodelling does not change the size or shape of the bones. Remodelling is more frequent in trabecular bone than in cortical bone, one of the reasons why a metabolic bone disease like postmenopausal osteoporosis affects primarily bones with proportionally increased amounts of trabecular bone, e.g. vertebrae, distal radius, and proximal femur. Remodelling is believed to be initiated by microcracks in the mineralized bone extracellular matrix and subsequent osteocytic apoptosis, which triggers osteoclast formation and resorption of the micro-damaged area [Martin and Seeman 2008]. The process causes release of "coupling factors" which attract and activate osteoblasts to form new bone under a canopy of bone lining cells [Martin and Sims 2005, Boyce et al. 2009, Martin et al. 2009]. When osteoblasts fill the resorption lacunae made by osteoclasts with new bone in the bone multicellular unit (BMU), remodelling is in balance and bone mass remains constant. This equilibrium involves bidirectional interactions between osteoclasts and osteoblasts to fine tune the balance between bone formation and bone resorption.

The skeleton is a support structure that serves as a reservoir for calcium, phosphate, and numerous other minerals, protects vital organs such as brain, heart, lung, and bone marrow, and recently has been implicated in glucose- and energy metabolism [Confavreux et al. 2009]. Three systemic hormones that play primary roles in calcium homeostasis and bone formation and resorption are parathyroid hormone (PTH), $1,25(OH)_2$-vitamin D_3, and calcitonin. PTH and $1,25(OH)_2$-vitamin D_3 stimulate bone resorption when serum calcium decreases, whereas calcitonin inhibits bone resorption when serum calcium is increased. Sex hormones also play important roles, with increased bone resorption and decreased bone formation occurring when levels of either estrogen or testosterone are decreased. Other agents known to play significant roles in bone turnover are the thyroid hormones, glucocorticoids, follicle stimulating hormone, and the retinoids. Interestingly, there is also a great deal of cross talk between bone cells and the immune system. This occurs during both normal physiological remodelling and in pathological inflammatory conditions involving bone, like rheumatoid arthritis and peridontitis [Takayanagi 2009].

3. Osteoclast differentiation

Osteoclasts are multinucleated giant cells found on bone surfaces that stain for tartrate resistant acid phosphatise (TRAP). They are formed by fusion of mononucleated progenitor cells derived from hematopoetic myeloid stem cells, which also give rise to macrophages and dendritic cells. For fusion of osteoclast precursors to occur, they must be differentiated specifically along the osteoclastic lineage [Lorenzo and Horowitz 2008, Edwards and Mundy 2011]. Formation of osteoclasts is controlled by osteoblasts at the bone surface. Thus, osteoblasts are responsible for not only bone formation, but regulate bone resorption as well. In addition to hematopoetic cells, bone marrow also contains pluripotent mesenchymal cells which are able to support differentiation of osteoclasts [Askmyr *et al.* 2009]; however, mature osteoclasts do not form within bone marrow, but enter the circulation as mononucleated osteoclast progenitors and home to periosteal and endosteal tissues. The details of this attraction are not known at present, but stomal cell-derived factor-1 (SDF-1 or CXCL12) produced by osteoblasts and CXCR4 expressed by osteoclast progenitors may play important roles [Kollet *et al.* 2006]. To what extent the circulating osteoclast progenitor cells are primed in the bone marrow, or to what extent priming occurs in the periosteum and endosteum is also not known at present. Nor is it known if osteoclast formation in trabecular bone in the close vicinity of bone marrow is different from osteoclast formation in periosteal tissues, which are always some distance from bone marrow. Recently, one group has presented evidence for the existence of a unique periosteal macrophage – osteomac which not only can form osteoclasts, but is also able to control bone formation [Chang *et al.* 2008]. Increasing evidence indicates that osteoclast formation does not follow a common pathway and that osteoclasts are different in different parts of the skeleton [Everts *et al.* 2009, Henriksen *et al.* 2011].

Crude bone marrow cultures, or co-cultures of periosteal osteoblasts and purified osteoclast progenitors from either bone marrow or spleens, have shown that osteoclast formation requires close physical contact of progenitor cells with either stromal cells in the bone marrow or osteoblasts. Molecularly, it has been found that macrophage colony-stimulating factor (M-CSF) and receptor activator of nuclear factor κB ligand (RANKL) are two products of stromal cells/osteoblasts that play key roles in regulating osteoclast formation. M-CSF supports progenitor cell proliferation and survival, and RANKL is responsible for progenitor differentiation to osteoclasts, rather than to macrophages or dendritic cells [Takayanagi 2009, Lorenzo and Horowitz 2008, Nakashima and Takayanagi 2009]. RANKL, which is a member of the TNF superfamily, functions by binding to RANK on osteoclast progenitor cells. Osteoprotegerin (OPG), a soluble protein released from stromal cells/osteoblasts, is another key factor regulating osteoclastogenesis. OPG functions as a decoy receptor for RANKL, blocking interaction between RANKL and RANK. The expression of RANKL is thought to be restricted to a relatively small number of cells: bone marrow stromal cells, osteoblasts, periodontal ligament cells, synovial fibroblasts, T-, B- and NK-cells, while OPG appears to be ubiquitously expressed. It is the relative expression of RANKL and OPG which determines whether osteoclast formation will take place. Enhancement of the RANKL/OPG ratio in stromal cells or osteoblasts by hormones and cytokines causes stimulation of bone resorption. Following RANKL binding to trimeric RANK, association of the cytoplasmic tail of RANK with TNF receptor-associated factor 6 (TRAF 6) leads to activation of several kinases, including IKKβ, MAPKs such as p38 and JNK, and PI3K (Fig. 2). Subsequently, transcription factors such as NF-κB, AP-1, MITF, NFATc1 and Akt are activated. Within the NF-κB family of transcription factors, p50 and p52 seem to be the most important subunits [Boyce et al. 2010]. RANK signaling leads to induction and activation of c-fos, which functions as a component of the transcription factor, activator protein-1 (AP-1). Mice with double knockouts of p50/p52 or with deletion of the c-Fos gene lack osteoclasts and exhibit osteopetrosis. The induction of the master transcription factor for osteoclastogenesis, NFATc1, is dependent on NF-κB and c-fos signaling by RANK [Negishi-Koga and Takayanagi 2009]. In cooperation with RANK, immunoglobulin-like receptors associated with adaptor proteins harboring the immunoreceptor tyrosine-based activation motif (ITAM) activate phospholipase Cγ, calcium signaling, and the formation of calcineurin required for activation of NFATc1 [Nemeth et al. 2011]. The activation of specific genes necessary for osteoclastogenesis and osteoclast function is regulated by NFATc1 cooperating with other transcription factors, such as AP-1, CREB, PU.1, and MITF. Important osteoclast genes include those encoding calcitonin receptor and TRAP, which serve as osteoclast markers, cathepsin K, which is involved in breakdown of bone matrix collagen, Atp6i and chloride chanel-7, involved in acidification and dissolution of bone mineral crystals, and the integrins α_v and β_3, which are important for attachments of osteoclasts to bone surfaces.

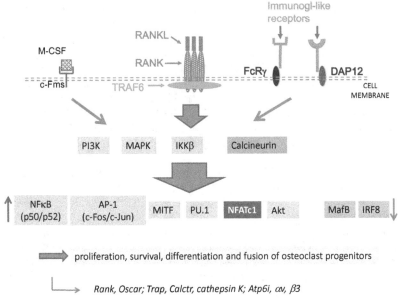

Fig. 2. Osteoclastogenic pathways, transcription factors, and genes stimulated by M-CSF and RANKL.

4. Retinoids and bone resorption in vitro

The effect of vitamin A on bone resorption has been studied the most thoroughly in rodent models. It has been known since the 1920´s that excess vitamin A has effects on the skeleton. In classical experiments in 1952 employing cultured fetal mouse limb bones, Dame Honor Fell showed that hypervitaminosis A stimulated osteoclast formation and bone resorption [Fell and Mellanby 1952]. Thirteen years later, Larry Raisz showed that vitamin A could stimulate bone resorption in organ cultures of fetal rat long bones [Raisz 1965]. Since those early experimental reports, there have been additional studies in organ cultures of fetal rat long bones [Scheven and Hamilton 1990], fetal rat calvariae [Delaissé et al. 1988] and calvarial bones from both fetal [Delaissé et al. 1988] and newborn [Raisz et al. 1977, Togari et al. 1991, Kindmark et al. 95, Conaway et al. 1997] mice confirming the osteoclastogenic effects of vitamin A and derivatives. An investigation indicating that ATRA increases mRNA expression of *RANKL* in primary human osteoblast-like cultures and decreases mRNA expression and protein formation of OPG in human MG-63 osteosarcoma cells [Jacobson et al. 2004] led to the suggestion that bone resorption stimulated by the retinoid is due to an increased RANKL/OPG ratio; however, until recently, there had been no data from bone or bone culture systems showing how vitamin A or derivatives stimulated bone resorption. In a recent investigation, we have reported that stimulation of osteoclastogenesis and bone resorption by retinoids in neonatal mouse calvarial bone is due to increased RANKL mRNA and protein expression. Supporting evidence for the role of RANKL was the observation that exogenous OPG administration blocked retinoid induced calvarial bone resorption [Henning et al. 2011].

Resorption in the bone organ culture systems depends on increased osteoclast formation and/or enhanced osteoclast activity. Attempts to elucidate effects of vitamin A on mature osteoclasts have generated conflicting results. It has been reported that bone resorbing activity of rabbit osteoclasts incubated on dentine slices is enhanced by ATRA [Saneshige et al. 1995]. Additionally, the vitamin A derivative isotretinonin has been observed to increase activity of rat osteoclasts incubated on cortical bone slices [Lakkakorpi and Väänänen 1991]. In contrast, bone resorbing activity of embryonic chicken osteoclasts on either bovine cortical bone or sperm whale dentine has been reported to be decreased by ATRA [O´Neill et al. 1992]. Furthermore, degradation of bone particles incubated with chicken osteoclasts is said to be enhanced by retinol and ATRA [Oreffo et al. 1988], which differs from experiments using osteoclast-like cell lines from human giant cell bone tumors, where Colucci et al. have found that ATRA inhibits degradation of bone matrix in rat bone particles [Colucci et al. 1996].

Evaluations of the effects of vitamin A on osteoclast formation have also generated conflicting data. In human bone marrow cultures, ATRA has been reported to stimulate formation of osteoclast-like multinucleated cells that are incapable of resorbing bone [Thavarajah et al. 1991]. Formation of multinucleated osteoclasts unable to resorb bone has also been reported following ATRA treatment of bone marrow cultures from egg laying hens [Chiba et al. 1996]. Scheven and Hamilton [1990] found no effect of ATRA on osteoclast formation in rat bone marrow cultures; however, when Hata et al. [1992] stimulated osteoclast formation in rat bone marrow cultures with $1,25(OH)_2$-vitamin D_3, they found inhibition with ATRA. Using an acyclic retinoid, geranylgeranoic acid, Wang et al. [2002] also found that osteoclast formation in mouse bone marrow cultures stimulated by $1,25(OH)_2$-vitamin D_3 was inhibited. Inhibition by the retinoid was most likely due to inhibition of osteoclast progenitor cells, since inhibition of osteoclast formation by geranylgeranoic acid was also observed in mouse bone marrow macrophage (BMM) cultures stimulated by RANKL. In agreement with these latter observations, we have recently shown that ATRA, as well as 9-cis retinoic acid, inhibit osteoclast formation in mouse bone marrow cell cultures stimulated with either $1,25(OH)_2$-vitamin D_3 or PTH [Conaway et al. 2009], an effect associated with decreased expression of the osteoclast genes Calcr, Acp5, and Catsk, which code for the calcitonin receptor, TRAP, and cathepsin K, respectively. ATRA did not affect 1, $25(OH)_2$-vitamin D_3 stimulated mRNA expression of Rankl, nor did the retinoid affect the decrease of Opg expression induced by $1,25(OH)_2$-vitamin D_3, suggesting that the inhibitory effect was at the level of osteoclast progenitors rather than stromal cells. Osteoclast formation in both crude bone marrow cultures and spleen cell cultures stimulated by RANKL was also inhibited by ATRA and 9-cis retinoic acid. Moreover, osteoclast formation stimulated by RANKL in highly purified mouse BMM cultures was inhibited by ATRA and 9-cis retinoic acid, providing good evidence that the retinoids inhibited osteoclastogenesis by directly affecting osteoclast progenitor cells.

Inhibition of osteoclast progenitor cell differentiation by ATRA was due to inhibition of AP-1 and Nfatc1 pathways, but did not involve the NF-κB pathway [Conaway et al. 2009]. ATRA inhibited mRNA and protein expression of the transcription factors c-Fos and Nfatc1 induced by RANKL. RANKL also enhanced the mRNA expression of Fra-1, Fra-2 and JunB in mouse BMM, but ATRA inhibited only Fra-2. The decrease of the macrophage transcription factor MafB caused by RANKL during osteoclastogenesis was blunted by ATRA, suggesting that ATRA arrested precursor cells at the macrophage stage. In agreement with these observations, it has been observed that ATRA inhibits Nfatc1 expression, translocation, and DNA-binding in RAW264.7 cells and mouse BMM [Balkan et al. 2011].

Mouse BMM express RARα and RARβ, but little RARγ. By use of different agonists and antagonists, it was demonstrated that ATRA induced inhibition of RANKL stimulated osteoclast formation in BMM was mediated by RARα [Conaway et al. 2009]. As discussed above, ATRA can also serve as a ligand for PPARβ/δ. However, ligands specific for this receptor did not mimic the inhibitory effect of ATRA.

Effects of retinoids on osteoclast formation have also been studied using osteoclast progenitor cells isolated from peripheral blood. Woods et al. [1995] found that monocytes from chicken peripheral blood spontaneously formed giant cells with osteoclast like features and that this process was inhibited by ATRA. Recently, it was shown that ATRA inhibited osteoclast formation in RANKL stimulated cultures of human CD14+ monocytes from peripheral blood [Hu et al. 2010]. In agreement with observations in RANKL stimulated mouse BMM, inhibition of osteoclast formation in human CD14+ cells was associated with decreased mRNA expression of osteoclastic genes such as ACP5 and CATSK, and the transcription factor NFATc1, indicating that retinoids inhibit osteoclast formation by inhibiting osteoclast differentiation rather than fusion of differentiated progenitor cells. The authors attributed the inhibition to decreased expression of RANK mRNA and protein; however, it remains to be shown if this is the primary event.

5. Retinoids and bone resorption in vivo

In short term in vivo studies where rodents were treated with increased concentrations of retinoids (ATRA or Ro 13-6298), it has been reported that thinning of cortical bone due to significant stimulation of periosteal resorption occurs at the same time that cancellous bone resorption is inhibited [Kneissel *et al.* 2005]. Furthermore, in a recent one week study where rats were fed increased vitamin A, increased cortical osteoclasts and cortical bone thinning were also observed; however, in these animals, endosteal osteoclasts disappeared because of impaired endosteal/marrow blood flow, which resulted in hypoxia and pathological endosteal mineralization [Lind *et al.* 2011]. This resulted in thinner, more brittle bones with little apparent affect on bone mass. Vitamin A and retinoids stimulate resorption in cultured fetal mouse and rat limb bones [Fell and Mellanby 1952, Raisz 1965, Scheven *et al.* 1990], but these studies are normally based on calcium release to medium and do not distinguish between cortical and cancellous bone breakdown. On the other hand, calvarial bone is considered to be a good model for periosteal resorption of cortical bone and it is established that vitamin A and ATRA are effective stimulators of osteoclastogenesis and bone resorption in calvarial bone [Raisz *et al.* 1977, Togari *et al.* 1991, Kindmark *et al.* 1995, Conaway *et al.* 1997]. As stated previously, retinoids are also good inhibitors of osteoclastogenesis in mouse bone marrow cell and BMM cultures. Thus, when comparing results of *in vitro* and *in vivo* experimental studies attempting to access the effects of increased vitamin A, it appears there may be good agreement regarding cortical osteoclast formation and function stimulated by vitamin A. In contrast, it seems a continuum of effects may occur in the endosteum, with increased vitamin A inhibiting endosteal osteoclast formation and function, and impaired blood flow and hypoxia promoting osteoclast death.

6. Conclusion

In developed countries, the diet is often supplemented with vitamin A and there is presently controversy over whether increased intake of vitamin A might promote skeletal fragility [Michaelsson *et al.* 2003, Melhaus *et al.* 1998, Feskanich *et al.* 2002, Promislow *et al.* 2002, Ribaya-Mercado and Blumberg 2007, Caire-Juvera *et al.* 2009]. If cortical bone thinning and suppression of osteoclastogenesis in cancellous bone play prominent roles in fracture incidence in humans following increased intake of vitamin A, this would be substantially different from conditions such as postmenopausal osteoporosis and glucocorticoid excess, where the increased incidence of fracture is due primarily to cancellous bone loss. These different paradigms for bone fragility may help explain some of the differing outcomes in studies evaluating vitamin A intake and fracture risk. It also seems possible that a duality of retinoid action on osteoclast precursors in cortical and cancellous bone might be manifest as different degrees of cortical resorption and cancellous inhibition, depending on other systemic and environmental factors. This would also affect bone mass and fracture risk, as would the development of hypoxia and death of endosteal osteoclasts. Our improving understanding of vitamin A action in bone cells is not only promising to be extremely valuable for future experimentation, but appears to warrant new evaluations of bone mass and fracture risk in patients with increased intake of vitamin A as well.

7. Acknowledgements

Studies performed in the author´s laboratories were supported by grants from the Swedish Research Council, Swedish Dental Society, the Royal 80 Year Fund of King Gustav V, the Swedish Rheumatism Association, Medical Faculty at Umeå University, Combine, ALF/LUA grants from the Sahlgrenska University Hospital and the County Council of Västerbotten.

8. References

Askmyr M, Sims NA, Martin TJ, Purton LE. (2009) What is the true nature of the osteoblastic hematopoetic stem cell niche? *Trends Endocrinol Metab* 20:303-309

Balkan W, Rodríguez-Gonzales M, Pang M, Fernandez I, Troen BR. (2011) Retinoic acid inhibits Nfatc1 expression and osteoclast differentiation. *J Bone Miner Metab* Epub ahead of print 2011

Bastien, J., and Rochette-Egly, C. (2004) Nuclear retinoid receptors and the transcription of retinoid-target genes. *Gene* 328, 1–16

Berry, D.C., and Noy, N. (2007) Is PPARβ/δ a retinoid receptor? *PPAR. Res.* 73256:1-5

Bocher, V., Pineda-Torra, I., Fruchart, J.C., and Staels, B. (2002) PPARs: transcription factors controlling lipid and lipoprotein metabolism. *Ann. N. Y. Acad. Sci.* 967:7-18

Boyce BF, Yao Z, Xing L. (2009) Osteoclasts have multiple roles in bone in addition to bone resorption. Crit Rev *Eukaryot Gene Expr* 19:171-180

Boyce BF, Yao Z, Xing L. (2010) Functions of nuclear factor κB in bone. *Ann NY Acad Sci* 1192:367-375

Caire-Juvera, G., Ritenbaugh, C., Wactawski-Wende, J., Snetselaar, L., G. and Chen, Z. (2009) Vitamin A and retinol intakes and the risks of fractures among participants of the Women's Health Observational Study. *Am. J. Clin. Nutr.* 89: 323-330

Chambon, P.(1996) A decade of molecular biology of retinoic acid receptors *FASEB J* 10, 940-954

Chang MK, Raggatt LJ, Alexander KA, Kuliwaba JS, Fazzalari NL, Schroder K, Maylin ER, Ripoll VM, Hume DA, Pettit AR. (2008) Osteal tissue macrophages are intercalated throughout human and mouse bone lining tissues and regulate osteoblast function in vitro and in vivo. *J Immunol* 181:1232-44

Chiba M, Teitelbaum SL, Cao X, Ross FP. (1996) Retinoic acid stimulates expression of the functional osteoclast integrin $\alpha_v\beta_3$: transcriptional activation of the β_3 but not the α_v gene. *J Cell Biochem* 62:467-475

Colucci S, Grano M, Mori G, Scotlandi K, Mastrogiacomo M, Mori C, Zambonin Zallone A. (1996) Retinoic acid induces cell proliferation and modulated gelatinases activity in human osteoclast-like cell lines. *Biochem Biophys Res Commun* 227:47-52

Conaway HH, Grigorie D, Lerner UH. (1997) Differential effects of glucocorticoids on bone resorption in neonatal mouse calvariae stimulated by peptide and steroid-like hormones. *J Endocrinol* 155:513-521

Conaway HH, Persson E, Halén M, Granholm S, Svensson O, Pettersson U, Lie A, Lerner UH. (2009) Retinoids inhibit differentiation of hematopoetic osteoclast progenitors. *FASEB J* 23:3526-3538

Confavreux CB, Levine RL, Karsenty G. (2009) A paradigm of integrative physiology, the crosstalk between bone and energy metabolism. *Mol Cell Endocrinol* 310:21-29

Delaissé JM, Eeckhout Y, Vaes G. (1988) Bone-resorbing agents affect the production and distribution of procollagenase as well as the activity of collagenase in bone tissue. *Endocrinology* 123:264-276

Edwards JR, Mundy GR. (2011) Advances in osteoclast biology: old findings and new insights from mouse models. *Nat Rev* Rheumatol EPUB ahead of print

Everts V, de Vries TJ, Helfrich MH. (2009) Osteoclast heterogeneity: lessons from osteopetrosis and inflammatory conditions. *Biochim Biophys Acta* 1792:757-765

Fell HB, Mellanby E. (1952) The effect of hypervitaminosis A on embryonic limb-bones cultivated in vitro. *J Physiol* 116:320-349

Feskanich, D., Singh, V., Willett, W.C. and Colditz, G.A. (2002) Vitamin A intake and hip fractures among postmenopausal women. *JAMA* 287:47-54

Frame, B., Jackson, C.E., Reynolds, W. A. and Umphrey, J. E. (1974) Hypercalcemia and skeletal effects in chronic hypervitaminous A. *Annals of Internal Medicine* 80:44-48

Frankel, T.L., Seshadri, M.S., McDowall, D.B., and Cornish, C.J. (1986) Hypervitaminosis A and calcium-regulating hormones in the rat. *J. Nutr.* 116:578-587

Hata K, Kukita T, Akamine A, Kukita A, Kurisu K. (1992) Trypsinized osteoclast-like multinucleated cells formed in rat bone marrow cultures efficiently form resorption lacunae on dentine. *Bone* 13:139-146

Henning P, Pirhayati A, Pettersson U, Svensson O, Conaway HH, Lerner UH. (2011) Stimulation of mouse calvarial periosteal resorption and inhibition of osteoclast formation in human peripheral CD14+ cells by vitamin A. Abstract at 3rd Joint Meeting European Calcified Tissue Society and International Bone and Mineral Society, Athens May 7-11, 2011.

Henriksen K, Bollerslev J, Everts V, Karsdal MA. (2011) Osteoclast activity and subtypes as a function of physiology and pathology – implications for future treatments of osteoporosis. *Endocr Rev* 32:31-63

Hough, S., Avioli, L.V., Muir, H., Gelderblom, D., Jenkins, G., Kurasi, H., Slatopolsky, E., Bergfeld, M.A. and Teitelbaum, S. L. (1988) Effects of hypervitaminosis A on the bone and mineral metabolism of the rat. *Endocrinology* 122:2933-2939

Hu L, Lind T, Sundqvist A, Jacobson A, Melhus H. (2010) Retinoic acid increases proliferation of human osteoclast progenitors and inhibits RANKL-stimulated osteoclast differentiation by suppressing RANK. *PLoS One* 5:e13305

Jacobson A, Johansson S, Branting M, Melhus H. (2004) Vitamin A differentially regulates RANKL and OPG expression in human osteoblasts. *Biochem Biophys Res Commun* 322:162-167

Johansson, S., Lind, P.M., Håkansson, H., Oxlund, H., Orberg, J., and Melhus, H. (2002) Subclinical hypervitaminosis A causes fragile bones in rats. *Bone* 31:685-689

Kindmark A, Melhus H, Ljunghall S, Ljunggren Ö. (1995) Inhibitory effects of 9-cis and all-trans retinoic acid on 1,25(OH)$_2$ vitamin D$_3$-induced bone resorption. *Calcif Tissue Int* 57:242-244

Kollet O, Dar A, Shivtiel S, Kalinkovich A, Lapid K, Sztainberg Y, Tesio M, Samstein RM, Goichberg P, Spiegel A, Elson A, Lapidot T. (2006) Osteoclasts degrade endosteal components and promote mobilization of hematopoetic progenitor cells. *Nat Med* 12:657-664

Kneissel, M., Studer, A. and Cortesi, M. S. (2005) Retinoid-induced bone thinning by subperiosteal osteoclast activity in adult rodents. *Bone* 36, 202-214

Lakkakorpi PT, Väänänen HK. (1991) Kinetics of the osteoclast cytoskeleton during the resorption cycle in vitro. *J Bone Miner Res* 6:817-826

Lind, T., Lind, P.M., Jacobson, A., Hu, L., Sundqvist, A., Risteli, J., Yebra-Rodriguez, A., Rodriguez-Navarro, A., Andersson, G. and Melhaus, H. (2011) High dietary intake of retinol leads to bone marrow hypoxia and diaphyseal endosteal mineralization in rats. *Bone* 48, 496-506

Lorenzo J, Horowitz M, Choi Y. (2008) Osteoimmunology: interactions of the bone and immune system. *Endocr Rev* 29: 403-440

Mangelsdorf, D.J., and Evans, R.M. (1995) The RXR heterodimers and orphan receptors. *Cell* 83:841-850

Mark, M., Ghyselinck, N.B., and Chambon, P. (2006) Function of retinoid nuclear receptors: lessons from genetic and pharmacological dissections of the retinoic acid signaling pathway during mouse embryogenesis. *Annu. Rev. Pharmacol. Toxicol.* 46: 451-480

Mark, M., Ghyselinck, N.B., and Chambon, P. (2009) Function of retinoic acid receptors during embryonic development. *Nuclear Receptor Signaling* 7, e002

Martin TJ, Seeman E. (2008) Bone remodeling: its local regulation and the emergence of bone fragility. Best Pract Res *Clin Endocrinol Metab* 22:701-722

Martin TJ, Sims NA. (2005) Osteoclast-derived activity in the coupling of bone formation to resorption. *Trends Mol Med* 11:76-81

Martin TJ, Gooi JH, Sims NA. (2009) Molecular mechanisms in coupling of bone formation to resorption. *Crit Rev Eukaryot Gene Expr* 19:73-88

Melhus, H., Michaelsson, K., Kindmark, A., Bergstrom, R., Holmberg, L., Mallmin, H., Wolk, A. and Ljunghall, S. (1998) Excessive dietary intake of vitamin A is associated with reduced bone mineral density and increased risk of hip fracture. *Ann. Intern. Med.* 129:770-778

Mic, F. A., Molotkov, A., Benbrook, D. M., and Duester, G. (2003) Retinoid activation of retinoid acid receptor but not retinoid X receptor is sufficient to rescue lethal defect in retinoic acid synthesis. *Proc. Natl. Acad. Sci. U. S. A.* 100, 7125–7140

Michaelsson, K., Lithell, H., Vessby, B. and Melhus, H. (2003) Serum retinol levels and the risk of fracture. *N. Engl. J. Med.* 348:287-294

Moise, A.R., Noy, N., Palcqewski, K., and Blaner, W.S. (2007) Delivery of retinoid-based therapies to target tissues. *Biochemistry* 46, 4449- 4458

Nakashima T, Takayanagi H. (2009) Osteoclasts and the immune system. *J Bone Miner Metab* 27:519-529

Negishi-Koga T, Takayanagi H. (2009) Ca^{2+}-NFATc1 signalling is an essential axis of osteoclast differentiation. *Immunol Rev* 231:241-256

Nemeth K, Schoppet M, Al-Fakhri N, Helas S, Jessberger R, Hofbauer LC, Goettsch C. (2011) The role of osteoclast-associated receptor in osteoimmunology. *J Immunol* 186:13-18

O'Neill RPJ, Jones JS, Boyde A, Taylor ML, Arnett TR. (1992) Effect of retinoic acid on the resorptive activity of chick osteoclasts in vitro. *Bone* 13:23-27

Oreffo RO, Teti A, Triffitt JT, Francis MJ, Carano A, Zallone AZ. (1988) Effect of vitamin A on bone resorption: evidence for direct stimulation of isolated chicken osteoclasts by retinol and retinoic acid. *J Bone Miner Res* 3:203-210

Peck, G.L.,Olsen, T.G., Yoder, F.W., Peck GL, Olsen TG, Yoder FW, Strauss JS, Downing DT, Pandya M, Butkus D, Arnaud-Battandier J.(1979) Prolonged remissions of cystic and conglobate acne with 13-cis-r retinoic acid . *N. Engl. J. Med.* 300: 329-333

Promislow, J.H.E., Goodman-Gruen, D., Slymen, D.J. and Barrett-Connor, E. (2002) Retinol intake and bone mineral density in the elderly: The Rancho Bernardo study. *J. Bone Miner. Res.* 17:1349-1358

Raisz LG. (1965) Bone resorption in tissue culture. Factors influencing the response to parathyroid hormone. *J Clin Invest* 44:103-116

Raisz LG, Simmons HA, Gworek SC, Eilon G. (1977) Studies on congenital osteopetrosis in microphthalmic mice using organ cultures: impairment of bone resorption in response to physiologic stimulators. *J Exp Med* 145:857-865

Ribaya-Mercado, J. D. and Blumberg, J. B. (2007) Vitamin A: Is it a risk factor for osteoporosis and bone fracture? *Nutr. Rev.* 65: 425-438

Saneshige S, Mano H, Tezuka K, Kakudo S, Mori Y, Honda Y, Itabashi A, Yamada T, Miyata K, Hakeda Y, Ishi J, Kumegawa M. (1995) Retinoic acid directly stimulates osteoclastic bone resorption and gene expression of cathepsin K/OC-2. *Biochem J* 309:721-724

Schug, T.T., Berry, D.C., Shaw, N.S., Travis, S.N. and Noy, N. (2007) Opposing effects of retinoic acid on cell growth result from alternate activation of two different nuclear receptors. *Cell* 129:723-733

Siddikuzzaman, Guruvayoorappan, C. and Berlin Grace, V., M. (2010) All trans retinoic acid and cancer. *Immunopharmacol. and Immunotoxicol.* EPUB ahead of print 1-9

Scheven BAA, Hamilton NJ. (1990) Retinoic acid and 1,25(OH)$_2$-vitamin D$_3$ stimulate osteoclast formation by different mechanisms. *Bone* 11:53-59

Takayanagi H. (2009) Osteoimmunology and the effects of the immune system on bone. Nat Rev Rheumatol 5:667-676

Thavarajah M, Evans DB, Kanis JA. (1991) 1,25(OH)$_2$D$_3$ induces differentiation of osteoclast-like cells from human bone marrow cultures. *Biochem Biophys Res Commun* 176:1189-1195

Togari A, Kondo M, Arai M, Matsumoto S. (1991) Effects of retinoic acid on bone formation and resorption in cultured mouse calvaria. *Gen Pharmacol* 22:287-292

Vestergaard, P., Rejnmark, L. and Mosekilde,L. (2010) High-dose treatment with vitamin A analogues and risk of fractures. *Arch. Dermatol.* 146:478-482.

Wald, G. (1968) Molecular basis of visual excitation. *Science* 162, 230-239

Wang X, Wu J, Shidoji Y, Muto Y, Ohishi N, Yagi K, Ikegami S, Shinki T, Udagawa N, Suda T, Ishimi Y. (2002) Effects of geranylgeranoic acid in bone: induction of osteoblast differentiation and inhibition of osteoclast formation. *J Bone Miner Res* 17:91-100

Wilson, T.M., Brown, P.J., Sternbach, D.D., and Henke, B.R. (2000) The PPARs: from orphan receptors to drug discovery. *J. Med. Chem.* 43:527-550

Woods C, Domenget C, Solari F, Gandrillon O, Lazarides E, Jurdic P. (1995) Antagonistic role of vitaminD3 and retinoic acid on the differentiation of chicken hematopoetic macrophages into osteoclast precursor cells. *Endocrinology* 136:85-95

Ziouzenkova, O., Orasanu, G., Sharlach, M., Adiyama T. E., Berger, J.P., Viereck, J., Hamilton, J. A., Tang, G., Dolnikowski, G. G., Vogel, S., Duester, G. and Plutzky, J. (2007) Retinaldehyde represses adipogenesis and diet-induced obesity. *Nature Med.* 13: 695-702

8

Monogenic Phosphate Balance Disorders

Helge Raeder, Silje Rafaelsen and Robert Bjerknes
Department of Clinical Medicine, University of Bergen,
Norway

1. Introduction

The last decade has seen that several of the dominant and recessive forms of hypo- and hyperphosphatemic bone disease have received their molecular explanation. This has led to new insight into the pathophysiology of hypo- and hyperphosphatemic bone disease, as well as the understanding of a bone-kidney axis which operates integrated and in parallel with the classical parathyroid-kidney axis in the regulation of phosphorus content in the body. In addition, it has led to the recognition of a Janus face of some of the involved genes, showing both hyper- and hypofunction, dependent on the nature of the mutation. In this book chapter, we will present an update on the emerging insight of monogenic hypo- and hyperphosphatemic disorders.

2. Genetic mechanisms and pathophysiology

Hypophosphatemia may lead to bone or dental disease resulting from decreased mineralization (calcification) of bone or dental matrix or osteoid. The simultaneous blood calcium levels will also influence the degree of mineralization. Hypophosphatemia leads to rickets in children or to osteomalacia in adults. In many of the hypophosphatemic conditions, there is also an impairment of renal activation of vitamin D, further aggravating disease. The mineralization of teeth can also be affected, and there are clinical forms where bone affection is minimal and the dental disorders dominate.

Hyperphosphatemia may lead to increased mineralization of both bone and non-bone tissues (ectopic calcification) due to an increase in the body content of phosphorus. This results in tumoral calcinosis with calcification of muscles, skin and vessels. The monogenic forms affect the renal handling of phosphorus by various mechanisms resulting from inactivation or activation of the involved genes.

With the advancement of genetic insight and the subsequent possibility to study subjects with mutations and a wide range of phenotypes, a broader phenotypic pattern is recognized. Consequently, we suggest the more appropriate terms of monogenic hypophosphatemia and monogenic hyperphosphatemia for these disorders, and that the specific disorders should be classified according to the affected gene, e.g. *PHEX*-hypophosphatemia and *FGF23*-hyperphosphatemia (Table 1).

We will now provide an overview of the genes directly implicated in monogenic phosphate balance disorders. Please refer to textbooks for a discussion of genes indirectly affecting phosphate balance (i.e. genes leading to defective parathyroid gland development or disrupted PTH receptor function).

Gene	Classical disease name	Suggested new name
PHEX	X-linked dominant hypophosphatemic rickets	*PHEX*-hypophosphatemia
DMP1	AR hypophosphatemic rickets	*DMP1*-hypophosphatemia
GALNT3	Familial hyperphosphatemic tumoral calcinosis	*GALNT3*-hyperphosphatemia
FGF23	AD hypophosphatemic rickets	*FGF23*- hypophosphatemia
	Familial hyperphosphatemic tumoral calcinosis	*FGF23*- hyperphosphatemia
FGFR1	Osteogophonic dysplasia with hypophosphatemia	*FGFR1*- hypophosphatemia
KL	Hypophosphatemic rickets and hyperparathyroidism	*KL*-hypophosphatemia
	Hyperphosphatemic tumoral calcinosis	*KL*-hyperphosphatemia
SLC34A1	Hypophosphatemic nefrolithiasis/osteoporosis	*SLC34A1*-hypophosphatemia
SLC34A3	HHRH	*SLC34A1*-hypophosphatemia
SLC9A3R1	Hypophosphatemic nephrolithiasis/osteoporosis	*SLC9A3R1*-hypophosphatemia
ENPP1	AR hypophosphatemic rickets, type 2	*ENPP1*-hypophosphatemia

Table 1. Overview of genes directly implicated in monogenic phosphate balance disorders AR, autosomal recessive; AD autosomal dominant, HHRH, Hereditary hypophosphatemic rickets with hypercalciuria.

2.1 PHEX

The *PHEX* (Phosphate-regulating endopeptidase homolog, XB; MIM* 300550) gene consists of 22 exons (Sabbagh, Boileau et al. 2003) and was positionally cloned in 1995 (HYP Consortium 1995). This gene is encoding a transmembrane protein and belongs to the type II integral membrane zinc-dependent endopeptidase family. The gene is expressed in a wide variety of tissues including the kidney with a higher expression in mature osteoblasts and odontoblasts. The substrate for the gene product is not known, but the pathogenesis seems to involve phosphate regulating humoral factors, phosphatonins, where the fibroblast growth factor-23 (FGFR-23) is central (Jonsson, Zahradnik et al. 2003; Juppner 2007; Bastepe and Juppner 2008). (See section 2.11 for a discussion on the physiological and pathophysiological mechanisms involved.) The protein is also believed to be involved in bone and dentin mineralization. Both the whole-body and bone-specific (osteocalcin-promoted inactivation) knockout mouse model of PHEX as well as the spontaneous Hyp mouse model display increased bone production, increased levels of serum FGF23, decreased kidney membrane NPT2 and osteomalacia (Yuan, Takaiwa et al. 2008). Cell studies indicate mechanistic defects both during protein processing in the endoplasmic reticulum and cell membrane (Sabbagh, Boileau et al. 2001) and as abrogated catalytic activity (Sabbagh, Boileau et al. 2003).

There are several mutations associated with PHEX-hypophosphatemia (see the PHEX mutation database: http://www.phexdb.mcgill.ca/) and most of the mutations are located in the region encoding the extracellular domain, but there are also examples of pathological mutations in the 5'UTR (Dixon, Christie et al. 1998) and 3'UTR (Ichikawa, Traxler et al. 2008) of the gene.

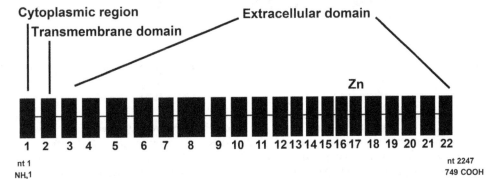

Fig. 1. *PHEX* gene structure and the corresponding encoded regions. Adapted from (Sabbagh, Boileau et al. 2003).

There is no clear genotype-phenotype correlation (Holm, Nelson et al. 2001). There is a slight dominance of familiar mutations (showing co-segregation with disease in a pedigree) to *de novo* mutations (sporadic) reported in literature (Holm, Nelson et al. 2001). The penetrance is high, although there are examples of non-penetrance (Gaucher, Walrant-Debray et al. 2009). The expressivity varies (Brame, White et al. 2004).

2.2 DMP1

The *DMP1* gene (dentin matrix acidic phosphoprotein 1; MIM* 600980) gene consists of 6 exons on chromosome 4q21, and was first implicated in a phosphate balance disorder in 2006 Lorenz-Depiereux, Bastepe et al. 2006). *DMP1* is highly expressed in osteocytes, and is a member of the 'SIBLING' (small integrin binding ligand n-linked glycoprotein) family of non-collagenous extracellular matrix proteins involved in bone mineralization (Huq, Cross et al. 2005). The *DMP1* knockout model displays rickets and osteomalacia with isolated renal phosphate wasting associated with elevated FGF23 levels and normocalciuria (Feng, Ward et al. 2006). In humans, homozygous or compound heterozygous mutations in *DMP1* leads to hypophosphatemic rickets with elevated FGF23, isolated phosphate wasting, and no evidence of hypercalciuria. The exact relation between DMP1 and FGF23 levels is not known, but in vitro studies have shown that vitamin D increases the expression of both (Farrow, Davis et al. 2009).

There are only a few reported mutations in the literature (Feng, Ward et al. 2006; Lorenz-Depiereux, Bastepe et al. 2006; Farrow, Davis et al. 2009; Koshida, Yamaguchi et al. 2010; Makitie, Pereira et al. 2010; Turan, Aydin et al. 2010), making *DMP1* mutations a rare cause of hypophosphatemic rickets (Gaucher, Walrant-Debray et al. 2009).

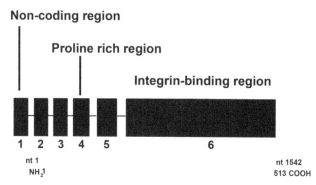

Fig. 2. *DMP1* gene structure and the corresponding encoded regions. Based on (Huq, Cross et al. 2005).

2.3 GALNT3

The O-glycosylation of serine and threonine residues on many glycoproteins depend on enzymatic catalyzation of the reaction UDP-GalNAc + polypeptide-(Ser/Thr)-OH to GalNAc-alpha-O-Ser/Thr-polypeptide + UDP. GalNAcT3 is one of 24 members in the UDP-GalNAc:polypeptide N-acetylgalactosaminyltransferase protein family involved in this process.

GalNAcT3 is encoded by the *GALNT3* gene (MIM *601756) on chromosome 2q24-q31, which contains 10 exons. GalNAcT3 is thought to protect FGF23 from proteolysis (Kato, Jeanneau et al. 2006) by O-glycosylation, and a deactivating mutation in *GALNT3* will thus lead to increased breakdown of FGF23. Mutations in *GALNT3* were the first to be associated with familial tumoral calcinosis (FTC) (Topaz, Shurman et al. 2004), and are also seen in the closely related disease, the hyperphosphatemic hyperostosis syndrome (HHS). These are the only diseases known to be caused by mutations in the family of UDP-GalNAc:polypeptide N-acetylgalactosaminyltransferases. Although the process of O-glycosylation is important in many tissues, mutations in *GALNT3* lead to a very restricted phenotype with hyperphosphatemia, periarticular calcifications and hyperostosis. This is thought to be explained by functional redundancy of this protein family. In addition to the effects on bone and renal phosphate handling caused by altered FGF23 metabolism, mutations in *GALNT3* are also thought to have direct effect in the process of ectopic calcification in extraosseous tissues (Chefetz and Sprecher 2009).

2.4 FGF23

The *FGF23* gene (MIM*605380) on chromosome 12 is composed of 3 exons, and encodes a member of the fibroblast growth factor family. The protein product, FGF23, acts via its receptor FGFR1 (fibroblast growth factor receptor 1, see 2.5), but is also dependent on the co-receptor Klotho (α-Klotho) to exert its functions (see below). Furthermore, FGF23 belongs to the FGF19 family where the two other family members, FGF19 and FGF21, (also binding to FGFR1) are dependent on ß -Klotho to exert their functions, illustrating the role of a co-receptor to ensure tissue specificity and function (Kurosu, Choi et al. 2007). FGF23 exerts its physiological effects on the kidney by the downregulation of the *CYP27B1* gene leading to a loss of compensatory increase in 1,25(OH)$_2$vitamin D levels, and by the endocytosis of the type IIa and IIc Na/phosphate (Pi) cotransporters (Npt2a and Npt2c) from the renal proximal tubular brush border membrane.

Heterozygous activating mutations in the cleavage site RXXR motif of exon 3 of *FGF23*, leads to stabilization and decreased degradation of the FGF23. The clinical phenotype is autosomal dominant hypophosphatemic rickets (Econs, McEnery et al. 1997; 2000).

Homozygous inactivating missense mutations in *FGF23* lead to hyperphosphatemic familial tumoral calcinosis, due to decreased renal excretion of phosphate and increased renal α-hydroxylation of vitamin D (Benet-Pages, Orlik et al. 2005; Ichikawa, Baujat et al. 2010).

2.5 FGFR1

The Fibroblast growth factor receptor 1 gene *FGFR1* (MIM*136315) located on chromosome 8p11 encodes a protein member of the FGFR (1-4) family, where the members are all receptor tyrosine kinases. FGFR1-3 are implicated in skeletal development, and various mutations in the corresponding genes are responsible for a number of skeletal dysplastic syndromes (Passos-Bueno, Wilcox et al. 1999). There are several subclasses of FGFRs, depending on the number of immunoglobulin-like loops and splicing differences in the third loop. FGFR1C combines with Klotho (*KL*) to become the functional receptor for FGF23 (Urakawa, Yamazaki et al. 2006).

Mutations in the *FGFR1C* lead to constitutive activation of the receptor and subsequent downregulation of the expression of the sodium-phosphate co-transporters NaPiIIa and NaPiIIc, as well as the downregulation of the *CYP27B1* gene leading to a loss of compensatory increase in 1,25(OH)$_2$vitamin D levels (Shimada, Hasegawa et al. 2004).

2.6 *KL*

Klotho (*KL*) (MIM*604824) is located to chromosome 13q12, comprises 5 exons, and encodes the protein Klotho (also known as α-Klotho), which in mice is considered a hormone with anti-aging properties (Kurosu, Yamamoto et al. 2005). *KL* knockout mice will go through a rapid aging process, and have decreased insulin secretion and increased insulin sensitivity (Kuro-o, Matsumura et al. 1997), while overexpression of *KL* leads to a prolonged life span in mice (Kurosu, Yamamoto et al. 2005). In addition, Klotho has been associated with disturbances of phosphate metabolism, as it is an obligate co-receptor for the binding of FGF23 to FGFR1C. In humans, there are two *KL* transcripts; one encoding a membrane bound protein and one encoding a secreted protein. Human *KL* is expressed mainly in the kidney, and the secreted variant seems to dominate (Matsumura, Aizawa et al. 1998). Recent findings from mouse studies suggest that Klotho has endocrine, paracrine and autocrine effects independent of FGF23 (Hu, Shi et al. 2010).

Inactivating mutations will lead to familial hyperphosphatemic tumoral calcinosis, similar to the phenotypes seen in *GALNT3*-hyperphosphatemia and *FGF23*-hyperphosphatemia (Ichikawa, Imel et al. 2007).

There is also one report of an activating translocation of the *KL* gene, leading to hypophosphatemic rickets with a phenotype similar to *PHEX*-hypophosphatemia but with additional distinctive dysmorphic features of the head (Brownstein, Adler et al. 2008).

2.7 SLC34A1

The solute carrier 34 (*SLC34*) gene family includes the three genes *SLC34A1*, *SLC34A2* and *SLC34A3*, all encoding sodium/phosphate cotransporters. *SLC34A2* encodes the intestinal NaPi-IIb, and will not be further discussed. *SLC34A1* and *SLC34A3* encode the two renal sodium/phosphate cotransporters, and the latter is described in 2.8 section.

The *SLC34A1* (MIM*182309) gene is expressed in the renal proximal tubule, and encodes the type IIa Na/Pi cotransporter (NaPi-IIa), which plays a central role in renal phosphate handling in various animal models. The expression of NaPi-IIa in the brush border membrane is regulated at the post translational level, by endocytosis and lysosomal degradation or microtubular recruitment (Tenenhouse 2005). Both PTH and FGF23 lead to increased endocytosis of NAPi-IIa, and thus decreased reabsorption of Pi from filtered urine, whereas hypophosphatemia and 1,25 dihydroxyvitamin D stimulate phosphate reabsorption (Tenenhouse 2005). There also seems to be a directly regulating effect of dietary Pi on Na/Pi cotransport in proximal tubules, and the existence of an intestinal-renal axis for phosphate regulation has been proposed [review: (Biber, Hernando et al. 2009)]. NaPi-IIa double knockout mice have hypophosphatemia, phosphaturia, elevated 1,25 dihydroxyvitamin D with resulting hypercalcemia, hypercalcuria and nephrocalcinosis/nephrolithiasis (Beck, Karaplis et al. 1998). This phenotype resembles hereditary hypophosphatemic rickets with hypercalcuria (HHRH) seen in humans, which interestingly is not caused by mutations in *SLCA34A1*, but rather by mutations in *SLC34A3* (NaPi-IIc) (see 2.8).

In man, a few cases have been described of heterozygous mutations in *SLC34A1*, leading to a syndrome of hypophosphatemia, osteoporosis and nephrolithiasis (Prie, Huart et al. 2002).

2.8 SLC34A3

The human *SLC34A3* (MIM*609826) gene, consists of 13 exons on chromosome 9q34, and homozygous mutations in this gene lead to hereditary hypophosphatemic rickets with hypercalciuria (HHRH) (Bergwitz, Roslin et al. 2006; Lorenz-Depiereux, Benet-Pages et al. 2006). The phenotype of HHRH resembles that of NaPi-IIa knockout mice, but the patients also display rickets or osteomalacia. In animal models the type IIc Na/Pi cotransporter (NaPi-IIc) has been shown to play a more minor role in proximal tubular phosphate resorption than NaPi-IIa. The opposite might be the case in man (Amatschek, Haller et al. 2010).

2.9 SLC9A3R1

The *SLC9A3R1* (MIM*604990) gene on chromosome 17 encodes the protein NHERF1 (sodium/hydrogen exchanger regulatory factor 1), which plays a part in maintaining the cytoskeleton in polarized cells with microvilli, such as renal tubular cells. Three different mutations in *SLC9A3R1* have recently been identified in 7 subjects with hypophosphatemia due to phosphaturia, nephrolithiasis and osteoporosis (Karim, Gerard et al. 2008).

2.10 ENPP1

The *ENPP1* (ectonucleotide pyrophosphatase/phosphodiesterase 1) (MIM*173335) gene on chromosome 6q22-q23 comprises 23 exones and encodes a type II transmembrane glycoprotein ectoenzyme responsible for the generation of inorganic pyrophosphate (PPi). PPi is an inhibitor of hydroxyapatite crystal growth, and also suppress chondrogenesis. In mice, *ENPP1* is expressed in plasma cells, on hepatocytes, renal tubules, salivary duct epithelium, epididymis, capillary endothelium in the brain, and chondrocytes (Harahap and Goding 1988). In man it has been shown that *ENPP1* is expressed in liver, cartilage and bone, and is thought to regulate physiological mineralization processes and pathological chondrocalcinosis (Huang, Rosenbach et al. 1994).

Homozygous mutations in *ENPP1* are known to cause generalized arterial calcifications of infancy (GACI) (Rutsch, Vaingankar et al. 2001; Rutsch, Ruf et al. 2003). Recently, homozygous mutations in *ENPP1* have been shown to cause autosomal recessive hypophosphataemic rickets (Levy-Litan, Hershkovitz et al. 2010). In some families, identical mutations cause GACI in some family members and hypophosphatemic rickets in other family members (Lorenz-Depiereux, Schnabel et al. 2010). Prolonged survival in GACI has been observed in subjects who have simultaneously displayed renal phosphate loss (Rutsch, Boyer et al. 2008).

Mutations in *ENPP1* have also been associated with susceptibility to insulin resistance and obesity (Goldfine, Maddux et al. 2008).

2.11 An integrated model for the physiological and pathophysiological mechanisms in the renal phosphate regulation

Figure 3 shows the integrated physiological and pathophysiological mechanisms in the renal phosphate regulation. The parathyroid-renal axis has been the traditional model explaining how PTH stimulates the renal tubular cells to phosphaturia as a negative feedback loop response to elevated phosphate levels (Figure 3A). In this model PTH acts via its receptor to block the sodium-phosphate co-transporters NaPiIIa and NaPiIIc encoded by the *SLC34A1* and *SLC34A3* genes, respectively. In addition, PTH stimulates the *CYP27B1* gene leading to a compensatory increase in 1,25(OH)$_2$vitamin D levels as a negative feedback loop to reduced serum levels of 1,25(OH)$_2$vitamin D and calcium. There is, however, also a PTH-independent pathway where hormonal substances from bone, phosphatonins, stimulate the renal tubular cells to phosphaturia in a negative feedback response to elevated serum phosphate and 1,25(OH)$_2$vitamin D levels. Recent emerging insight has laid the foundation for this model of a bone-kidney axis (Quarles 2003), where fibroblast growth factor 23 (FGF23) seems to be the central phosphatonin inhibiting phosphate reabsorption and hence inducing phosphaturia (Figure 3B). In contrast to PTH, FGF23 inhibits *CYP27B1* gene leading to an absent compensatory increase in 1,25(OH)$_2$vitamin D levels, recognized by clinicians as inappropriate normal 1,25(OH)$_2$vitamin D levels. In the normal state *PHEX* and *DMP1* gene products seem to inhibit FGF23 production, whereas the *GALNT3* gene product seems to stimulate FGF23 production. By interfering with the bone-kidney axis, increased FGF23 levels seem to play a central role in the pathogenesis of *PHEX*-hypophosphatemia (Jonsson, Zahradnik et al. 2003) (Figure 3C) and potentially also *DMP1*-hypophosphatemia (Lorenz-Depiereux, Bastepe et al. 2006; Turan, Aydin et al. 2010) and *FGF23*- hypophosphatemia (Imel, Hui et al. 2007), but the mechanisms are still poorly known (Strom and Juppner 2008). It is also poorly known how increased FGF23 levels in *FGF23*- hyperphosphatemia and *GALNT3*-

hyperphosphatemia explain the opposite condition of hyperphosphatemia (Topaz, Shurman et al. 2004; Benet-Pages, Orlik et al. 2005). A current model postulates that mutations in *PHEX* lead to increased FGF23 production by cancelled *PHEX*-mediated inhibition of FGF23 production (Figure 3 C).

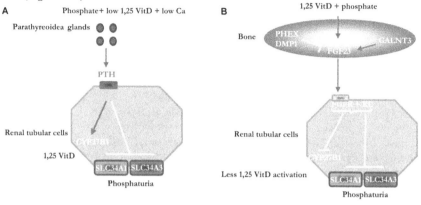

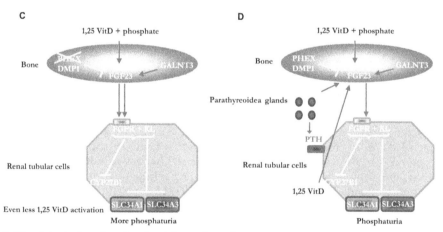

Fig. 3. Physiological and pathophysiological conditions in the phosphate regulation. For sake of clarity, only gene names are depicted and not the corresponding gene products. Adapted from (Bastepe and Juppner 2008; Strom and Juppner 2008).

Both the parathyroid-renal axis and the bone-kidney axis seem to be negative feedback loops where increased serum phosphate levels compared to a biological set value leads to phosphaturia. These two axes are different with respect to 1,25(OH)$_2$vitamin D: Whereas low 1,25(OH)$_2$vitamin D levels stimulating 1,25(OH)$_2$vitamin D activation is the major regulation in the parathyroid-renal axis, high 1,25(OH)$_2$vitamin D levels inhibiting 1,25(OH)$_2$vitamin D activation is the major regulation in the bone-kidney axis. Recent work also points to interactions between these feedback loops where FGF23 inhibits PTH, whereas PTH possibly stimulates FGF23 (Figure 3D). Mutations in genes encoding the sodium-phosphate co-transporters such as *SLC34A1*, *SLC34A3* and *SLC9A3R1* lead to increased phosphaturia but since the 1,25(OH)$_2$vitamin D activation is unaffected, there is a normal compensatory increase in 1,25(OH)$_2$vitamin D levels. Whether gene mutations lead to hypophosphatemia or hyperphosphatemia is dependent on the location of the gene product in the pathways outlined above and whether the mutation is activating or inactivating the affected gene.

3. Diagnostic considerations

The diagnosis of monogenic hypo- or hyperphosphatemia requires the demonstration of affected phosphate balance in patients in which acquired causes of phosphate disturbance have been excluded. A family history of rickets, kidney stones, soft tissue calcification, bone deformities or recurrent fractures, as well as an indication of monogenic inheritance pattern is usually found, unless the patient seems to represent a sporadic case. In the case of hypophosphatemia, there is typically low plasma phosphate, low renal tubular reabsorption of phosphate (% TRP) and tubular threshold maximum for phosphate for glomerular filtration rate (TmP/GFR), raised alkaline phosphatase, normal PTH, and inappropriate and normal 25(OH) and 1,25(OH)$_2$ vitamin D levels. Moreover, the urinary calcium excretion is normal, whereas X-ray changes may demonstrate rickets or osteomalacia. FGF23 levels are typically high, either due to overproduction or under-catabolism, and in children with rickets, the combined evaluation of FGF23 and PTH leads differential diagnosis in the direction of impaired phosphate homeostasis (high FGF23 and normal PTH) or altered metabolism of vitamin D, calcium or magnesium (low FGF23 and high PTH) (Alon 2010). In the case of hyperphosphatemia, there is usually high plasma phosphate, an inappropriate normal % TRP and TmP/GFR, a low or normal PTH and normal renal function. In some cases, the clinical picture and inheritance pattern will suggest a specific genetic diagnosis, and, in addition, the blood FGF23 levels and hypercalciuria may differentiate between different genetic disorders of phosphate balance, although the clinical role of blood FGF23 levels is at present not fully elucidated.

3.1 PHEX

PHEX-hypophosphatemia (X-linked dominant) is usually a progressive disorder with a typical onset at the age when the child starts to walk. The most common clinical manifestations include genu varus, radiological rickets, short stature, bone pain, dental abscesses and calcification of tendons, ligaments and joint capsules with boys being more severely affected than girls and a wide variation between families (Econs, Samsa et al. 1994; Carpenter 1997; Bastepe and Juppner 2008). Some patients may even have craniosynosteosis and spinal stenosis. Many patients suffer from long lasting dental problems, particularly tooth decay and recurrent spontaneous dental abscesses that occur in the absence of a history of trauma or dental decay. Histological findings include high pulp horns, globular dentin, and defects of dentin and enamel. The primary teeth are most commonly affected, as the mineralization process starts in utero. Permanent teeth develop after birth, and adequate treatment improve development in some cases (Batra, Tejani et al. 2006). In children with rickets, a low serum phosphorus level, combined with high serum alkaline phosphatase and normal serum calcium is typical (Carpenter 1997). Urinary leakage of phosphate is demonstrated by low % TRP and TmP/GFR, whereas urinary calcium is normal. The PTH levels are usually normal or slightly elevated, even before the onset of therapy. The 25(OH)vitamin D is normal, and there is no compensatory increase in 1,25(OH)$_2$vitamin D levels due to defective renal activation of vitamin D, and, hence, no hypercalciuria. The FGF23 levels are increased (Jonsson, Zahradnik et al. 2003), and since the lower extremities are more severely affected than the other parts of the skeleton, radiographs of the knees and ankles will demonstrate the extent of rickets. The diagnosis of *PHEX*-hypophosphatemia is confirmed by genetic analysis.

3.2 DMP1

DMP1-hypophosphatemia (autosomal recessive) is usually a progressive disorder with a typical onset at the age when the child starts to walk. The condition is rarer than *PHEX*-hypophosphatemia, but is phenotypically quite similar to *PHEX*- and *FGF23*-hypophosphatemie. There is no compensatory increase in 1,25(OH)$_2$vitamin D levels due to defective renal activation of vitamin D and hence no hypercalciuria. The circulation levels of FGF23 are increased (Feng, Ward et al. 2006). The degree of skeletal abnormalities varies between families (Makitie, Pereira et al. 2010). Some patients also have dental affection, with hypomineralization, enlarged pulp chambers, and decrease in the dentin and enamel layers, which can cause dental abscesses and loss of teeth (Koshida, Yamaguchi et al. 2010; Turan, Aydin et al. 2010).

3.3 GALNT3

GALNT3-hyperphosphatemia is the result of biallelic mutation in the *GALNT3*-gene, and leads to typical tumoral calcinosis (TC) (Topaz, Shurman et al. 2004) or hyperostosis-hyperphosphatemia syndrome (HHS). There are several mutations in the *GALNT3* gene, and the same mutation can lead to TC in some patients and HHS in other (Ichikawa, Baujat et al. 2010). TC is characterized by ectopic calcifications in soft tissues and around large joints, recognized clinically as palpable masses and/or on radiography. Calcifications may also be found in the retina, in blood vessels, as testicular microlithiasis, and there might be dental abnormalities. HHC is characterized by hyperostosis of long bones, seen radiographically as cortical hyperostosis, diaphysitis and periosteal apposition. The biochemical findings in TC and HHC are similar, with elevated serum phosphate levels, increased or normal 1,25(OH)$_2$vitamin D levels. The levels of serum calcium and parathyroid hormone are normal. Some authors suggest that TC and HHS are clinical variants of the same disease (Ichikawa, Baujat et al. 2010).

3.4 FGF23

FGF23-hypophosphatemia (autosomal dominant) shows a variable age at onset of disease.
The expression of disease varies, and some children may have fracture tendency without skeletal deformities, whereas other children may have only temporary renal phosphate loss (Econs and McEnery 1997). Tooth abscesses and loss also occurs (Imel, Hui et al. 2007).
FGF23-hyperphosphatemia (autosomal recessive) shows typical tumoral calcinosis , or more rarely the hyperostosis-hyperphosphatemia syndrome (Benet-Pages, Orlik et al. 2005).

3.5 FGFR1

FGFR1R-hypophosphatemia is characterized by osteoglophonic dysplasia and can be associated with hypophosphatemia (Farrow, Davis et al. 2006). Clinical features are skeletal abnormalities leading to dwarfism and facial abnormalities similar to achondroplasia. There is often failure of tooth eruption, and mandibular malformations. Patients may also have various degrees of craniosynostosis (White, Cabral et al. 2005).

3.6 *KL*

To date only one case of *KL*-hypophosphatemia has been described in the literature (Brownstein, Adler et al. 2008). A 1-year old girl suffered from poor linear growth and increasing head size. She had clinical and radiological signs of rickets, hypophosphatemia, renal phosphate wasting and elevated levels of parathyroid hormone and alkaline phosphatase. A balanced translocation between chromosomes 9 and 13 was detected (t(9,13)(q21.13;q13.1)). This translocation had led to upregulation of *KL*-transcription. After a few years she demonstrated dysmorphic features of the face, and also an Arnold-Chiari 1 malformation (Brownstein, Adler et al. 2008). Dental affection has not been described.

KL-hyperphosphatemia has also been described in only one report (Ichikawa, Imel et al. 2007). A 13 year old girl presented with severe calcifications in soft tissues and in the vasculature, including the dura and the carotid arteries. In addition to hyperphosphatemia and hypercalcemia, she presented with hyperparathyroidism and elevated levels of FGF23. She had no signs of premature aging, which is seen in *KL* knockout mice. Dental affection has not been described.

3.7 SLC34A1 and SLC34A3

In *SLC34A1*- and *SLC34A3*-hypophosphatemia, there is hypophosphatemic rickets with hypercalciuria without other tubular defects (Tieder, Modai et al. 1985). The inheritance pattern is autosomal recessive. Since there is normal renal activation of vitamin D (in contrast to *PHEX*-hypophosphatemia and *DMP1*-hypophosphatemia), hypophosphatemia leads to a normal compensatory increase in 1,25(OH)$_2$vitamin D levels and increased absorption of calcium and phosphate from the gut.

3.8 SLC9A3R1

A total of 7 cases of SLC9A3R1-hypophosphatemia (hypophosphatemia, nephrolithiasis/osteoporosis) have been described to date (Karim, Gerard et al. 2008). All patients were adults, and had either nephrolithiasis and/or bone demineralization combined with hypophosphatemia and hyperphosphaturia. 1,25 (OH)2 vitamin D levels were either elevated or in the upper normal range. Dental affection has not been described.

3.9 ENPP1

ENPP1-hypophosphatemia (autosomal recessive) has a variable age at onset and a variable phenotype including Generalized Arterial Calcification of Infancy (GACI). Also there seems to be phenotypic variation within the same family among affected subjects carrying the same mutation. Whereas the classic presentation is that of severe arterial calcification leading to death in infancy, some patients have renal phosphate wasting and hypophosphatemia. This phosphate loss seems to attenuate the tendency of arterial calcifications, and is associated with prolonged survival (Lorenz-Depiereux, Schnabel et al. 2010).

4. Management principles

4.1 Hypophosphatemia

Hypophosphatemic rickets is in childhood usually treated with elementary phosphorus at doses preferentially between 30 and 60 (100) mg/kg bodyweight and 24 hours, usually divided by 4-6 doses, whereas the deficient 1,25(OH)$_2$vitamin D production is treated with active vitamin D, e.g. alphacalcidol or calcitriol in doses of 20 to 70 ng/kg bodyweight and 24 hours, usually divided by 2 doses. It should, however, be emphasized that the dosage ranges for both phosphate and active vitamin D are wide, dependent on the severity of the disease, the compliance and the occurrence of complications. In *SLC34A1*- and *SLC34A3*-hypophosphatemia, activation of vitamin D is normal, and, consequently, there is no need for treatment with vitamin D.

It is important to adjust the drug doses individually and bear in mind that insufficient doses of elementary phosphorus and vitamin D may fail to prevent or correct skeletal deformities (rickets, osteomalacia) and can lead to growth retardation. On the other hand, excessive doses may lead to nephrocalcinosis (high phosphate doses), as well as hypercalciuria and hypercalcemia (high vitamin D levels). Secondary (and even tertiary) hyperparathyroidism is seen in patients with insufficient doses of vitamin D or excessive doses of phosphorus. We recommend aiming at normal levels of PTH, which in severe cases may be obtained by adding the calcimimetic drug cinacalcet to the treatment (Raeder, Bjerknes et al. 2008).

Close monitoring is necessary to balance the effects of phosphorus supplement and active vitamin D. Growth, serum calcium, phosphorus, alkaline phosphatase, PTH, as well as urinary calcium/creatinine ratio should be determined every 3-6 months, and X-rays of ankles, knees and wrist should be taken yearly. Renal ultrasound should be obtained yearly to assess nephrocalcinosis.

Supplementary treatment with growth hormone is currently not recommended for the growth retardation caused by hypophosphatemia (Huiming and Chaomin 2005), but may be warranted in selected cases. Corrective osteotomies are seldom necessary in childhood, and it should always be deferred until the rickets has healed. Future therapeutic possibilities may include direct targeting of blood FGF23 levels.

4.2 Hyperphosphatemia

Patients with hyperphosphatemia due to monogenic phosphate balance disorders, i.e. *GALNT3*-hyperphosphatemia, *FGF23*-hyperphosphatemia and *KL*-hyperphosphatemia, develop ectopic and vascular calcifications. Combined use of intestinal phosphate binders and the carbonic anhydrase inhibitor acetazolamide has been reported to lower serum phosphorus levels and reduce tumoral masses in some patients (Garringer, Fisher et al. 2006). However, other reports suggest that neither medical nor surgical treatment seems to be effective in controlling ectopic calcifications in these conditions (Carmichael, Bynum et al. 2009). Future therapeutic possibilities may include direct targeting of blood FGF23 levels.

4.3 Genetic diagnostics and predictive testing

Identification of a specific mutation has important therapeutic and prognostic implications and tailored follow-up as outlined above. Distinction between *PHEX*-hypophosphatemia and *DMP1*-hypophosphatemia can be done clinically based on the inheritance pattern, but in some cases there is an ambiguous inheritance pattern (Figure 4) and a genetic test will resolve this ambiguity.

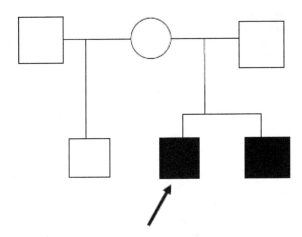

Fig. 4. An example of ambiguous inheritance pattern. Note that in this case, the pattern is compatible both with an X-linked disorder (i.e. *PHEX*-hypophosphatemia) and an AR disorder (i.e. *DMP1*-hypophosphatemia).

Monogenic phosphate balance disorders warrant genetic counseling, because of the known inheritance pattern and the high penetrance. This is also the case for novel gene variants where it is necessary to establish evidence for causality based on co-segregation studies and prediction tools (such as Polyphen http://genetics.bwh.harvard.edu/pph/)). Predictive genetic testing is less straightforward, and the legal regulations vary in different countries. Communicating genetic information can be difficult and it is important to take into account how well the individual understands both genetics in general and the disorder itself and the consequences of potentially diagnosing other family subjects. The basic fact that there is a 25% or 50% probability for a child to carry the family's mutation should be conveyed to the parents. In addition, the probability for the development of the disorder in the presence of a mutation (i.e. the penetrance) is not always 100%. The variable and in some cases unpredictable age of onset of some of the disorders should also be discussed. By increasing knowledge of the clinical spectrum of mutations, novel expected manifestations need to be discussed with the patient. A system for follow-up is required for children without a phenotype but with affected family members and where parents still request that their child be tested. This follow-up may include periodic testing for hypophosphatemia, with a frequency dependent on age and the suspected condition.

5. Research perspectives

We have established a national database of patients with hypophospahtemic bone disorder in order to study phenotype-genotype correlation in this disease and to be able to explore novel pathophysiologic pathways based on insight obtained from studies of families with no previously known genetic cause of monogenic hypophosphatemic bone disorder. We believe that a new classification of disease based on genetic etiology instead of clinical criteria may facilitate the finding of new phenotypes since it will facilitate the study of unobserved phenotypes, both in the patients and in their presumably unaffected relatives carrying mutations. In addition, it is possible that emerging new treatment options may vary based on the genetic diagnosis which warrants studies of associations between gene variants and therapeutic effects. Future studies of monogenic phosphate balance disorders will probably continue to include genomewide studies of families with genetically unexplained phosphate balance disorders. Animal and cell studies will probably also continue to contribute to the understanding of disease mechanism, and, in particular, the use of induced pluripotent stem cells (iPS) seems to be a promising new tool in the mechanistic and therapeutic studies (Rosenzweig 2010) as well as the use of small molecule screens in the search for new therapeutic options in monogenic disease (Shaw, Blodgett et al. 2011) .

6. Conclusion

As we have discussed in this book chapter, several of the dominant and recessive forms of hypo- and hyperphosphatemic bone disease have received their molecular explanation leading to new insight into the pathophysiology of hypo- and hyperphosphatemic bone disease. The major advancement in pathophysiological understanding has come from the understanding of a bone-kidney axis where the central bone phosphatonin FGF23 acts on FGFR1-receptors in the kidneys to promote phosphaturia and from the understanding of all the factors converging on this axis. In fact, this axis ties together the known monogenic forms of renal phosphate disorders. In addition, the understanding of the genetics and pathophysiology of these disorders has led to the recognition of the two faces of some of the involved genes, showing both hyper- and hypofunction, dependent on the nature of the mutation, which is in particular the case for mutations affecting the *KL* and *FGF23* genes.

We recommend the use of a genetic-oriented classification instead of the traditional disease-oriented classification since we believe that this will facilitate a broader understanding of the phenotype of monogenic phosphate balance disorders. Whereas increased molecular understanding has led to a more precise diagnosis, it has not yet led to new established treatment. We believe, however, that the molecular understanding will indeed facilitate the development of new treatment options with the use of the powerful tools including iPS cells and small molecular screens.

7. References

ADHR Consortium (2000). "Autosomal dominant hypophosphataemic rickets is associated with mutations in FGF23." Nat Genet 26(3): 345-348.

Alon, U. S. (2010). "Clinical practice : Fibroblast growth factor (FGF)23: a new hormone." European journal of pediatrics.

Amatschek, S., M. Haller, et al. (2010). "Renal phosphate handling in human--what can we learn from hereditary hypophosphataemias?" Eur J Clin Invest 40(6): 552-560.

Bastepe, M. and H. Juppner (2008). "Inherited hypophosphatemic disorders in children and the evolving mechanisms of phosphate regulation." Rev Endocr Metab Disord 9(2): 171-180.

Batra, P., Z. Tejani, et al. (2006). "X-linked hypophosphatemia: dental and histologic findings." J Can Dent Assoc 72(1): 69-72.

Beck, L., A. C. Karaplis, et al. (1998). "Targeted inactivation of Npt2 in mice leads to severe renal phosphate wasting, hypercalciuria, and skeletal abnormalities." Proc Natl Acad Sci U S A 95(9): 5372-5377.

Benet-Pages, A., P. Orlik, et al. (2005). "An FGF23 missense mutation causes familial tumoral calcinosis with hyperphosphatemia." Hum Mol Genet 14(3): 385-390.

Bergwitz, C., N. M. Roslin, et al. (2006). "SLC34A3 mutations in patients with hereditary hypophosphatemic rickets with hypercalciuria predict a key role for the sodium-phosphate cotransporter NaPi-IIc in maintaining phosphate homeostasis." Am J Hum Genet 78(2): 179-192.

Biber, J., N. Hernando, et al. (2009). "Regulation of phosphate transport in proximal tubules." Pflugers Arch 458(1): 39-52.

Brame, L. A., K. E. White, et al. (2004). "Renal phosphate wasting disorders: clinical features and pathogenesis." Seminars in nephrology 24(1): 39-47.

Brownstein, C. A., F. Adler, et al. (2008). "A translocation causing increased alpha-klotho level results in hypophosphatemic rickets and hyperparathyroidism." Proc Natl Acad Sci U S A 105(9): 3455-3460.

Carmichael, K. D., J. A. Bynum, et al. (2009). "Familial tumoral calcinosis: a forty-year follow-up on one family." The Journal of bone and joint surgery. American volume 91(3): 664-671.

Carpenter, T. O. (1997). "New perspectives on the biology and treatment of X-linked hypophosphatemic rickets." Pediatric clinics of North America 44(2): 443-466.

Chefetz, I. and E. Sprecher (2009). "Familial tumoral calcinosis and the role of O-glycosylation in the maintenance of phosphate homeostasis." Biochim Biophys Acta 1792(9): 847-852.

Dixon, P. H., P. T. Christie, et al. (1998). "Mutational analysis of PHEX gene in X-linked hypophosphatemia." J Clin Endocrinol Metab 83(10): 3615-3623.

Econs, M. J. and P. T. McEnery (1997). "Autosomal dominant hypophosphatemic rickets/osteomalacia: clinical characterization of a novel renal phosphate-wasting disorder." The Journal of clinical endocrinology and metabolism 82(2): 674-681.

Econs, M. J., P. T. McEnery, et al. (1997). "Autosomal dominant hypophosphatemic rickets is linked to chromosome 12p13." J Clin Invest 100(11): 2653-2657.

Econs, M. J., G. P. Samsa, et al. (1994). "X-Linked hypophosphatemic rickets: a disease often unknown to affected patients." Bone and mineral 24(1): 17-24.

Farrow, E. G., S. I. Davis, et al. (2006). "Extended mutational analyses of FGFR1 in osteoglophonic dysplasia." American journal of medical genetics. Part A 140(5): 537-539.

Farrow, E. G., S. I. Davis, et al. (2009). "Molecular analysis of DMP1 mutants causing autosomal recessive hypophosphatemic rickets." Bone 44(2): 287-294.

Feng, J. Q., L. M. Ward, et al. (2006). "Loss of DMP1 causes rickets and osteomalacia and identifies a role for osteocytes in mineral metabolism." Nat Genet 38(11): 1310-1315.

Garringer, H. J., C. Fisher, et al. (2006). "The role of mutant UDP-N-acetyl-alpha-D-galactosamine-polypeptide N-acetylgalactosaminyltransferase 3 in regulating serum intact fibroblast growth factor 23 and matrix extracellular phosphoglycoprotein in heritable tumoral calcinosis." The Journal of clinical endocrinology and metabolism 91(10): 4037-4042.

Gaucher, C., O. Walrant-Debray, et al. (2009). "PHEX analysis in 118 pedigrees reveals new genetic clues in hypophosphatemic rickets." Hum Genet 125(4): 401-411.

Gaucher, C., O. Walrant-Debray, et al. (2009). "PHEX analysis in 118 pedigrees reveals new genetic clues in hypophosphatemic rickets." Human genetics 125(4): 401-411.

Goldfine, I. D., B. A. Maddux, et al. (2008). "The role of membrane glycoprotein plasma cell antigen 1/ectonucleotide pyrophosphatase phosphodiesterase 1 in the pathogenesis of insulin resistance and related abnormalities." Endocr Rev 29(1): 62-75.

Harahap, A. R. and J. W. Goding (1988). "Distribution of the murine plasma cell antigen PC-1 in non-lymphoid tissues." J Immunol 141(7): 2317-2320.

Holm, I. A., A. E. Nelson, et al. (2001). "Mutational analysis and genotype-phenotype correlation of the PHEX gene in X-linked hypophosphatemic rickets." The Journal of clinical endocrinology and metabolism 86(8): 3889-3899.

Hu, M. C., M. Shi, et al. (2010). "Klotho: a novel phosphaturic substance acting as an autocrine enzyme in the renal proximal tubule." FASEB J 24(9): 3438-3450.

Huang, R., M. Rosenbach, et al. (1994). "Expression of the murine plasma cell nucleotide pyrophosphohydrolase PC-1 is shared by human liver, bone, and cartilage cells. Regulation of PC-1 expression in osteosarcoma cells by transforming growth factor-beta." J Clin Invest 94(2): 560-567.

Huiming, Y. and W. Chaomin (2005). "Recombinant growth hormone therapy for X-linked hypophosphatemia in children." Cochrane database of systematic reviews(1): CD004447.

Huq, N. L., K. J. Cross, et al. (2005). "A review of protein structure and gene organisation for proteins associated with mineralised tissue and calcium phosphate stabilisation encoded on human chromosome 4." Archives of oral biology 50(7): 599-609.

HYP Consortium. A gene (PEX) with homologies to endopeptidases is mutated in patients with X-linked hypophosphatemic rickets. Nature Genetics 1995;11:130-6

Ichikawa, S., G. Baujat, et al. (2010). "Clinical variability of familial tumoral calcinosis caused by novel GALNT3 mutations." Am J Med Genet A 152A(4): 896-903.

Ichikawa, S., E. A. Imel, et al. (2007). "A homozygous missense mutation in human KLOTHO causes severe tumoral calcinosis." J Clin Invest 117(9): 2684-2691.

Ichikawa, S., E. A. Imel, et al. (2007). "A homozygous missense mutation in human KLOTHO causes severe tumoral calcinosis." J Musculoskelet Neuronal Interact 7(4): 318-319.

Ichikawa, S., E. A. Traxler, et al. (2008). "Mutational survey of the PHEX gene in patients with X-linked hypophosphatemic rickets." Bone 43(4): 663-666.

Imel, E. A., S. L. Hui, et al. (2007). "FGF23 concentrations vary with disease status in autosomal dominant hypophosphatemic rickets." J Bone Miner Res 22(4): 520-526.

Jonsson, K. B., R. Zahradnik, et al. (2003). "Fibroblast growth factor 23 in oncogenic osteomalacia and X-linked hypophosphatemia." N Engl J Med 348(17): 1656-1663.

Juppner, H. (2007). "Novel regulators of phosphate homeostasis and bone metabolism." Therapeutic apheresis and dialysis : official peer-reviewed journal of the International Society for Apheresis, the Japanese Society for Apheresis, the Japanese Society for Dialysis Therapy 11 Suppl 1: S3-22.

Karim, Z., B. Gerard, et al. (2008). "NHERF1 mutations and responsiveness of renal parathyroid hormone." N Engl J Med 359(11): 1128-1135.

Kato, K., C. Jeanneau, et al. (2006). "Polypeptide GalNAc-transferase T3 and familial tumoral calcinosis. Secretion of fibroblast growth factor 23 requires O-glycosylation." The Journal of biological chemistry 281(27): 18370-18377.

Koshida, R., H. Yamaguchi, et al. (2010). "A novel nonsense mutation in the DMP1 gene in a Japanese family with autosomal recessive hypophosphatemic rickets." J Bone Miner Metab 28(5): 585-590.

Kuro-o, M., Y. Matsumura, et al. (1997). "Mutation of the mouse klotho gene leads to a syndrome resembling ageing." Nature 390(6655): 45-51.

Kurosu, H., M. Choi, et al. (2007). "Tissue-specific expression of betaKlotho and fibroblast growth factor (FGF) receptor isoforms determines metabolic activity of FGF19 and FGF21." The Journal of biological chemistry 282(37): 26687-26695.

Kurosu, H., M. Yamamoto, et al. (2005). "Suppression of aging in mice by the hormone Klotho." Science 309(5742): 1829-1833.

Levy-Litan, V., E. Hershkovitz, et al. (2010). "Autosomal-recessive hypophosphatemic rickets is associated with an inactivation mutation in the ENPP1 gene." Am J Hum Genet 86(2): 273-278.

Lorenz-Depiereux, B., M. Bastepe, et al. (2006). "DMP1 mutations in autosomal recessive hypophosphatemia implicate a bone matrix protein in the regulation of phosphate homeostasis." Nat Genet 38(11): 1248-1250.

Lorenz-Depiereux, B., A. Benet-Pages, et al. (2006). "Hereditary hypophosphatemic rickets with hypercalciuria is caused by mutations in the sodium-phosphate cotransporter gene SLC34A3." Am J Hum Genet 78(2): 193-201.

Lorenz-Depiereux, B., D. Schnabel, et al. (2010). "Loss-of-function ENPP1 mutations cause both generalized arterial calcification of infancy and autosomal-recessive hypophosphatemic rickets." Am J Hum Genet 86(2): 267-272.

Makitie, O., R. C. Pereira, et al. (2010). "Long-term clinical outcome and carrier phenotype in autosomal recessive hypophosphatemia caused by a novel DMP1 mutation." J Bone Miner Res 25(10): 2165-2174.

Matsumura, Y., H. Aizawa, et al. (1998). "Identification of the human klotho gene and its two transcripts encoding membrane and secreted klotho protein." Biochem Biophys Res Commun 242(3): 626-630.

Passos-Bueno, M. R., W. R. Wilcox, et al. (1999). "Clinical spectrum of fibroblast growth factor receptor mutations." Hum Mutat 14(2): 115-125.

Prie, D., V. Huart, et al. (2002). "Nephrolithiasis and osteoporosis associated with hypophosphatemia caused by mutations in the type 2a sodium-phosphate cotransporter." N Engl J Med 347(13): 983-991.

Quarles, L. D. (2003). "Evidence for a bone-kidney axis regulating phosphate homeostasis." J Clin Invest 112(5): 642-646.

Raeder, H., N. Shaw, et al. (2008). "A case of X-linked hypophosphatemic rickets (XLH): complications and the therapeutic use of cinacalcet." Eur J Endocrinol. 159 (Suppl. 1):101-105.

Rosenzweig, A. (2010). "Illuminating the potential of pluripotent stem cells." The New England journal of medicine 363(15): 1471-1472.

Rutsch, F., P. Boyer, et al. (2008). "Hypophosphatemia, hyperphosphaturia, and bisphosphonate treatment are associated with survival beyond infancy in generalized arterial calcification of infancy." Circ Cardiovasc Genet 1(2): 133-140.

Rutsch, F., N. Ruf, et al. (2003). "Mutations in ENPP1 are associated with 'idiopathic' infantile arterial calcification." Nat Genet 34(4): 379-381.

Rutsch, F., S. Vaingankar, et al. (2001). "PC-1 nucleoside triphosphate pyrophosphohydrolase deficiency in idiopathic infantile arterial calcification." Am J Pathol 158(2): 543-554.

Sabbagh, Y., G. Boileau, et al. (2003). "Structure and function of disease-causing missense mutations in the PHEX gene." The Journal of clinical endocrinology and metabolism 88(5): 2213-2222.

Sabbagh, Y., G. Boileau, et al. (2001). "Disease-causing missense mutations in the PHEX gene interfere with membrane targeting of the recombinant protein." Human molecular genetics 10(15): 1539-1546.

Shaw, S. Y., D. M. Blodgett, et al. (2011). "Disease allele-dependent small-molecule sensitivities in blood cells from monogenic diabetes." Proceedings of the National Academy of Sciences of the United States of America 108(2): 492-497.

Shimada, T., H. Hasegawa, et al. (2004). "FGF-23 is a potent regulator of vitamin D metabolism and phosphate homeostasis." J Bone Miner Res 19(3): 429-435.

Strom, T. M. and H. Juppner (2008). "PHEX, FGF23, DMP1 and beyond." Curr Opin Nephrol Hypertens 17(4): 357-362.

Tenenhouse, H. S. (2005). "Regulation of phosphorus homeostasis by the type iia na/phosphate cotransporter." Annu Rev Nutr 25: 197-214.

Tieder, M., D. Modai, et al. (1985). "Hereditary hypophosphatemic rickets with hypercalciuria." The New England journal of medicine 312(10): 611-617.

Topaz, O., D. L. Shurman, et al. (2004). "Mutations in GALNT3, encoding a protein involved in O-linked glycosylation, cause familial tumoral calcinosis." Nat Genet 36(6): 579-581.

Turan, S., C. Aydin, et al. (2010). "Identification of a novel dentin matrix protein-1 (DMP-1) mutation and dental anomalies in a kindred with autosomal recessive hypophosphatemia." Bone 46(2): 402-409.

Urakawa, I., Y. Yamazaki, et al. (2006). "Klotho converts canonical FGF receptor into a specific receptor for FGF23." Nature 444(7120): 770-774.

White, K. E., J. M. Cabral, et al. (2005). "Mutations that cause osteoglophonic dysplasia define novel roles for FGFR1 in bone elongation." Am J Hum Genet 76(2): 361-367.

Yuan, B., M. Takaiwa, et al. (2008). "Aberrant Phex function in osteoblasts and osteocytes alone underlies murine X-linked hypophosphatemia." The Journal of clinical investigation 118(2): 722-734.

9

Environmental Endocrinology: Endocrine Disruptors and Endocrinopathies

Eleni Palioura, Eleni Kandaraki and Evanthia Diamanti-Kandarakis
Medical School University of Athens,
Greece

1. Introduction

An endocrine disruptor (ED) is defined by the US- Environmental Protection Agency as "an exogenous agent that interferes with the production, release, transport, metabolism, binding, action, or elimination of natural hormones in the body responsible for the maintenance of homeostasis, reproduction, development, and/or behavior" (U.S. EPA., 1997). This definition encompasses a rather heterogeneous group of molecules from naturally occurring substances (e.g., phytoestrogens) to biochemically manufactured compounds such as plasticizers, pesticides, industrial solvents, pharmaceutical agents (diethylstilbestrol) and heavy metals.

Endocrine disruptors were originally considered to exert their biological action through nuclear steroid receptors by mimicking or antagonizing natural hormone's action (Waring & Harris, 2005) with the majority of them acting as pseudoestrogens and less possessing anti-androgenic or anti-estrogenic properties (McLachlan et al., 2006). Today, basic scientific research shows that the mechanisms are much broader than originally recognized and include interaction with transcriptional factors, non-nuclear steroid hormone receptors, gene regulation or even transgenerational effects by targeting germ cell lines (Anway & Skinner, 2006, 2008; Tabb & Blumberg, 2006).

In addition, targets for endocrine disruption extend beyond the traditional estrogen/androgen -mediated reproductive system. Within the last few years, scientists also have expressed concern about the potential role of EDs in increasing trends in obesity and diabetes, the major life-threatening diseases of modern word. At present, all hormone-sensitive physiological systems seem to be vulnerable to EDs, including brain and hypothalamic neuroendocrine systems; pituitary; thyroid; cardiovascular system; mammary gland; adipose tissue; pancreas; ovary and uterus in females; and testes and prostate in males (Diamanti-Kandarakis et al., 2009).

Undoubtedly, the issue of endocrine disruption has attracted considerable scientific attention with the weight of data obtained from wildlife populations, animal models and epidemiological studies growing extensively during the last years. After all, the unprecedented increase in the production and use of industrial and agricultural chemicals during last decades makes human exposure inevitable through multiple sources. Adults are exposed mainly through the ingestion of contaminated drinking water, food and breathing polluted air. Infants are exposed to EDs through breast milk, baby products, and polluted air while fetuses are exposed through the placenta and are more vulnerable to harmful, irreversible, pathological changes in adult life. People occupationally exposed to pesticides, fungicides and industrial chemicals are considered to be at highest risk for developing an endocrine abnormality as well as humans acutely exposed to an accidental release of an endocrine disrupting chemical.

This chapter reviews the evidence linking endocrine disrupting chemicals to a broad spectrum of clinical perturbations from reproduction and thyroid to metabolic regulation. A summarized review of literature focused on the strongest experimental data and human epidemiological studies targets to elucidate the underlying interactions between endocrine disruptors and endocrine abnormalities.

2. Reproductive function and endocrine disruptors

Reproductive health is traditionally considered as one of the well-studied fields in endocrine disruption. The effects of EDs on reproduction are amply documented in both wildlife and laboratory populations while interfering with human reproductive function is highly plausible. Establishing causality between human reproductive health and exposure to a certain environmental contaminant is challenging as several confounders need to be taken into account.

A critical concern is the potential lag between exposure to EDs and the manifestation of a reproductive disorder as in humans this period may be years or decades after initial exposure. The timing of exposure is key to human disease as the developmental periods from periconception and during pregnancy, infancy, childhood, and puberty are considered as critical and sensitive windows of susceptibility to environmental insults .Furthermore, chronic exposure to low amounts of mixtures of EDs than acute exposure to a single compound, as in many animal models, is the most possible scenario when studying human reproduction. In addition, as in other systems in the organism, EDs effects on human reproduction could be varied by individual differences in metabolism, body composition and susceptibility due to genetic polymorphisms (Diamanti-Kandarakis et al., 2009).

In the human female, the first evidence of endocrine disruption was provided almost four decades ago by diethylstilbestrol (DES), a synthetic oestrogen prescribed therapeutically in a large scale in the mid-20th century in order to prevent miscarriage in pregnant women. The observation of an uncommon gynecologic neoplasm, vaginal adenocarcinoma, in daughters born 15–22 yr earlier to women treated with this potent synthetic estrogen during pregnancy was the first clinical evidence of DES disruption on reproductive system (Herbst et al., 1971). Posterior studies have identified additional adverse effects in female off springs including increased risk for structural reproductive tract anomalies with a characteristic T-shaped uterus, infertility, menstrual irregularity and poor pregnancy outcomes manifested as spontaneous abortion, ectopic pregnancy, and preterm delivery (Kaufman et al., 1982, 2000; Palmer et al., 2001). Furthermore, DES grand-daughters born to mothers prenatally exposed to diethylstilbestrol exhibit irregular menstrual cycles and possible infertility (Titus-Ernstoff et al., 2006) .These robust clinical observations together with experimental data support the causal role of DES in female reproductive disorders.

Increasing data from wildlife and laboratory studies support a role of EDs in the pathogenesis of several other female reproductive disorders during a broad developmental spectrum from puberty onset to menopause (Diamanti-Kandarakis et al., 2010; McLachlan et al., 2006; Woodruff et al., 2008). The catalogue of reproductive aberrations possible related to

ED exposure is extending to include early/delayed puberty, polycystic ovarian syndrome (PCOS), impaired fertility and fecundity, premature ovarian failure, endometriosis, uterine fibroids, aneuploidy, pregnancy complications as well as breast and endometrial tumors (Caserta et al., 2008; Diamanti-Kandarakis et al., 2009).

To give few examples, earlier menarche onset has been observed in girls exposed to polychlorinated biphenyls(PCBs), polybrominated biphenyls (PBBs), phthalate esters and DDT while there are other data that link phthalates to premature thelarche and increased risk of endometriosis (Woodruff et al., 2008). With regard to human puberty, scientific interest is focused on the potential effect of environmental factors on puberty timing. This is based on the observation that since the 19th century there have been significant modifications in puberty timing with earlier age of thelarche and menarche in girls (Euling et al., 2008a).This puberty timing alteration has been associated, apart from apparent improvements in general health and nutrition, with a potential impact of endocrine-disrupting chemicals, particularly the estrogen mimics and antiandrogens (Euling et al., 2008b, Jacobson-Dickman & Lee, 2009).

Adult female reproductive functions are also disrupted by environmental chemicals with the strongest evidence incriminating heavy metals and especially lead exposure. Most modifiable risk appears to be associated with exposures in unique populations (contaminated fish consumers) or occupational groups (farmworkers) (Mendola et al., 2008). Furthermore, recent evidence imply a potential role of Bisphenol A (BPA) in the PCOS pathophysiology given that in women with PCOS, BPA levels were found to be higher compared to BMI-matched healthy women and also to be positively and strongly associated with androgen levels (Kandaraki et al., 2010). Serum BPA concentrations are significantly higher in men than in women (Takeuchi et al., 2002) and in women with ovulatory dysfunction compared to regularly ovulating women (Takeuchi et al., 2004). As PCOS pathogenesis remains partly unraveled, the role of environmental factors and in particular BPA could also been proposed in PCOS development.

With regard to male reproductive system, research has been mainly focused on three major health endpoints; impaired semen quality and infertility, urogenital tract abnormalities-cryptorchidism and hypospadias- and testicular germ cell cancer. This is probably related to the epidemiologic evidence that suggest a decline in human semen quality over the last 50 years (Carlsen et al., 1992) and temporal increasing trends in the prevalence of urogenital tract malformations such as cryptorchidism and hypospadias (Toppari et al., 2001). Interestingly, it is hypothesized that the above-mentioned abnormalities share a common embryogenic origin as parts of a pathogenic entity coined as "testicular dysgenesis syndrome" (TDS). This hypothesis proposes that a prenatal, synergistic, interaction between environmental, genetic and maternal factors lead to abnormal testis development (dysgenesis)(Skakkebæk et al., 2001) and secondarily to impaired androgen production and germ cell development due to Sertoli and Leydig cells' dysfunction (Sharpe & Skakkebæk, 2003). The existence of TDS as a distinct clinical entity and of possible associations with EDs is an area of active research.

Some substances that have been incriminated to have an aggravating impact on sperm parameters include polychlorinated biphenyls (Dallinga et al., 2002; Hauser et al., 2003), phthalates (Duty et al., 2003; Hauser et al., 2006) and non-persistent pesticides (Juhler et al., 1999; Padungtod et al., 2000).Epidemiologic evidence for EDC exposure and cryptorchidism or hypospadias are limited. Concerning ED exposure and cryptorchidism and/or hypospadias, the strongest epidemiological data are those suggesting an association between residency in agricultural areas and/or measures of direct parental exposure to non-organochlorine pesticides (Diamanti-Kandarakis et al., 2009).

Overall, the epidemiologic data on the environmental EDs suggest that there may be associations between exposure and adverse health outcomes in men. However, the limited human data highlight the need for further research on these chemicals. Future longitudinal epidemiology studies with appropriately designed exposure assessments are needed to determine potential causal relationships, to identify the most important time windows of exposure, and to define individual susceptibility factors for adverse effects on men's health in response to exposure.

3. Thyroid and endocrine disruptors

Thyroid hormones have been evolutionarily preserved as important regulators of development, tissue growth and metabolism among all vertebrates and in some invertebrate species (Heyland and Moroz, 2005). Given their importance for normal physiological processes, considerable concern has aroused regarding the clinical impact of environmental factors on thyroid function to the extent that human could be affected. This interaction is biologically plausible as a variety of heterogeneous synthetic chemicals has been recognized to interfere with thyroid homeostasis by acting on different points of regulation of thyroid hormone synthesis, release, transport through the blood, metabolism and clearance (Howdeshell, 2002) or directly at the receptor level (Zoeller, 2007).

Polychlorinated biphenyls (PCBs), Polybrominated diphenyl ethers (PBDEs), Bisphenol-A, dioxin, Perchlorate and furans have been incriminated as potential disruptors of thyroid homeostasis through their ability to affect the hypothalamic- pituitary- thyroid axis (Boas et al., 2006; Zoeller, 2010). Correlations between levels of these compounds in the body and circulating thyroid hormone levels, thyrotropin levels, thyroid volume and prevalence of thyroid antibodies have been reported by several researchers, however, inconsistency exists across studies (Hagmar et al., 2001; Langer et al., 2008; Meeker et al., 2007).

Literature on thyroid disrupting chemicals includes human epidemiological studies that indicate a potential association between exposure to endocrine disruptors and disturbance of thyroid function (Persky et al., 2001; Steinmaus et al., 2007; Takser et al., 2005) with most data pointing towards subtle alterations of the thyroid axis within normal ranges which may, in turn, be harmful especially for human fetus (Boas et al., 2006). Fetus' growth and brain development are very sensitive to modifications of thyroid homeostasis with a significant risk of neurological and cognitive deficiencies.

Overall, the literature on thyroid-disrupting effects of individual chemicals is rapidly increasing, as animal exposure studies and in vitro tests reveal a multitude of potential mechanisms of action. Quick and robust tools should be developed to identify potential thyroid disrupting chemicals and their multiple mechanisms of action. Furthermore, a better understanding of the mechanisms underlying disruption of the thyroid function may lead to changes in public policy in order to limit adverse outcomes for future generations.

4. Obesity epidemic and endocrine disruptors

A potential role of environmental contaminants on the escalating rates of human obesity has been hypothesized as an exogenous factor that may impair body's natural weight-control mechanisms (Baillie-Hamilton, 2002). As the current epidemic in obesity cannot be solely explained by alterations in food intake, physical activity and/or genetic predispotion, the contribution of environmental factors becomes suspicious.

Research on this field has been mainly focused on the identification of environmental "obesogens", molecules that inappropriately regulate lipid metabolism and adipogenesis and also on the molecular mechanisms underlying these metabolic alterations (Grün et al., 2006; Tabb & Blumberg, 2006). After all, recent epidemiology studies indicate that exposure to EDs during development is associated with overweight and obesity later in life. In a cross-sectional analysis of six urinal phthalates metabolites in a total sample of 4369 participants, positive correlations were observed between body mass index (BMI) and waist circumference and most of the metabolites in adult males (Hatch et al., 2008). High serum Polychlorinated Bisphenyls levels have been associated with high levels of total serum lipids and BMI in a Native American cohort (Goncharov et al., 2008) and prenatal and early life PCB exposures were associated with increased weight in boys and girls at puberty (Gladen et al., 2000).

So far, several experimental data have pointed to the effect of endocrine disrupting chemicals on lipid metabolism suggesting that adipocyte *per se* may represent a cell vulnerable to disruption. A characteristic example of such interaction is provided by the organotin tributyltin (TBT) that has been shown to modulate adipocyte differentiation by acting as an agonist for retinoid X receptor (RXR) and peroxisome proliferators-activated receptor γ (PPAR γ), the nuclear receptors that play important roles in lipid homeostasis and adipogenesis (Grün & Blumberg, 2006; Kanayama et al., 2005). Therefore, as it is speculated by Tabb & Blumberg, chronic life-time or developmental exposure to TBT could activate RXR and/or RXR:PPAR-γ signalling leading to long-term alterations of the total adipocyte number and/or a lipid haemostasis (Tabb & Blumberg, 2006).

Another chemical showed to display "obesogenic" properties *in vivo* is diethylstilbestrol. Female mice neonatally exposed to both low and high doses of this estrogenic compound exhibited increased body weight in adulthood. The low dose did not affect body weight during treatment but was associated with a significant increase in body weight in the adult animal by 4 to 6 months of age while the highest dose resulted in a significant decrease in mice weight during treatment followed by a "catch-up" before puberty and consecutively elevated body weight during adulthood (Newbold et al., 2008). Further studies indicated that the increase in body weight in DES-exposed mice was associated with an increase in the percent of body fat as determined by mouse densitometry (Newbold et al., 2007).

Bisphenol A is also postulated to play a role in the development of obesity by interacting with lipid homeostasis and body weight control mechanisms through pleiotropic modes of action. Micromolar concentrations of BPA were shown to enhance adipocyte differentiation and lipid accumulation in target cells in a dose-dependent manner (Masuno et al., 2002, 2005; Wada et al., 2007). From a molecular perspective, these effects are liked with up-regulation of gene expressions involved in lipid metabolism and adipogenic transcription factors (Phrakonkham et al., 2008; Wada et al., 2007). *In vivo* studies confirm the above observations. Perinatal exposure to low doses of BPA increases adipose storage in rodents in adult life (Rubin et al, 2001; Somm et al, 2009). A similar effect is observed when exposure takes place during gestation (Nikaido et al., 2004).

Many other environmental chemicals are suspected to be candidate obesogens including pesticides; for example, organochlorines such as DDT, endrin, lindane, and hexachlorobenzene; organophosphates; carbamates; polychlorinated biphenyls; other plastic components such as phthalates; perfluoroctanoic acid (PFOA); heavy metals such as cadmium, lead, and arsenic; and solvents (Newbold, 2010). Although the epidemiological link between specific obesogen exposure and obesity is highly suggestive, causality and overall significance currently remain ambiguous. New detailed longitudinal studies are merited as a high-priority investigative goal to establish the magnitude of the contributing risk by individual obesogens.

5. Metabolic disorders and endocrine disruptors

The issue of potential ED interference with metabolic imbalances is very timely especially in light of a recent cross-sectional study in the general adult population of the United States that reported an association between higher urinary BPA concentrations with diabetes, cardiovascular diagnoses and clinically abnormal concentrations of the liver enzymes γ-glutamyltransferase (Lang et al., 2008). An analysis of the posterior data from the US National Health and Nutrition Survey (NHANES) conducted by Melzer et al. confirmed the association between urinary BPA levels with coronary heart disease (Melzer et al., 2010).

These adverse effects of BPA on humans' metabolism appear to be confirmative of previously reported actions in animal models. Indeed, a series of studies by Alonso-Magdalena et al. have illustrated the potency of this estrogenic compound to directly affect pancreatic cells' function and to favor metabolic disorders (Alonso-Magdalena et al., 2005, 2006, 2010). Low doses of BPA acutely induced a change in glycemic balance characterized by a decrease in glycose levels that correlated with a rise of plasma insulin in adult male mice (Alonso-Magdalena et al., 2006). Furthermore, long term administration of BPA in β-cells from these rodents resulted to an increase in the insulin content and insulin secretion of the islets of Langerhans while BPA-treated mice appeared to be insulin resistant (Alonso-Magdalena et al., 2006). Pancreatic a-cells have also been implied as potential targets for endocrine disruption given that low doses of Bisphenol A were shown to impair the molecular signaling that leads to secretion of glycagon by suppressing intracellular calcium ion oscillations in a-cells in response to low blood glucose levels (Alonso-Magdalena et al., 2005).

Interestingly, gestational exposure to BPA has been recently linked to impaired glucose tolerance and reduced insulin sensitivity in adult mice' life when compared with non-exposed male offspring. Pregnant mothers were also affected as indicated by the aggravated insulin resistance during pregnancy and post-partum in this population in comparison to non-treated mothers (Alonso-Magdalena et al., 2010). As demonstrated in these rodent studies, BPA may contribute to metabolic disorders relevant to glucose homeostasis and, therefore, this altered blood glucose homeostasis may subsequently enhance the development of type 2 diabetes. Interestingly, human studies have also implied BPA to favor metabolic syndrome development through an inhibitory effect on adiponectin release from adipose depots of patients with morbidity obesity undergoing gastric bypass surgery (Hugo et al., 2008).

Other compounds that have been correlated with alterations in blood glucose homeostasis in humans are dioxins (Bertazzi et al., 2001; Henriksen et al., 1997) and arsenic (Lai et al., 1994; Meliker et al., 2007).

In conclusion, accumulating data are pointing to the potential role of endocrine disrupting chemicals either directly or indirectly in the pathogenesis of adipogenesis and diabetes ,the major epidemics of modern world.

6. Conclusion

Accumulative evidence from experimental and human studies imply that exposure to endocrine disruptors may have significant impact to all hormone-sensitive endocrine systems. The catalogue of endocrinopathies possible related to EDs is expanding to include a broad spectrum of disorders from reproductive function to metabolic regulation (see Table 1).

Human exposure to EDs is well-documented to occur through multiple sources, however, several parameters considerably complicate the assessment of EDs' interaction with human health. For instance, it is important to keep in mind that humans are continuously exposed to a multitude of pollutants which can act together, and lead to effects that are different from those of the individual pollutants that are usually studied in the laboratory. Furthermore,

the multiplicity of targets and the fact that many targets can be disrupted at the same time within an organism make difficult to truly evaluate the affect of an endocrine disrupting chemical to many endocrine systems. In addition, humans are not usually exposed to a single compound but to a mixture of EDs and as these chemicals may interact additively or antagonistically, the final clinical outcome may be variable. After all, human disorders are more likely the additive result of chronic exposure to low amounts of mixtures of EDs.

Another important parameter is timing of exposure as the biological effects of a compound vary depending not only on the nature of the chemical and dose, but on the susceptibility of the individual to this. The timing of exposure appears as a determining factor in the developmental programming hypothesis, which proposes that exposure of the developing tissues/organs to an adverse stimulus or insult during critical or sensitive times of development can permanently reprogram normal physiological responses leading to hormonal disorders later in life (Gluckman et al., 2005). In other words, when estimating the effect of a compound on human health the time of exposure may determine the clinical outcome. Importantly, the consequences of an exposure may not be apparent at the actual time of exposure, but may manifest later in life. Indeed, the potential lag between exposure to EDs and the manifestation of an endocrine disorder in humans may be years or decades after initial exposure.

Although direct causal links between exposures to EDs and disease states in humans are difficult to draw, results from basic research and epidemiological studies make it clear that more screening for exposures and targeting at-risk groups is a high priority. Innovative technologies designed to improve the assessment of human exposure and reproductive and endocrine health endpoints should be applied. Furthermore, scientific community should adopt a united approach with collaboration between different professional groups and government policy to prompt precautionary actions against excess exposure. After all, endocrine disruption is on the agenda of many experts' groups, steering committees and panels of governmental organizations, industry, and academia throughout the world.

Endocrine systems	Endocrine Disorders Possibly Related To Endocrine Disruptors' Exposure
Male reproductive system	Testicular Dysgenesis Syndrome Altered semen quality Hypospadias/ cryptorchidism Testicular cancer Prostate cancer
Female reproductive system	Precocious/delayed puberty Impaired fertility/fecundity Reproductive tract anomalies Endometriosis Menstrual and Ovarian dysfunction Pregnancy complication (Preterm delivery/Pregnancy lost) Premature menopause Impaired mammary gland differentiation / Breast cancer
Thyroid	Altered thyroid hormones
Adipose tissue	Promote adipogenesis Altered body weight Disturbed adipokine secretion
Pancreas	Diabetes mellitus Disturbed insulin secretion Disturbed glycagon secretion

Table 1. Endocrine system as a target for disruption: The potential impact of endocrine disruptors on endocrine system based on experimental and human data.

7. References

Alonso-Magdalena, P.; Vieira, E.; Soriano, S.; Menes, L.; Burks, D.; Quesada, I. & Nadal A. (2010). Bisphenol A exposure during pregnancy disrupts glucose homeostasis in mothers and adult male offspring. *Environ Health Perspect.*, Vol.118, No. 9, pp.1243-50

Alonso-Magdalena, P.; Laribi, O.; Ropero, AB.; Fuentes, E.; Ripoll, C.; Soria, B. & Nadal A. (2005). Low Doses of Bisphenol A and Diethylstilbestrol Impair Ca2+ Signals in Pancreatic α-Cells through a Nonclassical Membrane Estrogen Receptor within Intact Islets of Langerhans. *Environ Health Perspect,* Vol.113, No. 8, pp.969-77

Alonso-Magdalena, P.; Morimoto, S.; Ripoll, C.; Fuentes, E. & Nadal, A. (2006). The Estrogenic Effect of Bisphenol -A Disrupts Pancreatic β-Cell Function In Vivo and Induces Insulin Resistance. *Environ Health Perspect,* Vol.114, No. 1, pp.106-12

Anway, MD. & Skinner, MK. (2006). Epigenetic Transgenerational Actions of Endocrine Disruptors. *Endocrinology,* Vol.147, No.6, pp43-49

Anway, MD. & Skinner, MK. (2008). Transgenerational effects of the endocrine disruptor vinclozolin on the prostate transcriptome and adult onset disease. *Prostate* 2008; Vol.68, No.5, pp.517-529

Baillie-Hamilton, PF. (2002). Chemical toxins: a hypothesis to explain the global obesity epidemic. *J Altern Complement Med.,* Vol.8, No.2, pp.185-92

Bertazzi, PA.; Consonni, D.; Bachetti, S.; Rubagotti, M.; Baccarelli, A.; Zocchetti, C. & Pesatori, AC. (2001). Health Effects of Dioxin Exposure: A 20-Year Mortality Study. *Am J Epidemiol*, Vol.153, No.11, pp.1031–44

Boas, M.; Feldt-Rasmussen, U.; Skakkebæk, NE. & Main KM. (2006). Environmental chemicals and thyroid function. *Eur J Endocrinol.*, Vol.154, No.5,pp.599–611

Carlsen, E.; Giwercman, A.; Keiding, N. & Skakkebaek, NE.(1992). Evidence for decreasing quality of semen during past 50 years. *BMJ*, Vol.305, No.6854, pp.609-13

Caserta, D.; Maranghi, L.; Mantovani, A.; Marci, R.; Maranghi ,F. & Moscarini M. (2008). Impact of endocrine disruptor chemicals in gynaecology. *Hum Reprod Update,* Vol.14, No.1, pp.59–72

Dallinga, JW.; Moonen, EJ.; Dumoulin, JC.; Evers, JL.; Geraedts, JP. & Kleinjans JC. (2002). Decreased human semen quality and organochlorine compounds in blood. *Hum Reproduction*, Vol.17, No.8, pp.1973-9

Diamanti-Kandarakis, E., Bourguignon, JP., Giudice, LC., Hauser, R., Prins, GS., Soto, AM., Zoeller, RT. & Gore AC. Endocrine-disrupting chemicals: an Endocrine Society scientific statement. Endocr Rev. 2009;30(4):293-342.

Diamanti-Kandarakis, E.; Palioura, E.; Kandarakis, SA. & Koutsilieris, M. (2010) The impact of endocrine disruptors on endocrine targets. *Horm Metab Res.*, Vol.42, No.8, pp.543-52

Duty, SM.; Silva, MJ.; Barr, DB.; Brock, JW.; Ryan, L.; Chen, Z.; Herrick, RF.; Christiani, DC. & Hauser, R. (2003). Phthalate exposure and human semen parameters. *Epidemiology*, Vol.14, No.3, pp.269-77

Euling, SY.; Herman-Giddens, ME.; Lee, PA.; Selevan, SG.; Juu,l A.; Sørensen, TI.; Dunkel, L.; Himes, JH; Teilmann, G. & Swan, SH. (2008)a. Examination of US puberty-timing data from 1940 to 1994 for secular trends: panel findings. *Pediatrics.*, Vol.121, No.3, pp.172-91

Euling, SY.; Selevan, SG.; Pescovitz, OH. & Skakkebaek NE. (2008)b. Role of environmental factors in the timing of puberty. *Pediatrics.*, Vol.12, No.3, pp.167-71

Gladen, BC.; Ragan, NB. & Rogan, WJ. (2000). Pubertal growth and development and prenatal and lactational exposure to polychlorinated biphenyls and dichlorodiphenyl dichloroethene. *J Pediatr*, Vol.136, No.4, pp.490-496

Gluckman, PD.; Hanson, MA. & Pinal C. (2005). The developmental origins of adult disease. *Matern Child Nutr.*, Vol. 1, No.3, pp.130-141

Goncharov, A.; Haase, RF.; Santiago-Rivera, A.; Morse, G.; Akwesasne Task Force on the Environment; McCaffrey, RJ.; Rej, R. & Carpenter DO. (2008). High serum PCBs are associated with elevation of serum lipids and cardiovascular disease in a Native American population. *Environ Res*, Vol.106, No.2, pp.226-239

Grün, F. & Blumberg, B. (2006). Environmental obesogens: organotins and endocrine disruption via nuclear receptor signaling. *Endocrinology*, Vol. 147, No. 6, pp.50-5

Grün, F.; Watanabe, H.; Zamanian, Z.; Maeda, L.; Arima, K.; Cubacha, R.; Gardiner, DM.; Kanno, J.; Iguchi, T. & Blumberg, B. (2006). Endocrine-Disrupting Organotin Compounds Are Potent Inducers of Adipogenesis in Vertebrates. *Mol Endocrinol.*, Vol.20, No.9, pp.2141-55

Hagmar, L.; Bjork, J.; Sjodin, A.; Bergman, A. & Erfurth, EM. (2001). Plasma levels of persistent organohalogens and hormone levels in adult male humans. *Arch Environ Health,* Vol. 56, No.2, pp.138-143

Hatch, EE.; Nelson, JW.; Qureshi, MM.; Weinberg, J.; Moore, LL.; Singer M. & Webster TF. (2008). Association of urinary phthalate metabolite concentrations with body mass index and waist circumference: a cross-sectional study of NHANES data, 1999-2002. *Environ Health.,* Vol.7, pp.27

Hauser, R.; Chen, Z.; Pothier, L.; Ryan, L. & Altshul, L. (2003).The relationship between human semen parameters and environmental exposure to polychlorinated biphenyls and p,p'-DDE. *Environ Health Perspect,* Vol.111, No.12, pp.1505-11

Hauser, R.; Meeker, JD.; Duty, S.; Silva, MJ. & Calafat, AM. (2006). Altered semen quality in relation to urinary concentrations of phthalate monoester and oxidative metabolites. *Epidemiology,* Vol.17, No.6, pp. 682-91

Henriksen, GL.; Ketchum, NS.; Michalek, JE. & Swaby, JA. (1997). Serum dioxin and diabetes mellitus in veterans of Operation Ranch Hand. *Epidemiology,* Vol.8, No.3, pp.252-8

Herbst, AL.; Ulfelder, H. & Poskanzer DC. (1971). Adenocarcinoma of the vagina. Association of maternal stilbestrol therapy with tumor appearance in young women. *N Engl J Med,* Vol.284, No.15, pp.878-881

Heyland, A & Moroz, LL. (2005). Cross-kingdom hormonal signaling: an insight from thyroid hormone functions in marine larvae. *J Exp Biol.,* Vol.208, No.23, pp.4355-61

Howdeshell, KL. (2002). A model of the development of the brain as a construct of the thyroid system. *Environ Health Perspect,* Vol.110, No.3, pp.337-348

Hugo, ER.; Brandebourg, TD.; Woo, JG.; Loftus, J.; Alexander, JW. & Ben-Jonathan, N. (2008). Bisphenol A at environmentally relevant doses inhibits adiponectin release from human adipose tissue explants and adipocytes. *Environ Health Perspect.,* Vol.116, No.12, pp.1642-7

Jacobson-Dickman, E. & Lee, MM. (2009). The influence of endocrine disruptors on pubertal timing . *Curr Opin Endocrinol Diabetes Obes,* Vol.16, No.1, pp.25–30

Juhler, RK.; Larsen, SB.; Meyer, O.; Jensen, ND.; Spanò, M.; Giwercman, A. & Bonde JP. (1999). Human semen quality in relation to dietary pesticide exposure and organic diet. *Arch Environ Contam Toxicol,* Vol.37, No.3, pp.415-23

Kanayama, T.; Kobayashi, N.; Mamiya, S.; Nakanishi, T. & Nishikawa J. (2005). Organotin Compounds Promote Adipocyte Differentiation as Agonists of the Peroxisome Proliferator-Activated Receptor -γ /Retinoid X Receptor Pathway. *Mol Pharmacol.,* Vol. 67, No.3, pp.766-74

Kandaraki, E.; Chatzigeorgiou, A.; Livadas, S.; Palioura, E.; Economou, F.; Koutsilieris, M.; Palimeri, S.; Panidis, D. & Diamanti-Kandarakis E. Endocrine Disruptors and Polycystic Ovary Syndrome (PCOS): Elevated Serum Levels of Bisphenol A in Women with PCOS. *J Clin Endocrinol Metab.* 2010 Dec 30. [Epub ahead of print]

Kaufman, RH. (1982). Structural changes of the genital tract associated with in utero exposure to diethylstilbestrol. *Obstet Gynecol Annu.,* Vol.11, pp.187-202

Kaufman, RH.; Adam, E.; Hatch, EE.; Noller, K.; Herbst, AL.; Palmer, JR. & Hoover, RN. (2000). Continued follow-up of pregnancy outcomes in diethylstilbestrol-exposed offspring. *Obstet Gynecol,* Vol.96, No.4, pp.483-9

Lai, MS.; Hsueh, YM.; Chen, CJ.; Shyu, MP.; Chen, SY.; Kuo. TL.; Wu, MM. & Tai TY. (1994). Ingested inorganic arsenic and prevalence of diabetes mellitus. *Am J Epidemiol.,* Vol.139, No.5, pp.484-92

Lang, IA.; Galloway, TS.; Scarlett, A.; Henley, WE.; Depledge, M.; Wallace, RB. & Melzer D. (2008). Association of Urinary Bisphenol A Concentration With Medical Disorders and Laboratory Abnormalities in Adults. *JAMA.,* Vol.300, No.11, pp.1303-10

Langer, P.; Koban, A.; Tajtakova, M.; Koška, J.; Radikova, Z.; Kšinantova, L.; Imrich, R.; Hucková, M.; Drobná, B.; Gasperíková, D.; Seböková, E. & Klimes, I. (2008). Increased thyroid volume, prevalence of thyroid antibodies and impaired fastingand impaired fasting glucose in young adults from organochlorine cocktail polluted area: Outcome of transgenerational transmission? *Chemosphere*, Vol.73, No.3, pp.1145-1150

Masuno, H.; Iwanami, J.; Kidani, T.; Sakayama, K. & Honda K. (2005). Bisphenol a accelerates terminal differentiation of 3T3-L1 cells into adipocytes through the phosphatidylinositol 3-kinase pathway. *Toxicol Sci.*, Vol.84, No.2, pp.319-27

Masuno, H.; Kidani, T.; Sekiya, K.; Sakayama, K.; Shiosaka, T.; Yamamoto, H. & Honda K.(2002). Bisphenol A in combination with insulin can accelerate the conversion of 3T3-L1 fibroblasts to adipocytes. *J Lipid Res.*, Vol.43, No.5, pp.676-84.

McLachlan, JA.; Simpson, E. & Martin, M. (2006). Endocrine disrupters and female reproductive health. *Best Pract Res Clin Endocrinol Metab*, Vol.20, No.1, pp.63–75

Meeker, JD.; Altshul, L. & Hauser R. (2007). Serum PCBs, *p,p'*-DDE and HCB predict Thyroid Hormone Levels in Men. *Environ Res.*, Vol. 104, No.2, pp.296–304

Meliker, JR.; Wahl, RL.; Cameron, LL. & Nriag, JO. (2007). Arsenic in drinking water and cerebrovascular disease, diabetes mellitus, and kidney disease in Michigan: a standardized mortality ratio analysis. *Environmental Health*, Vol.6, pp.4

Melzer, D.; Rice, NE.; Lewis, C.; Henley, WE, & Galloway TS. (2010). Association of Urinary Bisphenol A Concentration with Heart Disease: Evidence from NHANES 2003/06. *PLoS One.*, Vol.5, No. 1, e.8673

Mendola, P.; Messer LC. & Rappazzo K. (2008). Science linking environmental contaminant exposures with fertility and reproductive health impacts in the adult female. *Fertil Steril.*, Vol.89, No.2, pp.81-94

Newbold RR. (2010). Impact of environmental endocrine disrupting chemicals on the development of obesity. *Hormones (Athens)*, Vol.9, No.3, pp.206-17

Newbold, RR.; Padilla-Banks, E.; Jefferson, WN. & Heindel JJ. (2008). Effects of endocrine disruptors on obesity. *Int J Androl*, Vol.31, No.2, pp.201-208, ISSN 0105-6263

Newbold, RR.; Padilla-Banks, E.; Snyder, RJ.; Phillips, TM. & Jefferson WN. (2007). Developmental exposure to endocrine disruptors and the obesity epidemic. *Reprod Toxicol*, Vol.23, No.3, pp.290-296

Nikaido, Y.; Yoshizawa, K.; Danbara, N.; Tsujita-Kyutoku, M.; Yuri, T.; Uehara, N. & Tsubura, A. (2004). Effects of maternal xenoestrogen exposure on development of the reproductive tract and mammary gland in female CD-1 mouse offspring. *Reprod. Toxicol*, Vol.18, No.6, pp.803–811

Palmer, JR.; Hatch, EE.; Rao, RS.; Kaufman, RH.; Herbst, AL.; Noller, KL.; Titus-Ernstoff, L. & Hoover RN. (2001). Infertility among women exposed prenatally to diethylstilbestrol. *Am J Epidemiol*, Vol.154, No.4, pp.316–21

Persky, V.; Turyk, M.; Anderson, HA.; Hanrahan, LP.; Falk, C.; Steenport, DN.; Chatterton, R Jr. & Freels, S.; Great Lakes Consortium. (2001). The effects of PCB exposure and fish consumption on endogenous hormones. *Environ Health Perspect.*, Vol.109, No.12, pp.1275-83

Phrakonkham, P.; Viengchareun, S.; Belloir, C.; Lombes, M.; Artur, Y. & Canivenc-Lavier MC. (2008). Dietary xenoestrogens differentially impair 3T3-L1 preadipocyte differentiation and persistently affect leptin synthesis. *J. Steroid Biochem. Molec. Biol*, Vol.110, No.1-2, pp.95–103

Rubin, BS.; Murray, MK.; Damassa, DA.; King, JC. & Soto, AM. (2001). Perinatal exposure to low doses of bisphenol-A affects body weight, patterns of estrous cyclicity and plasma LH levels. *Environ Health Perspect.*, Vol.109, No.7, pp.675–680

Skakkebæk, NE.; Rajpert-De Meyts, E. & Main KM. (2001). Testicular dysgenesis syndrome: an increasingly common developmental disorder with environmental aspects. *Hum Reprod Update*, Vol.16, No.5, pp. 972-978

Sharpe, RM. & Skakkebæk NE. (2003). Male reproductive disorders and the role of endocrine disruption: advances in understanding and identification of areas for future research. *Pure Appl Chem*, Vol.75, pp.2023-2038

Somm, E.; Schwitzgebel, VM.; Toulotte, A.; Cederroth, CR.; Combescure, C.; Nef, S.; Aubert, ML. & Hüppi PS. (2009). Perinatal Exposure to Bisphenol A Alters Early Adipogenesis in the Rat. *Environ Health Perspect*, Vol.117, No. 10, pp.1549-1555.

Steinmaus, C.; Miller, MD. & Howd, R. (2007). Impact of smoking and thiocyanate on perchlorate and thyroid hormone associations in the 2001-2002 national health and nutrition examination survey. *Environ Health Perspect.*, Vol.115, No.9, pp.1333-1338

Tabb, MM., & Blumberg, B. (2006). New Modes of Action for Endocrine-Disrupting Chemicals. *Mol Endocrinol.*, Vol.20, No.3, pp.475-482

Takeuchi, T. & Tsutsumi, O. (2002). Serum Bisphenol A Concentrations Showed Gender Differences, Possibly Linked to Androgen Levels. *Biochem Biophys Res Commun.*, Vol.291, No.1, pp.76-78

Takeuchi, T.; Tsutsumi, O.; Ikezuki, Y.; Takai, Y. & Taketani Y. (2004). Positive relationship between androgen and the endocrine disruptor, bisphenol A, in normal women and women with ovarian dysfunction. *Endocr J.*, Vol.51, No.2, pp.165-9

Takser, L.; Mergler, D.; Baldwin, M.; de Grosbois, S.; Smargiassi ,A. & Lafond, J. (2005). Thyroid hormones in pregnancy in relation to environmental exposure to organochlorine compounds and mercury. *Environ Health Perspect.*, Vol. 113, No.8, pp.1039-45

Titus-Ernstoff, L.; Troisi, R.; Hatch, EE.; Wise, LA.; Palmer, J.; Hyer, M.; Kaufman, R.; Adam, E.; Strohsnitter, W.; Noller, K.; Herbst, AL.; Gibson-Chambers, J.; Hartge, P. & Hoover RN. (2006). Menstrual and reproductive characteristics of women whose mothers were exposed in utero to diethylstilbestrol (DES). *Int J Epidemiol*, Vol.35, No.4, pp.862-868

Toppari, J.; Kaleva, M. & Virtanen HE.(2001). Trends in the incidence of cryptorchidism and hypospadias, and method0logical limitations of registry-based data. *Hum Reprod Update* Vol.7, No.3, pp.282-6

U.S. EPA. (1997). Special report on Environmental Endocrine Disruption: An Effects Assessment and Analysis. Office of Research and Development, 1997, EPA/630/R-96/012, Washington D.C.

Wada, K.; Sakamoto, H.; Nishikawa, K.; Sakuma, S.; Nakajima, A.; Fujimoto, Y. & Kamisaki Y. (2007). Life style-related diseases of the digestive system: endocrine disruptors stimulate lipid accumulation in target cells related to metabolic syndrome. *J Pharmacol Sci.*, Vol.105, No.2, pp.133-7

Waring, RH. & Harris RM. (2005). Endocrine disrupters: A human risk? *Mol Cell Endocrinol.*, Vol.244, No.1-2, pp.2-9

Woodruff, TJ.; Carlson, A.; Schwartz, JM. & Giudice, LC. (2008). Proceedings of the Summit on Environmental Challenges to Reproductive Health and Fertility: Executive Summary. *Fertil Steril*, Vol. 89, No.2, pp.281-300

Zoeller, RT. (2007). Environmental chemicals impacting the thyroid: targets and consequences. *Thyroid*, Vol.17, No.9, pp.811-817

Zoeller, TR. (2010). Environmental chemicals targeting thyroid. *Hormones (Athens).*, Vol.9, No.1,pp. 28-40

Permissions

The contributors of this book come from diverse backgrounds, making this book a truly international effort. This book will bring forth new frontiers with its revolutionizing research information and detailed analysis of the nascent developments around the world.

We would like to thank Prof. Dr. Evanthia Diamanti-Kandarakis, for lending her expertise to make the book truly unique. She has played a crucial role in the development of this book. Without her invaluable contribution this book wouldn't have been possible. She has made vital efforts to compile up to date information on the varied aspects of this subject to make this book a valuable addition to the collection of many professionals and students.

This book was conceptualized with the vision of imparting up-to-date information and advanced data in this field. To ensure the same, a matchless editorial board was set up. Every individual on the board went through rigorous rounds of assessment to prove their worth. After which they invested a large part of their time researching and compiling the most relevant data for our readers. Conferences and sessions were held from time to time between the editorial board and the contributing authors to present the data in the most comprehensible form. The editorial team has worked tirelessly to provide valuable and valid information to help people across the globe.

Every chapter published in this book has been scrutinized by our experts. Their significance has been extensively debated. The topics covered herein carry significant findings which will fuel the growth of the discipline. They may even be implemented as practical applications or may be referred to as a beginning point for another development. Chapters in this book were first published by InTech; hereby published with permission under the Creative Commons Attribution License or equivalent.

The editorial board has been involved in producing this book since its inception. They have spent rigorous hours researching and exploring the diverse topics which have resulted in the successful publishing of this book. They have passed on their knowledge of decades through this book. To expedite this challenging task, the publisher supported the team at every step. A small team of assistant editors was also appointed to further simplify the editing procedure and attain best results for the readers.

Our editorial team has been hand-picked from every corner of the world. Their multi-ethnicity adds dynamic inputs to the discussions which result in innovative outcomes. These outcomes are then further discussed with the researchers and contributors who give their valuable feedback and opinion regarding the same. The feedback is then collaborated with the researches and they are edited in a comprehensive manner to aid the understanding of the subject.

Apart from the editorial board, the designing team has also invested a significant amount of their time in understanding the subject and creating the most relevant covers. They scrutinized every image to scout for the most suitable representation of the subject and create an appropriate cover for the book.

The publishing team has been involved in this book since its early stages. They were actively engaged in every process, be it collecting the data, connecting with the contributors or procuring relevant information. The team has been an ardent support to the editorial, designing and production team. Their endless efforts to recruit the best for this project, has resulted in the accomplishment of this book. They are a veteran in the field of academics and their pool of knowledge is as vast as their experience in printing. Their expertise and guidance has proved useful at every step. Their uncompromising quality standards have made this book an exceptional effort. Their encouragement from time to time has been an inspiration for everyone.

The publisher and the editorial board hope that this book will prove to be a valuable piece of knowledge for researchers, students, practitioners and scholars across the globe.

List of Contributors

Duarte Pignatelli
Endocrinology, Hospital S. João, Porto, Portugal
Faculty of Medicine of the University of Porto, Portugal
IPATIMUP, University of Porto, Portugal

S.H.A. Brouns, T.M.A. Kerkhofs, I.G.C. Hermsen and H.R. Haak
Máxima Medical Center, Eindhoven, The Netherlands

Alberto Falorni and Stefania Marzotti
Department of Internal Medicine, Section of Internal Medicine and Endocrine and Metabolic Sciences, University of Perugia, Italy

Juan Manuel Busso
Instituto de Ciencia y Tecnología de Alimentos, Facultad de Ciencias Exactas, Físicas y Naturales (FCEFyN) – Universidad Nacional de Córdoba (UNC)/ Consejo Nacional de Investigaciones Científicas y Técnicas (CONICET), Argentina
Established investigators from the CONICET, Argentina

Rubén Daniel Ruiz
Instituto de Fisiología, Facultad de Ciencias Médicas, UNC, Argentina
Established investigators from the CONICET, Argentina

Gonzalo Díaz-Soto and Manuel Puig-Domingo
Servicio de Endocrinología y Nutrición, Hospital Clínico de Valladolid, Centro de Investigación de Endocrinología y Nutrición Clínica (IEN), Facultad de Medicina de Valladolid, Spain
Servei de Endocrinologia i Nutrició. Hospital Germans Trias i Pujol, Badalona,Universitat Autònoma de Barcelona, Spain

Benjamin U. Nwosu
University of Massachusetts Medical School Worcester, Massachusetts, USA

H. Herschel Conaway
Department of Physiology and Biophysics, University of Arkansas for Medical Sciences, USA

Ulf H. Lerner
Department of Molecular Periodontology, Umeå University
Center for Bone and Arthritis Research at Institute of Medicine, Sahlgrenska Academy at University of Gothenburg, Sweden

Helge Raeder, Silje Rafaelsen and Robert Bjerknes
Department of Clinical Medicine, University of Bergen, Norway

Eleni Palioura, Eleni Kandaraki and Evanthia Diamanti-Kandarakis
Medical School University of Athens, Greece

Printed in the USA
CPSIA information can be obtained
at www.ICGtesting.com
JSHW011354221024
72173JS00003B/278